Giving Blood

Giving Blood represents a new agenda for blood donation research. It explores the diverse historical and contemporary undercurrents that influence how blood donation takes place and the social meanings that people attribute to the act of giving blood. Drawing from empirical studies conducted in the United States, Canada, France, Australia, China, India, Latin America, and Africa, the book's chapters turn our attention to the evolution of blood donation worldwide, examining:

- the impact of technology advances on blood collection practices
- the shifting approaches to donor recruitment and retention
- the governance and policy issues associated with the establishment of blood clinics
- the political and legal challenges of regulating blood systems.

This innovative examination moves the focus from individual explanations of rates of blood donation to a social, structural explanation. It will appeal to international scholars and students working in the areas of sociology, medical anthropology, healthcare, public policy, socio-legal studies, comparative politics, organizational management, health and illness, the history of medicine, and public health ethics.

Johanne Charbonneau is Professor at the Université INRS – Centre Urbanisation Culture Société, Québec, Canada.

André Smith is Associate Professor of Sociology at the University of Victoria, British Columbia, Canada.

Routledge studies in the sociology of health and illness

Giving Blood

The institutional making of altruism

**Edited by Johanne Charbonneau
and André Smith**

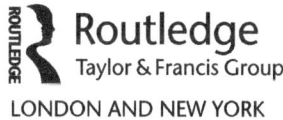

Routledge
Taylor & Francis Group

LONDON AND NEW YORK

First published 2016
by Routledge
2 Park Square, Milton Park, Abingdon, Oxon OX14 4RN

and by Routledge
605 Third Avenue, New York, NY 10017

First issued in paperback 2021

Routledge is an imprint of the Taylor & Francis Group, an informa business

Publisher's Note
The publisher has gone to great lengths to ensure the quality of this reprint but points out that some imperfections in the original copies may be apparent.

British Library Cataloguing in Publication Data
A catalogue record for this book is available from the British Library

Library of Congress Cataloging in Publication Data
Giving blood: the institutional making of altruism/edited by Johanne Charbonneau and André Smith.
  p. cm. – (Routledge studies in the sociology of health and illness)
  Includes bibliographical references.
  I. Charbonneau, Johanne, editor. II. Smith, André (Professor of sociology), editor. III. Series: Routledge studies in the sociology of health and illness.
  [DNLM: 1. Blood Donors. 2. Blood Transfusion. 3. Culture. 4. Sociological Factors. WH 460]
  RM172
  362.17′84–dc23   2015002971

ISBN 13: 978-0-367-34145-9 (pbk)
ISBN 13: 978-1-138-91194-9 (hbk)

Typeset in Times New Roman
by Wearset Ltd, Boldon, Tyne and Wear

Contents

Figures

Tables

Contributors

Vincanne Adams, Ph.D., is Professor and Vice Chair in the Department of Anthropology, History, and Social Medicine at the University of California, San Francisco. She has written extensively on Asian medicine, modernization and development, global public health, and disaster recovery based on field research in Nepal, Tibet, China, and the USA.

Johanne Charbonneau has been Professor at Université INRS – Centre Urbanisation Culture Société since 1993, having received a Ph.D. in political sciences from Université Laval in 1991. She is Chairholder of the Research Chair on the Social Aspects of Blood Donation financed by Héma-Québec, the Héma-Québec Foundation, and the Social Sciences and Humanities Council of Canada, since 2009. She began her career by working on such topics as the circulation of the gift within families, social and family solidarities, organ donation, as well as on immigrant communities.

Sophie Chauveau, Ph.D. in history, is Professor of History of Sciences and Technology and a Research Fellow for the Institut de recherche sur les Transports, l'Énergie et la Société at the Technological University of Belfort-Montbeliard, France. She is an honorary member of the Institut Universitaire de France and has worked on the history of the relationships between the French state and the pharmaceutical firms in the twentieth century. Her most recent works include research on blood transfusion organizations in France, sanitary scandals, and the study of human body parts' medical uses.

Jacob Copeman, Ph.D., is a lecturer in social anthropology, School of Social and Political Studies, at the University of Edinburgh. His main areas of interest are South Asian studies, contemporary social reform/politics of "superstition," medical anthropology, and studies of biological exchange/bioeconomy.

Renaud Crespin is a senior research fellow at the French National Center for Scientific Research (CNRS) in the Centre for the Sociology of Organizations (CSO-UMR 7116) of Sciences Po Paris, which is a joint program of Sciences Po Paris and the CNRS (UMR 7116). Prior to joining the CNRS in 2007, he received a Ph.D. in political science from the University of Paris I-Pantheon-Sorbonne in

2003. Lecturing/teaching locations have been at Sciences Po Paris, the French School of Public Health (EHESP), and the French National School of Administration (ENA), University of Paris-Dauphine.

Bruno Danic has been an MD since 1990 and has had a practice in transfusion medicine since 1991 in the French national blood establishment (EFS). He obtained a master's degree in 2000, focusing on molecular and cellular biology and health sciences. He has been Deputy of the blood transfusion establishment of Bretagne, France, since 2004. As national referent at medical direction of EFS, he participates in working groups on blood safety in the French health products safety agency (ANSM) and the Institute of Health Surveillance (InVS).

Kathleen Erwin, Ph.D., is Director of UC Research Initiatives at the University of California, Office of the President. An anthropologist by training, her research specializations include China, Asian medicine, gender, sexuality and the body, and cultural constructions of health and illness.

Jean-Paul Lallemand-Stempak is a certified professor and instructor at Université Paris Diderot. His Ph.D. research, conducted at the EHESS, focuses partly on the history of blood's segregation in the United States from the 1930s to the 1970s. In a perspective borrowed from both the social history of medicine and political history, his work focuses more largely on the setting up of a "socio-medical racism" and its questioning in the political sphere.

Phuoc Le graduated from Dartmouth in 2000 with a double major in biochemistry and molecular biology and Asian and Middle Eastern languages and literature. He earned his MD in Stanford Medical School. He also obtained a Master's degree in Public Health from UC Berkeley with a focus on global health. Currently, he is Assistant Professor in Internal Medicine and Pediatrics at UCSF and Assistant Professor of Public Health at UC Berkeley.

Vishala Parmasad is a Ph.D. candidate at the University of British Columbia (UBC), Canada. She is studying the socio-cultural dimensions of chronic diseases, specifically type 2 diabetes mellitus, in Trinidad, the West Indies. She pursued a master's degree in science in medical anthropology at University College London (UCL), gaining Distinction. She is also trained as a physician in Trinidad and Tobago. She has been a guest lecturer at her alma mater, Faculty of Medical Sciences at the University of the West Indies, Trinidad. She is also a Vanier Canada Graduate Scholar (2012) and Killam Doctoral Scholar (2012).

Anne Quéniart is a professor in the Department of Sociology at Université du Québec à Montréal. Since 2009, she has been an active member of the research chair on the social aspects of blood donation and has led research on youth and blood donation and on the transmission of blood donation values and practices within the family. Her current research also examines multiple forms of activism; after having focused on militant youth within political parties and alternative groups; she has become interested in the social and political involvement of older women and socially conscious consumerism as a form of implication.

Carlos Alberto Sanchez is a student of Psychology at the University San Sebastian of Concepción, Chile. He is also President of the Biovida Foundation, aiming to promote voluntary blood donation in Chile.

William H. Schneider is Professor of History and Philanthropic Studies and adjunct Professor of Medical and Molecular Genetics at Indiana University, where he also directs the program in medical humanities and health studies. He has received grants from the National Endowment for the Humanities, National Institutes of Health, National Science Foundation, and Fulbright Fellowships. His books on the history of medicine and global health include *History of Blood Transfusion in Sub-Saharan Africa* (Ohio University Press).

André Smith is Associate Professor of Sociology at the University of Victoria, British Columbia, Canada. His research interests concern the areas of ageing, mental health, and blood donation. His research examines how regulatory environments and organizational cultures influence healthcare practices. His articles have appeared in the *Journal of Aging Studies*, *Transfusion*, the *Canadian Review of Sociology*, and the *Journal of Deviant Behaviour*.

Kylie Valentine is Senior Research Fellow at the Social Policy Research Centre, University of New South Wales. Her research interests include the politics of (and policies for) families, children, and mothers; marginalized communities and individuals; and the translation of research into politics and practice.

María Cristina Martínez Valenzuela has been Director of the Blood Centre Concepción, Chile, since 2008. A doctor with over 30 years' experience in the field of blood transfusion, she is responsible for the creation, planning, design, implementation, and continuing development of the institution. She is the group leader responsible for the elaboration of National Standard Quality for Chilean Transfusion Centers and the technical coordinator of the Ministry National Blood Program. She is also in charge of the international relationship with other centers and hospitals, allowing doctors and other health professional to increase technical and theoretical information about blood transfusion. She also has teaching and training experience at many levels.

Introduction

Blood donation and the range of historical and institutional trajectories

Johanne Charbonneau and André Smith

In 1971, Richard Titmuss published *The Gift Relationship*, in which he argued in favour of an anonymous, voluntary, non-remunerated blood collection system as opposed to one based on the payment of blood donors. He felt confident that there were enough people intrinsically motivated to donate blood without compensation to ensure both the quality and viability of such a system, even in market economies. In the decades since Titmuss' book was published, major international health organizations, such as the Red Cross and the World Health Organization (WHO), have encouraged governments worldwide to establish voluntary blood donor programs and to eliminate paid donation. They believe that voluntary donation is the best way to guarantee blood products' safety.

The need for blood transfusion for the treatment of serious illnesses and injuries has increased over the years. "About 234 million major operations are performed worldwide every year, with 63 million people undergoing surgery for traumatic injuries, 31 million more for treating cancers and another 10 million for pregnancy-related complications" (WHO/IFRCRCS 2010, 9). According to the WHO (2011), approximately 92 million blood donations are collected annually around the world, half of these in high-income countries where only 15 percent of the world's population live. In contrast, the African Region accounts for 4 percent of donations worldwide, with 12 percent of the global population. The United States, China, India, Japan, Germany, the Russian Federation, Italy, France, the Republic of Korea, and the United Kingdom are, in order of magnitude, the ten countries with the largest volume of blood collected. Forty-seven percent of the countries with the fewest collections are in the WHO African Region.

Despite the intensive promotion of voluntary and non-remunerated blood donation by international health organizations, only 62 countries collect 100 percent – or almost 100 percent – of their blood supplies from voluntary unpaid blood donors (WHO 2011). Forty countries collect more than 75 percent of their blood supply from family/replacement or paid donors. Family/replacement donors are those who give blood when it is required by a member of their own family or community. In recent years, India has reported the greatest increase in the amount of voluntary unpaid blood collected.

Blood collection services which rely on voluntary unpaid blood donation are generally able to meet the demand for blood and blood products. However, apheresis components (plasma, platelets) are still procured from compensated donors in many high-income countries, such as Germany and the United States. This USA alone provides 55 percent of the world's supply of plasma derivatives (Farrugia *et al.* 2010). Blood can meet the needs of more patients when separated into components (red cells, plasma, platelets, etc.). In high-income countries, 91 percent of the blood collected is separated as compared to 31 percent in low-income countries.

There are also significant differences in how efficiently countries collect blood: the average annual collection per blood centre is 30,000 in high-income countries, but only 3,700 in low-income countries (WHO 2011). The 2008 WHO report based on responses received from 164 countries, covering 92 percent of the world's population, states that 39 countries still do not routinely test blood donations for transfusion-transmissible infections. Thirty-four countries also reported lacking a national blood policy.

Treatment of complications during pregnancy and childbirth, severe childhood anaemia, trauma, and the management of congenital blood disorders accounts for the largest proportion of transfusion prescriptions in countries where treatment options are limited (WHO/IFRCRCS 2010). In high-income countries, sophisticated medical and surgical procedures, trauma care (e.g., for road traffic injuries), and the management of blood disorders (thalassemia and sickle-cell disease) have produced a growing demand for blood and blood products. In many countries, the health needs of an older population are placing pressure on blood supplies, while stricter donor selection criteria and an aging donor base are reducing the pool of eligible blood donors.

The increasing need for blood and blood products across the world and the conviction that in systems based on voluntary blood donation, patients have improved access to safe blood transfusion are two of the most important factors motivating research on the social leverages of blood donation. Scholars have first confirmed the important role altruism plays in the motivation of blood donors. However, this type of research has overwhelmingly emphasized individual-level determinants of blood donation. Considerably less attention has been given to understanding the influence of broader factors influencing blood donation, including the role blood collection agencies play in leveraging social resources to recruit donors, although we know from epidemiological research that blood donation rates vary significantly by community, ethnicity, age, gender, education, social class, occupation, and religion (Alessandrini 2007; Zou *et al.* 2008).

In 2006, Kieran Healy partly addressed this gap in knowledge with a comparative study of blood collection regimes in Europe and the United States. The observation of discrepancies between blood donation rates across different countries suggests the advantages of a structural approach to researching the phenomena of blood donation and donor recruitment. According to Healy, one must go beyond psychosocial analyses of individual motivations to get a better handle on the cultural and institutional factors that guide the practice of blood donation. He hypothesizes that differences in the nature of institutional regimes for supplying blood products impact not only the size and socio-demographic characteristics of donor populations but also the nature of the donations themselves and the meanings attributed to donating. Healy does not deny that individuals have their own reasons for donating blood, but he nonetheless argues that organizations contribute to defining a set of available and widely accepted reasons for donation, from among which donors are able to pick and choose. Healy invites researchers to study the institutional context that gives rise to the conditions surrounding the practice of blood donation, as well as the rhetoric of altruistic donation. In a sense, this was the invitation that prompted us to write this book. Our chief objective is to demonstrate the importance of institutions (be they medical, political, legal, or administrative) in shaping blood collection systems and in constructing a rhetorical discourse aimed at reinforcing donor motivation.

In her analysis of charitable giving, Barman (2007) states that donors' behaviour may be accounted for by studying their personal attributes, by examining the social relationships between donors and fundraising organizations, or – as she has chosen to do herself – by looking instead at the dynamic of the organizational field, in which there exist defined strategies of solicitation, i.e., the opportunities and constraints surrounding donation. As Barman points out, organizations do not act in isolation. A surrounding organizational field structures them. Barman goes so far as to hypothesize that variations in charitable giving practices may be better explained by the dynamic of relationships between the organizations existing in the field than by the relationships between individuals and organizations.

As readers will see, each author has chosen a distinct set of theoretical instruments, depending on the topic addressed. However, to organize the overall content of this book, interpreting blood donation and transfusion as an organizational field seems a useful approach. In doing so, we draw from various institutional theories from sociology and organizational studies (DiMaggio and Powell 1983; Fligstein and McAdam 2012; Meyer and Rowan 1977; Scott and Meyer 1983).

An institutionalist analytical framework

Field theory has its roots in Lewin's (1951) and Bourdieu's (1984) ideas that fields operate as mesolevel social orders, and constitute the basic structural foundation of modern political/organizational life in society. A field is an arena of action and of power relationships; each field is organized according to a logic determined by specific issues or circumstances (Bourdieu 1984). According to DiMaggio and Powell (1983), organizational fields "constitute a recognized area of institutional life: key suppliers, resource and product consumers, regulatory agencies, and other organizations that produce similar services or products" (148). For Fligstein and McAdam (2012), each field is part of a broader environment that contains other fields, whether distant or proximate, with which it interacts. Powell (2007) further remarks that organizations may themselves be embedded in social and political environments. Geographical borders may also have some importance in defining the limits of a field, although this is increasingly uncommon, as social relationships are developed and maintained at a variety of territorial levels. In particular, Drori and colleagues (2006) emphasize how organizational fields stretch across national borders.

A field is constructed in such a way that social actors must share its institutional logic, which involves an understanding of what is at stake within the field (Bourdieu 1984; Scott 2001). Dynamic processes animate all fields, as participants constantly vie for material advantages, for recognition, or for the achievement or maintenance of dominance in their field (Emirbayer and Johnson 2008; Martin 2003). According to Hoffman (1999), fields should be seen as contested centresa of debate. They are characterized by a power structure dominated by a small number of actors who set rules and agendas (Bourdieu and Wacquant 1992; Powell 2007). But in each field, there are also "challengers" (Fligstein and McAdam 2012), or "institutional entrepreneurs," as DiMaggio (1988) defines them. The interactional dynamic between social actors often involves competition, but also cooperation (Mahoney and Thelen 2009; Powell 2007). As Mahoney and Thelen (2009, 8) point out:

> In some cases, the power of one group (or coalition) relative to another may be so great that dominant actors are able to design institutions that closely correspond to their well-defined institutional preferences. But institutional outcomes need not reflect the goals of any particular group; they may be the unintended outcome of conflict among groups or the result of "ambiguous compromises" among actors who can coordinate on institutional means even if they differ on substantive goals.

All participants in a specific field try to leverage resources to transform or create new institutional arrangements and to define the "rules of the game." As Barman (2007) notes, citing Geertz (1973) and Lamont (1992), the corporate elite holds ownership of the cultural models that serve as a reference: "A cultural model, in a general sense, refers to a shared conceptualization of a set of goals and the legitimate means by which to achieve them" (1433). Defining the rules of the game also means defining the logic behind actions and cultural frames.

The cultural approach of the institutionalist current of sociology, presented by Hall and Taylor (1996, 939), emphasizes the role of cultural logics played by institutions:

> Institutions provide moral or cognitive templates for interpretation and action. The individual is seen as an entity deeply embedded in a world of institutions, composed of symbols, scripts and routines, which provide the filters for interpretation, of both the situation and oneself, out of which a course of action is constructed. Not only do institutions provide strategically useful information, they also affect the very identities, self-images and preferences of the actors.

The logics of action produced by the dominant social actors within an organizational field are therefore composed not only of formal rules, procedures, and norms but also of symbolic systems, cognitive scripts, and moral reference models. According to DiMaggio and Powell (1983), individual efforts at managing uncertainty and constraints tend to create homogeneity in structures, cultures, and results. Organizational fields are consequently fraught with strong pressure toward conformism and rationality. To counter a sense of uncertainty, organizations strive to copy the models of other, seemingly more legitimate organizations (e.g., Western ones) and to conform to norms, for instance, under the influence of professional networks associated with the academic world or of the agencies that provide their funding.

Meyer and Rowan (1977, 343) consider such norms of rationality to be deeply embedded in social reality:

> Many of the positions, policies, programs, and procedures of modern organizations are enforced by public opinion, by the views of important constituents, by knowledge legitimated through the educational system, by social prestige, by the laws, and by the definitions of negligence and prudence used by the courts. Such elements of formal structure are manifestations of powerful institutional rules which function as highly rationalized myths that are binding on particular organizations.

The part played by the state in the dynamics of organizational fields has retained the attention of many scholars (DiMaggio and Powell 1983; Hall and Taylor 1996; Scott and Meyer 1983). The modern state is a very influential actor, owing to the promulgation of laws and rights or the creation of regulatory authorities. Changes in rules, normative systems, or cognitive beliefs may contribute to redefining an organizational field (Powell 2007). As noted by DiMaggio and Powell (1983), the state and professions are great rationalizers. In some cases, states can also form alliances with groups from other fields in order to achieve their own goals.

As Powell (2007) pointed out, research demonstrated that "regulation and legal mandates were as much an endogenous force as an exogenous constraint" (4). Professionals inside organizations may help construct laws and create regulations. In this regard, Fligstein and McAdam (2012) used the term "internal governance units" in describing organizations whose purpose is to ensure order and stability within a strategic action field, and which are strongly influenced by the interests and views of the dominant actors.

Studying an organizational field reveals a constant and dynamic movement spurred by changes in issues or in actors' positions, but also sometimes by crises and major changes resulting from them. A field can emerge as a result of technological advances, population growth, or the intrinsic development of social organizations. Nation-states, by means of their authoritarian actions, may themselves contribute to the creation of a new field (Hall and Taylor 1996; Scott 2001). The stabilization of the field is achieved when most actors share its institutional logic. According to Fligstein and McAdam (2012), this outcome depends on skilled social actors' abilities to assert their dominance over an emerging field. The importance of resources in the process of a field's emergence brings to mind the structuration theory of Giddens (1977, 1984). For this author, rules and resources define a social structure. An organizational field's stability rests on the dominant actors' powers and social skills in using the resources at their disposal to maintain their position and domination within the field. In this regard, the actors can use various forms of resources: group size, access to government, existing law, professional expertise, knowledge of organizing technologies, and external allies.

External events, the arrival of new actors, or changes in internal dynamics can all destabilize a field. Critical junctures open up opportunities for historic agents to alter the trajectory of organizations (Mahoney and Thelen 2009). According to Giddens (1984), uncertainty leads to social change, when trust in organizations is broken down. "Internal participants and external constituents alike call for institutional rules that promote trust and confidence in outputs and buffer organizations from failure" (Meyer and Rowan 1977, 358). The uncertainty that arises in a field is conducive to the redefining of power rules and relations, as well as to the use of innovative forms of action.

In short, the institutionalist analytical framework offers us many tools for an organizational analysis of blood donation.

Blood donation: an organizational field?

The first question to ask in this regard is whether blood donation and transfusion indeed constitute an organizational field in their own right. The answer is undoubtedly in the affirmative. Doctors, hospitals, and charitable associations like the Red Cross were leading social actors in the field's emergence, and in fact, they contributed to creating the agencies, whether private (commercial) or public, that have become responsible for the supply of blood products. These agencies have become dominant social actors in the field. Over time, other actors have also become involved, namely the plasma industry, regulatory bodies, and civic associations. Donors and recipients alike are essentially individual actors in this context, but they can also be represented by associations seeking to defend their interests. This was the case, in particular, in the context of the contaminated blood scandal.

Actors from other distant or proximate fields – in particular, the state (health, political, and legal systems), international organizations, professional groups, and the media – influence the field of blood donation and transfusion. It is a field in which controlling the rules of the game is a key issue – certain internal governance units have in fact been created to do this – but the functions of regulation and certification are also shared by the state and by certain international authorities.

The dominant actors in this field constantly seek to ensure the field's stability in order to reassure the population (donors and recipients); yet the history of blood transfusion has been marked by periods of crisis – such as the contaminated blood scandal – that have led to a profound redefinition of the field and to substantial changes in its power relations.

In Western countries, the field appears to be relatively stable in spite of its ongoing debates, which include the question of blood donor remuneration and body commodification. In other countries, however, the field is still emergent or under transformation, and a number of cultural action models for donor recruitment and blood donation practices are competing with one another, even while the World Health Organization and the Federation of Red Cross and Red Crescent Societies attempt to impose a universal model inspired by the one established in Western countries.

This is a field in which the rules of the game are quite formal and well known but are not necessarily accepted by all the actors involved: one might take the example of the associations representing homosexual interests and challenging the rules excluding them from blood donation.

As a result, the actors in this organizational field find themselves confronted with a number of issues and concerns: risk control, body commodification, the defining of social solidarity and of the donation dynamic, and relationships of trust/mistrust between the health and political systems and the population. The foremost concern for those dominating this field is to demonstrate that the system, as they have defined it, is functional (Meyer and Rowan 1977) and hence that blood products are safe and available:

> Institutionalized organizations must not only conform to myths but also maintain the appearance that the myths actually work.... The more an organization's structure is derived from institutionalized myths, the more it maintains elaborate displays of confidence, satisfaction, and good faith, internally and externally.
>
> (Meyer and Rowan 1977, 356–358)

The proof of the reference model's efficiency is tied to the decisions and viewpoints which those dominating the field are able to impose upon others. These decisions and viewpoints are largely made in connection with body issues, risk, trust, and solidarity, and they translate into technologies, physical facilities, rules and norms, logics, strategies, and cultural frames of action.

Book sections and chapters

The analytical framework suggested by authors belongs to the institutionalist sociological current and is highly relevant to analyzing the rules and institutional dynamics that define the world of blood donation. It also allows the grouping the chapters of this book into three parts:

1   Technology and the evolution of blood clinics.
2   The institutional politics of donor recruitment.
3   The governance of blood donation: the authority of state control.

Part I Technology and the evolution of blood clinics

Part I brings together four chapters on the emergence of the field of blood donation and transfusion in four different territorial contexts: the United States, Africa, China, and France. However, the third and fourth chapters, which deal with China and France, do not examine the period that initially enabled the development of the countries' blood transfusion system. Instead, their primary aim is to understand how the field, as it stands today, emerged following the contaminated blood crisis of the early 1980s in France, and in the early 1990s in China.

The history of blood transfusion and the development of blood clinics show, first and foremost, the role that certain pioneering physicians played in the emergence of these novel medical practices. The development and dissemination of innovative technologies was also an extremely important factor in structuring and organizing activities. One might cite the example of conservation techniques for blood products, which have enabled the development of blood banks. Although some countries have been more advanced in developing new technologies, importing these into foreign countries lacking the basic infrastructure to accommodate them has, in some cases, represented a major challenge for local social actors.

In many countries, the vital issue of supplying blood products to soldiers during World War II drove the emergence of this field of medical practice. Blood donation was often a political and patriotic act. This was the case in the United States, China, and France, but not so much in Africa, where the main issue has most often been simply to meet patient needs. In Africa, as in other developing countries, expertise has come from abroad – more specifically, from Western countries. The colonial powers imported their model from European countries in order to develop the field in Africa.

In all countries, the field of blood donation and transfusion rapidly spread from hospitals, new collection centres, volunteer associations such as the Red Cross, and public administrations. Populations needed to be convinced to donate blood. In each country, this goal led to alliances between hospitals and the Red Cross, or to depending on donations from institutions such as the army, schools, and prisons. In China, work units were also swiftly leveraged for the cause. In addition, the media, which have often been called upon in order to recruit donors, have also constituted important disseminators of the arguments of the various groups that have defended distinct development models for blood collection and production activities, i.e., voluntary donation, replacement donation (from family and friends), and commerce.

In all countries, the state has acted as arbiter, very often to protect against health hazards but also sometimes to guarantee the promotion or preservation of values deemed to be fundamental. This was the case in the United States when the state sought to end the segregation of blood products from white or black donors, and in France when the state strove to reassert the importance of voluntary, unpaid donation in spite of pressure from the plasma industry to develop a commercial model.

For their part, politicians have not always played a positive role in the history of the emergence and establishment of this strategic action field. In certain American states, some have defended the policy of segregating the blood of whites and blacks, while in many African countries, blood transfusion systems have been continually disrupted as a result of political instability.

The study of the African situation clearly shows the influence of many internal and external events on the development of blood collection and transfusion systems, be these events the end of colonization, economic crises, or epidemics, such as AIDS. As in the case of the contaminated blood scandal, these events have acted as catalysts for changes to power relations in the field of blood transfusion. New social actors have emerged, such as human rights organizations or supranational authorities disseminating new guidelines. New hierarchies have become established, and some organizations find themselves bestowed with new powers in order to control health hazards or to better guarantee the circulation of blood products.

The field of blood donation and transfusion began to be structured during World War II. In the 1980s and 1990s, the contaminated blood scandal marked a major break in the organization of national systems for blood transfusion. Authorities implemented substantial efforts to diminish public uncertainty in these systems, contributing to restoring some measure of order. As we will see in Part III of this book, this field has always been characterized by dynamic processes of change resulting from both new issues and from the variations dependent on countries' different characteristics and situations. In this respect, geographic borders continue to hold great importance in the dynamic of the field's structuring, in spite of the strong presence of international organizations.

Part I chapters

In Chapter 1, Jean-Paul Lallemand-Stempak tackles the history of blood donation and transfusion in the United States, from the beginning of the nineteenth century to the early 1980s, focusing on two major issues that have intersected at various moments in its evolution: the questions of institutionalization (Boltanski 2009; Boltanski and Thévenot 1991) and racialization (Wieviorka 1996). Although historically defined by their status as, respectively, a healthcare technique and a commodity within medicine, transfusion and donated blood appear in Lallemand-Stempak's analysis as political tools that reflect the racialized attitudes predominant in American society during these periods.

In Chapter 2, William H. Schneider argues that there were important historical circumstances in Africa that distinguished blood donation there from donation elsewhere. Schneider highlights the differences across French and British colonial administrations in their efforts to establish modern, centralized transfusion centers. After independence, central coordination became increasingly difficult. Several factors played a role, including the world economic crisis and political instability, which were followed by the AIDS epidemic ten years later.

In Chapter 3, Vincanne Adams, Kathleen Erwin, and Phuoc Le argue that there is an important role for strong national public health programs. Their exploration of China's donation system is haunted by the public health crisis that emerged from China's initial inattention to HIV/AIDS prevention, and the mushrooming of HIV transmission from contaminated blood in the early 1990s. The success of the Public Health Bureau campaign arises in part from strategies used in China to publicize the marketing of blood donation as a public good in ways that make cultural sense to Chinese donors.

In Chapter 4, Sophie Chauveau draws our attention to France in the early 1980s and the reasons why the country sustained one of the highest rates of HIV – and hepatitis C – contaminated transfusion recipients and hemophiliacs in Europe. The nation-wide scandal sparked a major transformation in the economy of blood transfusion in France. The result is the co-existence of a moral gift economy (Godbout and Caillé 1992; Bourdieu 2000), which accommodates the obtaining of blood as raw material, and that of a market economy (Healy 2006; Scheper-Hughes and Wacquant 2002; Waldby and Mitchell 2006), which determines the availability, safety, and quality of all blood products.

Part II   The institutional politics of donor recruitment

In the second part of the book, the authors turn to cases in which the field is relatively stable. In this environment, what is examined is how the current institutional context creates the conditions needed for the field to work. The authors seek to establish how the system supplies a context conducive to the practice of blood donation and how it produces an effective rhetoric to convince the population to give blood. As Meyer and Rowan (1977) point out, institutional organizations need to convince populations that their "myths" work. This is the condition needed for them to foster trust, satisfaction, and good faith, both internally and externally. It is essential for the dominant social actors in a relatively stable field to use all the resources at their disposal to maintain the established order. The blood collection and transfusion system therefore needs to prove that it is able to supply safe blood products that can meet the growing needs of hospitals and health institutions.

Of the three examples presented in the second part of the book, two describe situations in Canada. These, however, involve the responsibility of distinct suppliers of blood products. The third example describes a situation in India, where maintaining or increasing the number of blood donors has become a focal issue following the implementation of legislation prohibiting remunerated blood donation.

In Canada, the organizational structure of the field of blood donation and transfusion was overhauled in the 1980s in the wake of the contaminated blood crisis. Government powers authoritatively created two organizations to oversee the supply of blood products: Héma-Québec for the province of Québec and Canadian Blood Services (CBS) for the rest of Canada. All rules governing blood product safety and health hazard prevention are nevertheless supervised and defined by Health Canada, a federal organization. Some internal governance units were also created by government authorities to oversee the activities of Héma-Québec and CBS, which were further required to acquire certification from international regulatory organizations. The geographical scope of territory covered by CBS has raised an issue that is not prevalent in Québec, namely the co-existence of homogeneous, centralized national guidelines and of concrete donor recruitment practices intended to be adapted to local contexts.

CBS headquarters in Ottawa, a dominant social actor, can use all the resources at its disposal to impose its rules and maintain its position in the field. Employees at local collection centers are certainly not always able to resist these imposed rules, but they are also adept at using all the resources to fulfill their own mission of maintaining and increasing the number of blood donors. How can they develop their donor recruitment and reception activities in spite of the constraints imposed by national authorities? They can forge alliances with other social actors, such as businesses, schools, local associations, and volunteers from the community. Those in charge of organizing local blood drives (at CBS and Héma-Québec) understood long ago that such alliances are very efficient for recruitment purposes. Other factors are just as important, however, in ensuring the system's effectiveness. For example, building up a meaningful rhetorical dis-course is a requisite condition for reinforcing positive donor identity. Employees at local blood drives must also develop a measure of "collective creativity" to make the donation experience as satisfying as possible for donors; this will ensure that they become regular donors in the long run.

The situation is rather different in India. With the end of the remunerated donation system, the main social actors in the country's blood donation field (doctors, blood organizations, hospitals, the Red Cross, politicians, political parties, and the media) had to make tremendous efforts to convince the popula-tion to donate blood under the new reference model – strongly suggested by the WHO – of voluntary, unpaid, anonymous donation. Replacement donation (offered by family members or friends), however, still remains highly prevalent. The new cultural frame, imported from the Western world, has come up against dominant social values and generalized fears associated with blood donation. Doctors have nonetheless understood that to make the system work and to show the model's efficiency, an alliance with religious leaders (gurus) could be the best strategy. The rhetorical discourse must also adapt to local conditions. While promoting voluntary, unpaid blood donation, the organizations in charge of blood donation marketing can incorporate other messages that are better associ-ated with the country's extant cultural values.

Part II chapters

In Chapter 5, André Smith argues that finding effective ways to recruit blood donors is vitally important in the context of a rising demand for blood due to an aging population, strict donor deferral criteria, and the limited shelf life of blood products. In this case study, the author sought to understand how clinic practices, which are guided by national policies, professional standards, and regulations, also reflect unique local beliefs, ideologies, and organizational cultures (Geertz 1973; Lee 2000; Powell and DiMaggio 1991). The blood donation clinic is conceptualized as an environment where employees construct and legitimate their activities in the context of shifting structural contingencies (Meyer and Rowan 1977), and where "social relations [are] deliberately created, with the explicit intention of continuously accomplishing some specific goals or purposes" (Stinchcombe 1965, 142). The author shows how the activities at one CBS clinic, in a community with substantially higher rates of donation, are shaped by specific organizational dynamics and local belief systems about how best to recruit blood donors and enhance their donation experience.

In Chapter 6, Johanne Charbonneau and Anne Quéniart identify the processes by which blood collection organizations influence blood donation motivations and practices (Giddens 1984; Healy 2006; Henrion 2003; Piliavin and Callero 1991). Their research is based on interviews with current and former donors in Québec about their blood donation experiences. It examines the reasons leading these donors to develop and maintain the practice, or to abandon it, over time. The authors explore how blood collection agencies influence motivation with appeals that reinforce the positive aspects of blood donation and the altruistic identity of donors. The analysis sheds light on the fact that certain institutional conditions are essential at every step of the blood donor's career.

In Chapter 7, Jacob Copeman explains that the 1998 banning of paid donation in India forced blood banks and other health institutions to find innovative strategies to radically increase levels of voluntary blood donation. The author highlights how the reluctance of people to partake in anonymous blood donation is tied to a cultural understanding of blood as rare and precious, and to the view that giving blood permanently depletes the donor's blood supply and can result in a loss of vital energy. In this context, family-based replacement donations continue to account for more than half of the total blood donations given in many regions of India. Appeals for voluntary donations have not been very successful, with one notable exception: that of campaigns targeting religious movements, in particular those led by gurus, which have now become important providers of voluntarily donated blood throughout India. The successive setting and surpassing of world records has turned the collection of blood by religious movements in India into something akin to a system of "alternating disequilibrium," as described by Strathern (1971), one group achieving the record and being dominant until another group breaks it, and so on.

Part III   The governance of blood donation: the authority of state control

The final part of the book comprises four chapters that look at situations of instability and transformation in the field of blood donation and transfusion. The Australian and French systems, analyzed in the first two chapters of Part III, may certainly be considered as relatively stable fields; however, these spaces always remain dynamic. Certain social actors may wish to contest the established order and the rules defined by the dominant actors, or to acquire more power or recognition. The issues examined in Australia and France relate to risk prevention and relationships of trust/mistrust within the field. The authors look into the processes that have led to defining selection and exclusion criteria, as well as the actions undertaken by groups that have challenged exclusion policies. While the authors whose contributions are featured earlier in the book concentrate on cultural frames and institutional rhetoric, the focus here is the processes of producing instruments, standards, and techniques that are also part of the action frame in the field of blood donation, namely in connection with the issue of risk control. The analyses also indicate that such technical and regulatory choices can introduce strong social meanings that can go so far as to redefine the meaning of citizenship and civic participation.

In both France and Australia, as in many other countries, a substantial paradigm shift has taken place in the relationship between blood organizations and the population since the contaminated blood crisis. From trusting blood donors, the system has progressively developed a new action framework based on a relationship of mistrust of all potentially "at risk" donors. The French state, for example, has encouraged the creation of a number of internal governance units to control this risk. However, some "institutional entrepreneurs" – epidemiologists – have also succeeded in asserting themselves in this process. They hold very socially legitimate skills based on academic and scientific knowledge. These "skilled individual actors" have been able to create coalitions with other dominant actors in the field. This redefinition of power relations appears, in fact, to reinforce standardization and homogenization in practices, consistent with a seemingly unavoidable phenomenon already observed by DiMaggio and Powell (1983).

The reinforcement of risk control actually leads to an increase in exclusion criteria. The organizations in charge must therefore develop a rhetoric aimed at convincing more people to engage in the practice. This discourse emphasizes the importance of civic participation, reinforcing a sense of exclusion among those who have been denied the possibility of donating blood. The social actors who are excluded from donating do, however, also have resources at their disposal to challenge these policies. Tensions remain high, since they struggle to impose their views in an organizational field where alliances between the dominant actors have built up a system that is very difficult to transform.

The two final chapters of the book underline that the field of blood donation and transfusion is far from stable in all countries across the world. In some cases, it actually seems to be in a state of permanent instability. It is as if the conditions are not in place for this field to emerge or to be restabilized after major disturbances. Sometimes, it appears that no social actor is capable of dominating the field and imposing ground rules in addition to an institutional logic that could be recognized by all the other actors in the field. Hierarchies do not emerge, and coalitions remain fleeting. To illustrate these situations of permanent instability, two different angles are considered: first, a macrosocial analysis that compares the general features of blood transfusion systems in Latin American countries;

and second, a case study of the conditions leading up to a failed transformation of the blood collection system in Trinidad.

The macrosocial analysis serves as a reminder of the importance of many economic, health, social, and political factors in the process of structuring this field. Its arguments echo those of Schneider in the first part of this book. In the absence of commitment on the part of political, judicial, and health authorities – who fail to supply the necessary resources and structure – the active organizations in the field generally continue to operate at largely decentralized levels, in an uncoordinated fashion and with uneven results. Some countries, such as Nicaragua, are more successful than others, bearing out that the influence of the political and social conditions specific to each country impact upon implementation and results. The case study, for its part, describes how the government authorities that wanted to establish a voluntary, non-remunerated, anonymous system had to abandon this goal and return to their previous system of replacement donation. The inability to bring about an acceptance of new forms of social solidarity that do not reflect the social values of the population is associated with, among other things, an absence of skilled individual actors capable of imposing their viewpoints, yet it is also part of the same decentralized and uncoordinated context described above. In these two chapters, the authors point out that no one seems to take into serious consideration the need to meet these populations' blood needs.

Part III chapters

In Chapter 8, Renaud Crespin and Bruno Danic examine the implementation of donor selection and deferral criteria since the contamination of the French blood supply in the 1980s. They approach this history as that of a dynamic of instrumentation (Lascoumes and Le Galès 2007). This approach allows them to expose the steps taken by successive government regimes in developing and implementing the standards that are used for the selection and exclusion of donation candidates, and this, in turn, invites us to focus on the spaces, players, knowledge, and techniques mobilized by this production process (Hacking 2001). The authors argue that these criteria reflect a logic of anticipating risks that is in truth likely to harm the health of the populations for whom they have – to borrow a term from Peter Conrad (1992) – "healthicized" the process of blood donation. The authors show how actors external to the transfusion system have played a determining role in the formulation of the exclusion policies which transfusion professionals have an obligation to defend in order to ensure blood supply safety.

In Chapter 9, Kylie Valentine focuses on Australia's national systems of blood donation, their governance arrangements, and their deferral policies. She examines the impact and political meanings of deferral policies, especially as they relate to marginalized groups. The author argues that the social solidarity and altruism so highly valued in blood donation have a concomitant devaluing effect on those who are excluded from donation. In recent years, the civil and political significance of blood donation has become particularly visible in Australia, in part because of the contesting of deferral policies for gay men. This activism – which is medically engaged, relationally historical, and a form of bio-logical citizenship (Rose and Novas 2005) – is at odds with the blanket exclusion of sexually active gay men, a top-down, bureaucratic, un-negotiated rule.

In Chapter 10, Maria Cristina Martínez Valenzuela and Carlos Alberto Sanchez focus on the management of blood donation across Latin America. As the authors argue, the sufficiency of the blood supply not only depends on the altruistic motivation of blood donors but also on how responsive and effective blood collection systems are in accommodating donors and processing donated blood. Despite facing major economic challenges, a number of Latin American countries have invested substantially in centralized, well-coordinated blood services and have been able to achieve high rates of voluntary blood donation. Unfortunately, several other Latin American countries remain hampered by the unwillingness of their respective governments to tackle the many economic, political, and organizational challenges associated with creating a safe, non-remunerated, voluntary blood donation system.

In Chapter 11, Vishala Parmasad draws upon qualitative and ethnographic research conducted between 2008 and 2013 to explore blood donation in Trini-dad in the context of chronic blood supply insufficiency. Her research shows that blood donation and procurement in Trinidad are subject not only to health sector inadequacies but also to complex networks of social meaning, exchange, and trust (Cohen 1999; Mauss 1923; Scheper-Hughes 2000). Successive govern-ments have failed in their efforts to develop a fully integrated national blood transfusion system that would allow blood to be managed as a national resource. In this country, replacement donation has been the main mode of blood procure-ment since the inception of transfusion, and this practice is entangled with the prevailing notions of reciprocity and kinship (Bourdieu 1977; Mauss 1923; Strathern 1992) that facilitate social cohesion.

In the concluding chapter, André Smith and Johanne Charbonneau revisit the institutionalist analytical framework in relation to the varied insights and find-ings that are presented in this book. The authors argue that these theoretical insights permit a sophisticated encapsulation of the complex institutional dynamics and risk management strategies that have influenced and transformed the organization of blood donation and transfusion. The concluding chapter finally offers a reflection on new issues in blood donation, including the ever-important question of exclusion, the development of the plasma industry, the growing influence of pharmaceutical laboratories, and the promotion of special-ized medicine for rare phenotypes, as well as the revival of racial identity issues that have been present since the beginning of blood transfusion development. The authors argue that we ought to disentangle these issues from technology and technical discourses and reinsert them into the lived experience of donors, into the complex organizational and regulatory dynamics of blood systems, and ulti-mately, into the social structure itself.

This new collection of cutting-edge research thus improves our understanding of how blood donation, as a fundamentally social act, is linked to diverse personal, political, and cultural meanings, as well as to the populations' trust of the state, which are themselves intersected by structural constraints that influence the willingness of some to donate and limit the legitimacy and ability of others to do so.

References

Alessandrini, M. 2007. "Community volunteerism and blood donation: altruism as a lifestyle choice." *Transfusion Medicine Reviews* 21(4): 307–316.

Allain, J.-P. 2010. "Volunteer safer than replacement donor blood: a myth revealed by evidence." *ISBT Science Series* 5: 169–175.

Barman, E. 2007. "An institutional approach to donor control: from dyadic ties to a field-level analysis." *AJS* 112(5): 1416–1457.

Boltanski, L. 2009. *De la critique: Précis de sociologie de l'émancipation.* Paris: Gallimard.

Boltanski, L. and Thévenot, L. 1991. *De la justification: les économies de la grandeur.* Paris: Gallimard.

Bourdieu, P. 1977. *Outline of a Theory of Practice.* Translated by Richard Nice. Cambridge: Cambridge University Press.

Bourdieu, P. 1984. *Distinction: A Social Critique of the Judgement of Taste.* Cambridge, MA: Harvard University Press.

Bourdieu, P. 1998. *Les règles de l'art : genèse et structure du champ littéraire.* Paris: Seuil.

Bourdieu, P. 2000 [1972]. *Esquisse d'une théorie de la pratique.* Paris: Le Seuil.

Bourdieu, P. and Wacquant, L. 1992. *An Invitation to Reflexive Sociology.* Chicago, IL: University of Chicago Press.

Cohen, L. 1999. "Where it hurts: Indian material for an ethics of organ transplantation." *Daedalus* 128(4): 135–165.

Conrad, P. 1992. "Medicalization and social control." *Annual Review of Sociology* 8: 209–232.

DiMaggio, P.J. 1988. "Interest and agency in institutional theory." In *Institutional Patterns and Culture*, edited by L. Zucker, 3–22. Cambridge, MA: Ballinger Publishing.

DiMaggio, P.J. and Powell, W.W. 1983. "The iron cage revisited: institutional isomorphism and collective rationality in organizational fields." *American Sociological Review* 48(2): 147–160.

Drori, G.S., Meyer, J.W., and Hwang H. (eds) 2006. *Globalization and Organization: World Society and Organizational Change.* New York: Oxford University Press.

Emirbayer, M. and Johnson, V. 2008. "Bourdieu and organizational analysis." *Theory and Society* 37: 1–44.

Farrugia, A., Penrod, A.J., and Bult J.M. 2010. "Payment, compensation and replacement – the ethics and motivation of blood and plasma donation." *Vox Sanguinis* 99(3): 202–211.

Fassin, D. 2000. *Les enjeux politiques de la santé: études sénégalaises, équatoriennes et françaises.* Paris: Karthala.

Fligstein, N. and McAdam, D. 2012. *A Theory of Fields.* New York: Oxford University Press.

Geertz, C. 1973. *Interpretation of Cultures.* New York: Basic Books.

Giddens, A. 1977. *Studies in Social and Political Theory.* London: Hutchinson.

Giddens, A. 1984. *The Constitution of Society Outline of the Theory of Structuration.* Berkeley: University of California Press.

Godbout, J. and Caillé, A. 1992. *L'esprit du don.* Paris: La Découverte.

Hacking, I. 2001. *Entre science et réalité: la construction sociale de quoi?* Paris: La Découverte.

Hall, P.A. and Taylor, R.C.R. 1996. "Political science and the three new institutionalisms." *Political Studies* 53: 936–957.

Healy, K. 2006. *Last Best Gifts. Altruism and the Market for Human Blood and Organs.* Chicago, IL: The University of Chicago Press.

Henrion, A. 2003. *L'énigme du don de sang. Approche ethnographique d'un don entre inconnus.* Liège: Université de Liège, faculté de philosophie et lettres, mémoire.

Hoffmann, A.J. 1999. "Institutional evolution and change: environmentalism and the US chemical industry." *Academy of Management Journal* 42(4): 351–371.

Lamont, M. 1992. *Money, Morals, and Manners: The Culture of the French and American Upper-Middle Class.* Chicago, IL: University of Chicago Press.

Lascoumes, P. and Le Galès, P. 2007. "Introduction: Understanding public policy through its instruments – from the nature of instruments to the sociology of public policy instrumentation." *Governance: An International Journal of Policy, Administration, and Institutions* 20: 1–21.

Lee, O. 2000. "The constitution of meaning: on the practical conditions of social understanding." *Current Perspectives in Sociological Theory* 20: 27–64.

Lewin, K. 1951. *Field Theory in Social Science: Selected Theoretical Papers.* New York: Harper.

Mahoney, J. and Thelen, K. 2009. "A theory of gradual change." In *Explaining Institutional Change: Ambiguity, Agency, and Power*, edited by J. Mahoney and K. Thelen, 1–37. New York: Cambridge University Press.

Martin, J.L. 2003. "What is field theory?" *AJS* 109(1): 1–49.

Mauss, M. 1990 [1923]. *The Gift: The Form and Reason for Exchange in Archaic Societies.* Translated by W. Halls. London: Routledge.

Meyer, J.W. and Rowan, B. 1977. "Institutionalized organizations: formal structure as myth and ceremony." *AJS* 83(2): 340–363.

Piliavin, J.A. and Callero, P.L. 1991. *Giving Blood: The Development of an Altruistic Identity.* Baltimore, MA: Johns Hopkins University Press.

Powell, W.W. 2007. "The new institutionalism." *The International Encyclopedia of Organization Studies.* Thousand Oaks, CA: Sage (preprint). www.stanford.edu/group/song/papers/NewInstitutionalism.pdf (last accessed December 16, 2014).

Powell, W.W. and DiMaggio, P.J. 1991. *The New Institutionalism in Organizational Analysis.* Chicago, IL: University of Chicago Press.

Rose, N. and Novas, C. 2005. "Biological citizenship." In *Global Assemblages. Technology, Politics and Ethics as Anthropological Problems*, edited by A. Ong and S.J. Collier, 439–463. Oxford: Blackwell.

Scheper-Hughes, N. 2000. "The global traffic in human organs." *Current Anthropology* 41(1): 191–224.

Scheper-Hughes, N. and Wacquant, L. (eds) 2002. *Commodifying Bodies.* London: Sage.

Scott, W.R. 2001. *Institutions and Organizations.* Thousand Oaks, CA: Sage.

Scott, W.R. and Meyer, J. 1983. "The organization of societal sectors." In *Organizational Environments: Ritual and Rationality*, edited by J. Meyer and W.R. Scott, 108–140. Beverly Hills, CA: Sage.

Stinchcombe, A.L. 1965. "Social structure and organizations." In *Handbook of Organizations*, edited by J.G. March, 142–193. Chicago, IL: Rand McNally.

Strathern, A. 1971. *The Rope of Moka: Big-men and Ceremonial Exchange in Mount Hagen, New Guinea.* Cambridge: Cambridge University Press.

Strathern, A. 1992. *After Nature: English Kinship in the Late Twentieth Century.* Cambridge: Cambridge University Press.

Titmuss, R.M. 1972. *The Gift Relationship: From Human Blood to Social Policy.* New York: Vintage Books.

Waldby, C. and Mitchell, R. 2006. *Tissue Economies. Blood, Organs and Cell Lines in Late Capitalism.* Durham, NC: Duke University Press.

Wieviorka, M. 1996. "Racisme, racialisation et ethnicisation en France." *Hommes et migrations.* Documents: 27–33.

World Health Organization (WHO). 2011. *Global Database on Blood Safety. Summary Report 2011.* www.who.int/bloodsafety/global_database/GDBS_Summary_Report_2011. pdf (last accessed December 16, 2014).

World Health Organization (WHO) and International Federation of Red Cross and Red Crescent Societies (IFRCRCS). 2010. *Towards 100% Voluntary Blood Donation. A Global Framework for Action.* www.who.int/bloodsafety/publications/9789241599696_ eng.pdf (last accessed December 16, 2014).

Zou, S., Musavi, F., Notari, E.P., Rios, J.A., Trouen-Trend, J., and Fang, C.J. 2008. "Changing age distribution of the blood donor population in the United States." *Transfusion* 48(2): 251–257.

Part I
Technology and the evolution of blood clinics

1 "What flows between us"

Blood donation and transfusion in the United States (nineteenth to twentieth centuries)[1]

Jean-Paul Lallemand-Stempak

Introduction

Long circumscribed to a "technician" history of medicine, the history of blood donation and transfusion was a history without actors – aside from doctors, of course – and especially without any stakes involved other than a certain idea of constant progress in medicine. Historiography may therefore have appeared to be out of step, and even belated, in examining these subjects. Since the emergence of what is today called the new social history of medicine, historians have focused on the social construction of medicine, understood as a *field* (Bourdieu 1998) in which interactions among various actors (patients, politicians, doctors, etc.) contribute to the emergence of new public health models (Fassin 2000). This shift in perspective today allows us to consider the history of blood donation and transfusion practices from a new angle. The history of blood transfusion in the United States must be examined in terms of two major problems that have intersected at various moments in their evolution: the question of its institutionalization (Boltanski 2009; Boltanski and Thévenot 1991) and of its racialization (Wieviorka 1996). This chapter seeks to provide a historical synthesis focused on the evolution of transfusion and blood donation in the United States, from the beginning of the nineteenth century to the start of the 1980s. The aim is to capture the ambivalence of blood donation.[2] Indeed, defined by their status as a healthcare technique and a commodity, blood donation and transfusion also appear, reading between the lines, as political tools that define belonging to a community (Anderson 1983; Douglas 1966).

The synthesis will hinge on four key periods in the history of transfusion and blood donation. If, during its genesis phase in the nineteenth century, this history does not seem to be pervaded by the political realm, it is above all because it appears to be the sole product of a hesitant medicine, of doctors who conducted experiments single-handedly and in an almost "homemade" fashion. In sum, this subject mainly interested physicians, who discussed it with other physicians. The development of transfusion and blood donation would later be facilitated by technical innovations at the turn of the 1930s. During this period, transfusion-related matters attracted attention from both the state (mainly the army) and members of the general public who became involved through associations (political, church, unions, civil rights, etc.).

World War II produced a strong demand for blood products. This period is crucial for understanding the evolution of the American transfusion system. The "spirit of the gift" underwent transformation and became a political gesture, namely participating in the war effort to save democracy and humanistic ideals. This period also saw the state become involved in the transfusion system. With the support of the Red Cross, the American government then developed the first network of blood banks to be established over a large stretch of its territory. During this expansion of the transfusion model, two visions of medicine clashed and sparked discussion among numerous actors. First, a racialized medicine versus a medicine blind to race, scientifically speaking; and second, a medicine governed by a mercantile logic versus a social medicine. While the state succeeded, at least temporarily, in putting aside the issue of race, the issue of commerce would never be entirely settled. In many ways, these debates are still alive today.

From the miracle of medicine to flourishing commerce

During its first phase of development between the second third of the nineteenth and the beginning of the twentieth century, transfusion in the United States was a rare and expensive medical operation, practiced only by an elite of pioneering doctors and, consequently, for the benefit of a minority of well-to-do patients (Schmidt 1968). W.B. Drinkard recorded only four transfusions performed on American soil prior to 1871 (Drinkard 1872). The transfusion centre at New York's Mount Sinai Hospital only registered some 20 transfusions each year at the dawn of the twentieth century. Transfusion was most often performed in emergency situations to counter significant blood loss, generally caused by major surgery or complications in childbirth (Lederer 2008).

The lack of scientific knowledge – blood groups had not yet been discovered – as well as the difficulty of finding blood required doctors to call upon the close acquaintances of their patients to donate. Relying on acquaintances seemed to be justified by both practical (speed and compatibility) and symbolic (kinship) considerations. Some doctors considered that they were limiting the risks of adverse physiological and psychological reactions among patients by calling upon their families. When family members declined, some surgeons gave their own blood or sought out remunerated donors whom they recruited in the immediate vicinity. It was not uncommon to see doctors recruit donors at hospital doors, among passers-by or ambulance drivers (Lederer 2008). Until the 1910s, the practice of transfusion nevertheless remained limited and marginalized in medicine and surgery. The establishment of new "direct" transfusion techniques by George Washington Crile, at the dawn of the twentieth century, caused a take-off in the practice and changed the very nature of blood donation. The invention of a specialized cannula considerably lowered the technical skill needed for a surgeon to perform a transfusion, as well as the duration of the operation (Schneider 1997; Nathoo et al. 2009). Whereas entire teams previously needed to be mobilized for one day or more, transfusions could now be performed quickly (in emergency medicine), and by only one doctor and one assistant (Crile 1909).

An ensuing climb in the number of transfusions led to the first shortages of donors. Transfusion was still a source of numerous fears and, in spite of pharmacopoeia used to reduce the anxiety of patients/donors (morphine, cocaine, etc.), certain transfusions failed for technical reasons or simply never took place because the donors changed their minds. To address the lack of donors, Crile (1909) was the first medical specialist to systematically appeal to donors with the promise of compensation. This was a departure from the first phase in the history of transfusion, when blood had almost no monetary value, insofar as it was obtained as an *altruistic gift* (Godbout 2000) from within a restricted group (family, friends, and doctors). As need continued to grow, blood became a rare and sought-after commodity in the context of transfusion.

The first remunerated donors were recruited through advertisements in newspapers or from among medical students and hospital staff. Because information on the product was scarce and the market unstable, prices for donated blood were volatile and established by the doctor or hospital. While Bertram Bernheim at Johns Hopkins Hospital in Baltimore paid up to US$100 for a blood donation in the 1910s, at Bellevue Hospital in New York, one obtained little more than US$10 (Bernheim 1942). Even so, potential donors abounded, sometimes in their hundreds, in hopes of selling their blood. When it spoke of men who sold their blood in 1915, the *New York Sun* did not hesitate to suggest the birth of a new profession. It was not long before overworked doctors were forced to delegate the management of donors to specialized agencies. In New York, the Mixon Blood Donor Agency had a list of 300 potential donors. A dozen donors were permanently present on their premises and in fact literally lived on site. In Baltimore, Dr. Bernheim obtained provisions from two specialized establishments in the area, namely Levering House and Wayfarer's Rest (Lederer 2008). Those who responded to his advertisements were mainly passers-by intrigued by the new miracle of medicine that was transfusion (Bernheim 1942).

In spite of the existence of a market for blood and donors, not everyone considered the commerce of blood to be morally acceptable. A medical student at Johns Hopkins, when interviewed by a journalist, admitted that he would have preferred to give blood without compensation, but needed money to pay for his wedding. Likewise, during a spike in blood prices in 1920, medical students at Flower Hospital in New York took the initiative of offering their blood to those who lacked the resources to obtain private donors (Lederer 2008). Scandalized by the practice of commercial blood donation, some 100 workers from the working class (janitors, chauffeurs, factory workers, etc.) united in St. Louis, Missouri in 1935 under the banner of the Blood Donors Benevolent Association, seeking to demonstrate a certain magnanimity, as a class, by showing that they preferred to make an altruistic donation to the poorest members of society (Lederer 2008). Other blood donors garnered media coverage by the number of voluntary donations they made. In the American press, Rose McCulli, a native of Philadelphia, became "the world champion of blood donors," with more than 300 donations made throughout the country in the 1930s (Lederer 2008).

If reactions to the commercial nature of blood donation became more critical in the 1930s, it is because, as the United States sank deeper into crisis, the number of professional donor offices was rapidly growing. The New York City Health Department also showed concern about this issue. Appealing to poverty-stricken donors was common, and the risks of transmitting certain diseases (syphilis, jaundice, etc.) were increasing. A number of centres were also found to be "somewhat negligent" in managing their donor lists: it was not unusual to see people give blood dozens of times each year (Bulletin of the NewYork Academy of Medicine 1930). To improve blood transfusion practices, the Blood Transfusion Betterment Association (BTBA) was created in 1929 by a group of leading specialists in the discipline (including Alexis Carrel). After a lengthy and in-depth study, the association submitted several recommendations to health authorities in their city. These recommendations led to the development of the first safety standards for transfusion. Among other things, the association created a donor passport to control the number of donations and the medical history of patients. It also established a recommended price for a pint of blood, which contributed to rapidly lower prices (Bulletin of the New York Academy of Medicine 1930).

It is important to note that at the time there was no national legislation on transfusion and blood donation, and that the American College of Surgeons – the chief authority on recommendations for hospital standards – did not address the issue until after World War II (ACS Committee On Blood and Allied Problems 1951).

Blood transfusion and fear of miscegenation

Thanks to its spectacular nature, transfusion was a favourite subject of the American press, which headlined this new medical miracle from its inception. Press articles provide a snapshot of popular representations and fears surrounding blood donation from its early days. Representations of blood played a major role in the symbolic (Douglas 1966; Héritier 2010; Roux 1988) and often legal (Gross 2008) definition of race. Between the 1910s and 1930s, as blood transfusion and, de facto, the fear of miscegenation developed in the USA, a dozen states established their own hypodescent laws defining as black anyone with any black ancestry (also known as the "one drop rule" (Gross 2008)).

As Susan Lederer has clearly shown, before World War II, transfusions that were seen as constituting a form of social infringement by breaking the color line nourished the press columns of sensationalist media, both nationally and locally (Lederer 2008). Generally, these accounts involved patients who, following a transfusion, wondered about the new blood circulating in their veins and feared physiological transformation or symbolic miscegenation (Douglas 1992; Héritier 2010). Such accounts point to an "imaginary network" associated with representations of blood based on national, ethnic, religious, moral, sexual, or racial identity.

In 1909, the fact that a white man gave blood to a "Negress" at Bellevue Hospital was dubbed "a case without precedent" by the New York press. Likewise, following a double transfusion in 1921, famed tenor Enrico Caruso was upset at the prospect of losing his Italian identity and wondered about his own nature: "I have no more my pure blood Italian ... what now am I?" (Lederer 2008) Before the advent of blood banks, transfusions were made directly from the donor to the recipient. A thin curtain usually separated the two patients, but, at one moment or another, they could always meet. It was therefore possible for a patient to refuse a donor, since the latter was never anonymous. In 1938, a young Orthodox Jewish woman who reportedly refused the blood of a non-Jewish donor asked her doctor to find her a Jewish donor. Embarrassed, the doctor made arrangements with the agency that usually supplied him with donors so that he could find a "kosher substitute." The agency proposed one Isaac Goldberg, a blond man of Swedish origin with a strong Minnesota accent, who was accepted by the patient (Lederer 2008). The importance given to these accounts of donations and transfusion in the press and popular culture suggests that such cases were rare and defied a certain social order.

At the start of the 1930s, with the invention and use of citrate solutions enabling longer conservation of blood without coagulation, doctors, for the first time, were able to keep separate the donor from the patient during transfusion. This practice transformed transfusion from a surgical standpoint, but in reality, at least at first, the common practice was still to call upon agencies whose donors could be identified. Only at the end of the 1930s, with the creation and development of blood banks, was anonymity introduced. This factor would profoundly change the patient–donor relationship, as well as the symbolism of blood donation (Godbout 2000).

The emergence of blood banks

In 1937, after having studied works published by Soviet doctors, Bernard Fantus came up with the idea to create a system at Cook County Hospital in Chicago that would ensure the permanent availability of ready-to-use blood reserves. This would eliminate the risk of a shortage, which loomed over transfusion centers relying on lists from donor agencies. Although he was not the first to have the idea of conserving previously collected blood, he did father the concept of the blood bank. The principle was simple, the method was efficient, and the concept struck a chord and caught on (Fantus 1938a, 1938b). The functioning of such a blood bank required formalized management practices. Donor management therefore had to comply with a rationality of accounting, which participated in the development of the commerce of blood products. In a matter of months, Fantus's model had inspired surgeons across the United States.

During the 1930s, blood transfusion thrived, particularly with the discovery that it could be used in cases of trauma. From almost 3,000 transfusions per year in 1930, the Blood Transfusion Betterment Association recorded three times more in 1937. In 1938, Philadelphia's General Hospital and John Gaston Hospital in Memphis opened their own banks based on Fantus's model. One year later, they were followed by Johns Hopkins Hospital in Baltimore, Presbyterian in New York, Children's Hospital in Washington, DC, and Jefferson Davis in Houston (Lederer 2008). The appearance of these blood banks established a practice which, a few years later, would lead to the greatest controversy in the history of transfusion in the United States: the segregation of African Americans' blood.

The new way to manage blood donation followed a logic that dehumanized blood donation. The emphasis was no longer on recruiting donors through agencies, but rather on managing blood stock. Thus in this anonymous pattern of donation (Titmuss 1971; Godbout 2000), blood should not be refused because of a donor's ethnic, religious, or racial background.

But while ethical, religious, or gender-related considerations could easily be set aside by science, the same could not be said for race. The link between blood and race always produced major debates in the scientific community (Kenny 2006). However, most doctors, and in particular those in charge of blood banks, agreed that there was no difference between blood from a black person or a white person, and that there was no risk of miscegenation. How then can it be explained that as blood banks appeared, the first practices of racial blood segregation arose? While the first blood bank created by Bernard Fantus in 1937 at Cook County Hospital in Chicago recorded patients' race, it is unknown whether the blood was segregated in practice. The memoirs of Fantus' daughter suggest that the surgeon opposed such segregation in the name of humanistic ideals (Gendron and Brubeck 2007). However, this practice appeared to be more frequent elsewhere. Lemuel Diggs, who founded the blood bank at John Gaston Hospital in Memphis in 1938, made no secret of the fact that he segregated blood donations. Once the donor's race (white or colored) was noted in a register, Diggs would store donated blood on different shelves of refrigerators. He took care to note that patients should receive blood corresponding to their race. Diggs nevertheless specified that, in case of a medical emergency, any type of blood could be used (Diggs 1939). Mark Ravitch, who was in charge of the blood bank at Johns Hopkins Hospital in Baltimore the following year, did not hesitate to declare in the leading American medical journal (Ravitch 1940) that "the considerable proportion of Negro patients at the Johns Hopkins Hospital constituted one of the primary problems for establishing the bank" because this blood couldn't be transfused to white patients who usually attended this hospital. Even if he admitted that no biological or physiological arguments justified this segregation, he always made sure that no bottles of blood could ever cross the color line. This brings us to the core of the racial issue in the United States; certain historians, such as Susan Lederer, hypothesize that doctors, who cited the danger represented by syphilis, a disease considered to primarily affect black populations, promoted the purity of blood and health safety. However, this argument is not very convincing, since all collected blood samples were screened for syphilis using the Kline or Wassermann test.

The segregation of African American donors therefore followed two complementary trends. The first was institutional: the entire medical community in the United States was segregated; black doctors and surgeons belonged to different medical organizations than white doctors and surgeons (National Medical Association vs. American Medical Association). They were trained and practiced in establishments that were differentiated by race (Byrd 2000). The segregation of blood may thus have appeared as an obvious practice to these doctors, since refraining from such segregation would have fundamentally contradicted the way in which American hospitals were managed (Gamble 1995).

This institutional explanation is insufficient to account for this phenomenon, since most doctors also offered reasons that could be described as social. In fact, the introduction of new anonymous practices for managing donors offered the possibility of blind miscegenation. No one could know any longer whether they had received blood from a black donor, which at the time represented the ultimate infringement, along with interracial marriage. It could be said that the system refused to fully implement the pattern of purely anonymous donation (Godbout 2000). While all the elements defining identity disappeared (name, religion, gender, etc.), the one identity-related element that had to remain, in American society, was the unsurpassable issue of race.

Brothers of blood

In June 1940, as Europe spiralled into war, the American government considered supporting its British ally by exporting plasma for the injured. In a meeting between the Army, the Marines, the BTBA, the National Research Council, and the Rockefeller Institute, a decision was made to establish a "Blood for Britain Project" aiming to supply the English with plasma collected at a pilot center in New York. Plasma (a blood fluid from which red blood cells have been removed) was then preferred over blood in that it was less fragile, suitable for freezing, and therefore easier to carry and preserve over long distances. Two hematologists, Charles Drew and John Scudder, who managed the blood bank at Presbyterian Hospital in New York City, were appointed to lead the project. Between August 1940 and January 1941, almost 15,000 New Yorkers gave blood in support of this initiative. Once the experimental phase was completed in January 1941, it was decided that the project should be extended to the entire country and that the mission would be handed over to the American Red Cross (Report of the Blood Transfusion Association 1941).

The choice of the Red Cross was an obvious one in view of the agency's vast network of volunteers, who were dispersed across the USA and could easily be mobilized (Stetten 1941). The Red Cross also enjoyed a very positive image among civil populations. Detailed specifications were given to the agency. The first Red Cross blood donation centre opened in February 1941; 35 others followed by 1945. In total, during the war, 14 million Americans gave blood at Red Cross centres. To achieve this level of success, the Red Cross launched a communications campaign that used all available media. Advertisements on the radio, in newspapers, and even in movie theatres appealed to the American citizens to give blood to fight the Nazi threat and save democracy. Communications mainly targeted the civic sense of donors (DeKleine 1950). Giving blood meant asserting one's faith in democracy and in humanistic ideals. It is in the context of this citizen mobilization that controversy arose over the segregation of African American donors.

During the establishment of the pilot blood bank at Presbyterian Hospital, all donors were accepted. When the Red Cross launched its own centres, it sided with the American Army and Marines in refusing the participation of black donors in the project. In New York and Philadelphia, the blood of black donors was sent to local hospitals that were less strict about the origins of transfused blood (ARC Archives RG200).

It was the development of Red Cross donation centres and their policy of refusing black donors that led to the first indignant reactions. In July 1941, when five African Americans presented at the Red Cross centre in Baltimore to give blood, they were told that their blood would not be used by the Red Cross but sent to local hospitals. They left without making a donation, and a few days later, *The Afro-American*, a local newspaper, published a series of articles denouncing this segregation policy. In a few months, the Red Cross faced large-scale opposition from major black associations and from doctors' associations (NAACP, NUL, NMA, AAPA, etc.). The Red Cross's action was deemed scandalous, not only because it was scientifically unfounded but also because it challenged the ultimate gift: the gift of life. Refusing the blood of blacks amounted to denying their citizenship and their desire to save democracy (Valentine 2005; Chapter 9, this volume; Fassin 1996, 2000). Opponents often compared this Red Cross policy to the Nazis' ideology of racial purity (ARC Archives RG200). The wave of criticism and indignation produced no change in the Army's policy on this matter (the Army was in fact facing opposition over its broader policy of segregation), but the Red Cross decided in January 1942 to accept black donors, although it labeled their donations (N for Negro or AA for *Africanus Americanus*) so that they could only be distributed to black soldiers (Guglielmo 2010). In a private response to Eleanor Roosevelt, who had requested an explanation, Red Cross President Norman H. Davis said:

> It must be recognized that there are many people in this country who object to having Negro blood used for transfusion of white persons. This is a matter of tradition and sentiment rather than of science, as there is no known difference in the physical properties of white and Negro blood.... Neither the American Red Cross nor the Medical Departments of the Armed Forces have considered that this feeling can be disregarded.
>
> (ARC RG200)

In spite of strong popular opposition and objections from the NAACP to the National Urban League, the Red Cross maintained its national policy of segregation until 1947.

Blood banks confronted with desegregation

World War II had created a link between medicine, the fight against Nazism, and democracy. Black participation in the war effort contributed to producing new views on race and health, raising questions of inequality, democracy, and citizenship. The segregation of blood exemplified the weakness of segregationist positions on the health system. It was perceived as a superstition that was bound to disappear in a scientific era, but also as a principle that ran contrary to promoting democracy in the face of the racist ideology that had pervaded the war (Wailoo 2001).

In the South, where public spaces were more segregated than in the North, blood segregation was an important issue. Up until then, "Jim Crow" laws had not addressed segregation in transfusion, only in interpersonal relationships (marriage, adoption, sexuality) and in public spaces. Blood donation centres were partly segregated: entrances, bathrooms, and waiting rooms were differentiated, but not treatment rooms. In situations with greater legislative constraints, specific days were set aside for blacks. At the Birmingham Alabama Center, for example, Thursdays were reserved for black donors. In Mississippi, specifications at certain blood banks clearly stated that in case black donors occupied the centre, sheets had to be changed and specific dishes be used (ARC RG200).

Following the decision in *Brown v. Board of Education*, which was the starting point for the Civil Rights Movement, segregationists in the South rallied to fight desegregation and to preserve a certain Southern tradition. Although opposition to desegregation primarily concerned schools, it also addressed blood segregation.

In January 1958, a law was tabled in the Georgia Senate to the effect that the social origin of donors had to be written on blood samples and that patients had to be informed of this origin. Failure to respect the law could lead to an 18-month prison sentence and a US$1,000 fine. The law was passed by the Senate but was rejected by the House of Representatives. Similar laws were proposed every few years in eight Southern states: Louisiana, Mississippi, Virginia, South Carolina, Arkansas, Georgia, Alabama, and Florida. The reasoning was clear: as George S. Harrel declared before the House of Representatives in South Carolina in 1959:

> The Supreme Court and Eisenhower are going to beat you on integrating the schools … but that is no reason why we should mix the blood in South Carolina.

> (Lederer 2008)

In just a few years, blood segregation became a major political issue for segregationists in the South. Faced with the Civil Rights Movement and the growing issue of medical integration in these states, legislating on blood transfusion became a way to oppose desegregation on a practical level, but also, and especially, on a symbolic level. While these laws were adopted only in Arkansas and Louisiana, they were certainly discussed, and representatives defended them vehemently in both the local and national press.

In 1964, the absence of legislation on blood segregation came to an end with the passing of the Civil Rights Act. Immediately after its adoption, the Public Health Service ordered hospitals to end segregation in blood banks, barring which they would lose their federal funding (Medicare, Medicaid, Hill-Burton

Fund). In spite of opposition from its governor, Arkansas was required to repeal its law in 1969. Blood segregation persisted in Louisiana despite repeated warnings from the government, as illustrated by a statement made by Archie Davis to the House of Representatives in 1960:

> I would see my family die and go to eternity before I would see them have a drop of nigger blood in them.
>
> (Lederer 2008)

> The issue was too important to be dropped. Finally, in June 1972, the governor urged congressmen to change the law amid fears of financial reprisals from the federal government.
>
> (Lederer 2008)

The same year, American blood banks collectively came under the authority of the Food and Drug Administration (FDA). The FDA decreed new rules and regulations, beginning with an official ban on segregation. The American transfusion system was in a state of chaos, and the Nixon Administration undertook to completely overhaul the sector. This decision profoundly altered the American blood donation system, which had previously relied on the principles of the private sector and was generally organized at the regional level. To understand how the FDA came to oversee blood, we must backtrack several decades to the period immediately following World War II.

Opposition between two models of transfusion medicine

In the aftermath of the War, the Red Cross was to a certain extent divested of its functions by the Army and had to close down its centres. The cost of managing the National Blood Program had also left the Red Cross in a critical financial situation that had to be addressed without delay in order for activities to resume. The American government owed the organization almost US$16 million (Starr 1998).

With the beginning of the Cold War and rising fears of a nuclear attack on American soil, the Army thought that the system established by the Red Cross could help to meet a large portion of blood-related needs in case of an attack. Following a number of meetings, the Red Cross, in agreement with the Army, decided in 1947 to pursue its mission during peacetime. During the War, it had acquired an enviable image, upon which it now hoped to capitalize. Moreover, transfusion could be a way to stabilize its finances.

But at that same moment, a group of doctors led by John Scudder realized the importance of transfusion and the system of blood banks for the American health system. The group founded the American Association of Blood Banks (AABB) in Dallas, Texas. The idea was to establish a vast system of cooperation among blood banks across the country, under the management and supervision of competent doctors. The suggested model would be based on a loan system. Patients who became ill would be loaned blood on the condition that they pay back the loan via an equivalent blood donation or financial repayment (Starr 1998).

This marked the beginning of a long conflict between the two institutions. The two models were utterly at odds on the meaning to give to donation. From this opposition emerged two visions of medicine and its functioning. The AABB criticized the Red Cross for its lack of competence and its close ties with the government. Indeed, Red Cross centres depended on a national headquarters and were not managed by doctors, unlike the AABB. John Scudder saw this as a will to "nationalize blood banks by the government": in a word, it was a "socialist project" managed by "incompetents" who had no understanding of medicine.

The Red Cross, for its part, considered the AABB model a commercial project that was both morally and ethically unacceptable. Internal reports of the American College of Surgeons and the Red Cross suggest that these organizations feared John Scudder and his colleagues might use the AABB for profit (Committee On Blood Banks 1954). In the absence of national legislation on blood transfusion and blood banks, the United States therefore inherited a patchwork system of non-remunerated donation (ARC), semi-commercial donation (AABB), and purely commercial and independent blood banks. In 1962, in a context of 4,000 blood banks in the United States, almost 40 percent of the transfusion market was managed by the Red Cross, 35 percent by the AABB, and the rest by private groups (Committee On Blood Banks 1962). In some hospitals, patients had to pay large sums for transfusions that they could have obtained freely at a hospital just a few blocks away.

Private and commercial banks led to scandals, which in turn led the public and the American government to rethink the legal status of blood. The most iconic example may be found in the World Blood Bank, founded in 1954 in Kansas City, Missouri. Its marketing slogan "cash for blood," along with its offer of transfusion insurance to anyone interested in participating, mainly attracted the homeless and the marginalized. The World Blood Bank did not hesitate to send out its sales agents to pressure medical interns on night shifts to buy its surplus blood. These *modus operandi* and recruitment methods scandalized local doctors, who founded their own bank, the Community Blood Bank, which was soon joined by most local hospitals. Deeming this organization to contravene the law of free competition, the World Blood Bank accused the Community Blood Bank of economic boycotting and attempting to create a monopoly. Despite the mobilization of the AABB and ARC, which had formed a sacred union, the Federal Trade Commission ultimately upheld the World Blood Bank and required the Community Blood Bank to work with it or face a fine of US$5,000 per day. Two senate proposals in 1964 and 1967, seeking to exempt blood banks from antitrust laws, failed. The judgments handed down by the federal government considered that blood was a good like any other. More specifically, insofar as it was not pure – because it was enriched with sodium citrate to avoid agglutination – blood was a medical commodity rather than a body tissue. Blood donation consequently came down to a contractual relationship, as with any remunerated labour (Starr 1998). In the early 1970s, commercial blood banks faced an almost simultaneous three-pronged attack from different sectors in American society. The first came from journalists, who denounced several major scandals, including the backdating of blood samples by the Dallas Blood Bank (1969). A series of articles (awarded by the Pulitzer Prize) were published in the *National Observer* in 1972. Entitled "The Blood that Kills," the articles showed each week how commercial blood banks primarily recruited donors on the margins of society: drug addicts, alcoholics, prisoners, the homeless, etc. (Lederer 2008). This pointed to the high risk of transmitting hepatitis, which could not be detected in blood samples at the time (Starr 1998).

The second wave of criticism came from the scientific community. Richard Titmuss, who underscored the loss of a sense of community, a drop in scientific standards, the introduction of market logic in medicine, and the social and financial cost of this system, launched an initial attack. While his critique was aimed at the American transfusion system at large, it must be recognized that his study excluded nearly 75 percent of the market represented at the time by the ARC and AABB (Titmuss 1971). The same year, the National Institute of Health (NIH) published a study demonstrating that almost 30 percent of blood donations were destroyed each year, that their prices were disproportionate and unequal, and especially that the transfusion system was not exempt from danger. The NIH advanced that 850 deaths were caused by hepatitis infections (NIH 1971).

Aware of the limits of the system and fearful of legal proceedings, President Richard Nixon declared in 1972 that blood was a "unique national resource" and that it would henceforth be managed under the supervision of the Food and Drug Administration (Lederer 2008). In 1978, the FDA decided to label blood samples according to their origin (commercial or non-remunerated donation), which contributed, in the space of a few years, to gearing the market of commercial blood banks toward activities other than medicine. Most of them joined forces with major players in the pharmaceutical industry that managed the production of plasma needed to develop various medicinal products. At the same time, the blood banks of the AABB and ARC were faced with the greatest health crisis in their history: the discovery of HIV and the contamination of blood products (Starr 1998).

Conclusion

The history of blood transfusion and donation in the United States is a history fraught with controversies, whether racial, economic, or health-related. With each new crisis, the "spirit of the gift" has undergone transformation. The original and miraculous donation, almost magical, would give way to a citizen act marking belonging to a community (Fantauzzi 2008). The emergence of the post-war medical industry in no way spared the special gift that is blood donation. Still, today, it is at the heart of major controversies (discrimination, health hazards) that, in many ways, are comparable to the crises of yesterday.

Even though indicating race on blood samples was abolished in the 1960s in the name of a race-blind science, this new position was not tenable for long, and

American health authorities soon had to re-evaluate their policies. Indeed, the discovery of diseases affecting specific ethnic groups (sickle-cell anemia, thalassemia, etc.) constrained doctors to use blood with similar phenotypes. In 1998, the American Red Cross therefore established banks of rare donors, which today count almost 45,000 potential donors. To avoid encouraging a certain community centredness, the Red Cross has avoided emphasizing the "ethnic" character of this donation, which, just like other blood donations, remains anonymous, free, and voluntary. It is worth noting that, although blood transfusion is no longer segregated in the United States, health-related exclusions for certain population categories (homosexuals and foreigners in particular) are similarly perceived, by these peoples, as a form of discrimination that jeopardizes their recognition by society.[3]

The advent of new surgical techniques (bloodless surgery) and the development of blood substitute products (Hemopure, Biopure) are increasingly challenging the altruistic, voluntary, and non-remunerated model that the WHO called for in 2008. While most members of the medical community agree on the usefulness and need for such a model, others are concerned about its costs and about potentially greater dependency on pharmaceutical laboratories. If medicine is one day able to dispense with blood donation by using these substitutes, an altruistic and non-remunerated system of transfusion will ultimately never have been established, thus reinforcing risks of unequal access to care. It is the very "spirit of the gift" which founds and structures societies that is at stake.

Notes

1 A previous version of this chapter has been published in Johanne Charbonneau and Nathalie Tran (eds). 2012. *Les Enjeux du Don de Sang dans le Monde*. Rennes: Presses de l'EHESP. However, this chapter, originally published in French, has been updated, and additional ideas have been included in the analyses and conclusions.
2 This chapter draws from recent historiography on the subject and from a diversified corpus of primary sources (personal archives of doctors; archives from institutions, states, and associations; and a press review). A list may be found in the bibliography of this chapter.
3 See Chapters 8 and 9, this volume.

References

Primary sources

1930. Bulletin of the NewYork Academy of Medicine.
1941. Report of the Blood Transfusion Association.
1951. ACS Committee On Blood and Allied Problems.
1954, 1962. Committee on Blood Banks.

34   *J.-P. Lallemand-Stempak*

Secondary sources

Anderson, B.R. 1983. *Imagined Communities: Reflections on the Origin and Spread of Nationalism*. New York: Verso.

Bernheim, B.M. 1942. *Adventure in Blood Transfusion*. New York: Smith & Durrell.

Boltanski, L. 2009. *De la critique: Précis de Sociologie de L'Émancipation*. Paris: Gallimard.

Boltanski, L. and Thévenot, L. 1991. *De la Justification: Les Economies de la Grandeur*. Paris: Gallimard.

Bourdieu, P. 1998. *Les Règles de L'Art : Genèse et Structure du Champ Littéraire*. Paris: Seuil.

Byrd, W. 2000. *An American Health Dilemma, Vol. 2*. New-York: Routledge.

Crile, G.W. 1909. *Hemorrhage and Transfusion; An Experimental and Clinical Research*. New York and London: D. Appleton.

DeKleine, W. 1950. *The History of the American National Red Cross, Vol. 33b*. Washington, DC: American Red Cross.

Diggs, L.W. 1939. "Problems in Blood Banking." *American Journal of Clinical Pathology* 9: 591–603.

Douglas, M. 1966. *Purity and Danger: An Analysis of Concepts of Pollution and Taboo*. New-York: Praeger.

Douglas, M. 1992. *De la souillure: essai sur les notions de pollution et de tabou*. Paris: La Découverte.

Drinkard, W.B. 1872. "History and Statistics of the Operation and Transfusion of Blood." *National Medical Journal* 2: 181–194.

Fantauzzi, A. 2008. "Une intéressante problématique: Ethno-anthropologie du Don du Sang chez les Immigrés Marocains de Turin." *Revue du MAUSS permanente* [online]. www.journaldumauss.net/spip.php?article423 (last accessed December 16, 2014).

Fantus, B. 1938a. "Cook County's Blood Bank." *Modern Hospital* 50: 57–58.

Fantus, B. 1938b. "The Therapy of the Cook County Hospital." *Journal of the American Medical Association* 111(4): 317–321.

Fassin, D. 1996. *L'Espace Politique de la Santé: Essai de Généalogie*. Paris: PUF.

Fassin, D. 2000. *Les Enjeux Politiques de la Santé: Études Sénégalaises, Équatoriennes et Françaises*. Paris: Karthala.

Gamble, V. 1995. *Making a Place for Ourselves: The Black Hospital Movement 1920–1945*. New York: Oxford University Press.

Gendron, V. and Brubeck, N.S. 2007. *Blood of Life: A Biography of the Life of Bernard Fantus M.D.* Baltimore, MD: N.S. Brubeck.

Godbout, J.T. 2000. *Le don, la dette, l'identité: homo donator vs homo oeconomicus*. Paris: La Découverte.

Gross, A. 2008. *What Blood Won't Tell: A History of Race on Trial in America*. Cambridge, MA: Harvard University Press.

Guglielmo, T. 2010. "Red Cross Double Cross: Race and America's World War II-Era Blood Donor Service." *Journal of American History* 97(1): 63–90.

Héritier, F. 2010. *Hommes, Femmes: La Construction de la Différence*. Paris: Le Pommier.

Kenny, M.G. 2006. "A Question of Blood, Race, and Politics." *Journal of the History of Medicine and Allied Sciences* 61: 456–491.

Lederer, S. 2008. *Flesh and Blood: Organ Transplantation and Blood Transfusion in 20th Century America*. New-York: Oxford University Press.

Mauss, M. and Weber, F. 2007. *Essai sur le Don: Forme et Raison de L'Échange dans les Sociétés Archaïques*. Paris: Presses Universitaires de France.

Nathoo, N., Lautzenheiser, F.K., and Barnett, G.H. 2009. "The First Direct Human Blood Transfusion: The Forgotten Legacy of George W. Crile." *Neurosurgery* 64(3 Suppl.): ons20–26; discussion ons26–27.

Ravitch, M.M. 1940. "The Blood Bank of the Johns Hopkins Hospital." *Journal of the American Medical Association* 115(3): 171–178.

Roux, J.-P. 1988. *Le Sang: Mythes, Symboles et Réalités*. Paris: Fayard.

Schmidt, P.J. 1968. "Transfusion in America in the eighteenth and nineteenth centuries." *The New England Journal of Medicine*. 279(24): 1319–20.

Schneider, W.H. 1997. "Blood Transfusion in Peace and War, 1900–1918." *Social History of Medicine* 10(1): 105–126.

Starr, D. 1998. *Blood: An Epic History of Medicine and Commerce*. New York: Harper.

Stetten, DeW. 1941. *The Blood Plasma for Great Britain Project*. New York: Bulletin.

Titmuss, R. 1971. *The Gift Relationship: From Human Blood to Social Policy*. New York: Vintage Books.

Valentine, K. 2005. "Citizenship, Identity, Blood Donation." *Body and Society* 11(2): 113–128.

Wailoo, K. 2001. *Dying in the City of the Blues: Sickle Cell Anemia and the Politics of Race and Health*. Chapel Hill: The University of North Carolina Press.

Waldby, C. and Mitchell, R. 2006. *Tissue Economies: Blood, Organs, and Cell Lines in Late Capitalism*. Durham, NC: Duke University Press.

Wieviorka, M. 1996. "Racisme, Racialisation et Ethnicisation en France." *Hommes et Migrations. Documents:* 27–33.

2   History of transfusion in Africa

Who gave blood?[1]

William H. Schneider

Introduction

In Africa, as elsewhere, the question of who gives blood is of great importance for at least two reasons. First, in order to secure an adequate supply of blood, it is crucial to know who gave and, even more importantly, why blood was given. Second, who donates blood is very relevant to the safety of blood transfusion because, quite simply, people in certain circumstances have higher risk of transmitting infections. Thus an overview of who gave blood in the history of transfusion in Africa is valuable in order to understand the historical and cultural origins of securing an adequate and safe blood supply (Schneider 2013).

As may be expected, taboos, superstitions, and cultural traditions prevented many Africans from donating blood (Musambachime 1988; White 2002). Yet, despite the rumours and misunderstandings or the warnings of old colonials, ultimately, Africans were persuaded to give up blood and agreed to place the blood of another person in their bodies. In this sense, they were generally not so different from potential donors in Europe or America who had reservations and questions about giving blood. A review and assessment of the record shows that lack of donors was not the biggest hindrance to the growth of blood transfusions in Africa. In fact, Africans gave blood and welcomed blood transfusions, eventually almost to the fault of overuse.

Along with these similarities, there were some important circumstances in Africa that made blood donation different from that undertaken in Europe or America. These included greater poverty as well as different diseases that affected blood safety. For example, greater poverty in Africa made payment for blood much more significant than in the developed world. A payment and meal or other refreshments given to most Africans meant far more than small payments given in some European countries for donating blood. Payment for blood in Africa was not a token compensation for inconvenience, as it was often described in France, for example. It was a source of cash not otherwise readily available to Africans, who responded very well when such payments were offered.

From the start, all evidence shows that men gave blood overwhelmingly more frequently than women, with little difference between regions and, until recently, at all times. Younger donors also gave in higher numbers in Africa than in

Europe and America. Both of these features were partly the result of the early, organized recruitment at military barracks, prisons, and schools by transfusion services that could store blood. As time went by and disease risk rose, especially for HIV/AIDS, the donors in the military and prisons were excluded and the importance of students rose accordingly. Although there were more boys in schools, the girls who were enrolled provided by far the largest source of female donors in Africa.

Among the other consequences of practicing transfusion in poor countries, besides the generally more precarious nature of health, were the frequent shortages of supplies (i.e., bottles, bags, and blood-drawing sets), as well as the lack of sufficient infrastructure such as widely available and reliable electricity, needed for refrigeration and storage. Just to take one of the many consequences, these conditions made it difficult to maintain adequate supplies of stored blood outside the big cities in Africa. The result was that most donors were recruited for immediate transfusion. This was not so different from what happened initially in Europe and America between the World Wars, where the local Red Cross branches in Britain and the continental hospital transfusion services established lists (or panels) of pre-tested and willing donors who could be called when needed to give blood (Schneider 2003). In Africa, when the supply of blood was insufficient, hospitals encouraged patients to bring in family and friends who, in many cases, whether known or not by the hospitals, were paid to give blood by the family of the patient. This occurred especially in transfusions for maternity and pediatric cases in Africa, because there it was much more likely that there would be family members with a strong sense of obligation to provide the blood for the patient. This circumstance also gave rise to the practice of "replacement" donation. Although never formalized like the "chit" system in Trinidad described elsewhere in this volume,[2] the underlying practice, whereby families were told to provide blood donations equal to or in excess of that planned for their family members' transfusion, became widespread in sub-Saharan Africa. This is quite controversial because it directly contradicts the "voluntary, non-remunerated blood donor" system advocated by the WHO (Allain 2010; Bates and Hassal 2010).

Early blood donation before independence

Blood donors in Africa were initially recruited by or found in the hospitals where transfusions were given, and thus were part of the original "hospital based" transfusion system. Not surprisingly, donors were first sought within the hospital itself. For example, an early experiment in the *Hôpital de l'Etoile* in Katanga province of the Belgian Congo treated 238 African patients suffering from pneumonia with blood drawn from other, recovering patients. (Spedener 1924) Likewise, a 1940 report on transfusions done at Katana Hospital in Kivu province of eastern Belgian Congo indicated that blood was taken from recovering patients (Lambillon and Denosoff 1940). In fact, a main conclusion of the report was: "in the colonial setting blood transfusion is very easily done, thanks to the large number of chronic patients that are in all the native hospitals who can serve as donors" (Lejeune 1921; Spedener 1924; Lambillon and Denisoff 1940).

The outbreak of World War II greatly stimulated interest in transfusion, but there are conflicting reports and mixed results of attempts to obtain larger quantities of blood in Africa. For example, the report of a study of African troops in Kenya at the end of the war began, "Considerable difficulty has been experienced in getting voluntary East African blood donors" (Dewhurst 1945). To explain why there were difficulties in obtaining blood, the report described a study of 2,000 troops, selected from three "intelligence" groups, classified according to their ability to speak English and whether individuals came from trades or lower classes. The methods reveal much about British prejudices, but the results also provide some indication about Africans' views of blood transfusion in 1945. For example, initially, those in the study were given a simple lecture on the facts of transfusion that stressed safety; made the promise of tea, cigarettes, and a donor badge afterwards; and assured the audience that the blood would be used only for treating Africans. This was followed by a demonstration of blood taken from a European and a call for volunteers. Only ten of the 2,000 soldiers agreed, and, according to the report, "all belonged to intelligence group A," the upper-class English speakers. When asked who would give blood to their own tribe, only an additional five agreed, all from the two "lower intelligence" groups.

The rest of the study relied on answers to questions, and when initial, poorly phrased ones such as "are you afraid of venepuncture?" or "are there any tribal superstitions that prevent you giving blood?" elicited no response, extended interviews eventually revealed what appear to be more informative responses. Thus, 15 percent stated that they would not give blood because of poor army conditions (e.g., bad food). A larger group (31%) admitted perceptively that their blood was "bad," due to bilharzia, dysentery, malaria, hookworm, or syphilis. The most common reason for not giving blood (54%), according to the report, came "chiefly from the low intelligence groups," who feared their pint of donated blood would be "irrevocably lost." The study offered the following as a typical rationale: "I was born with a certain amount of blood and I don't want to lose any now."

The French in West and North Africa had a different experience with African blood donors during World War II. When French colonial doctor Gaston Ouary went to Algiers from Senegal in 1944 to study the latest transfusion techniques with Edouard Benhamou, he had already done numerous transfusions in Dakar, which he likened to "a minor surgical intervention." He noted a bigger problem was finding adequate donors (Ouary 1944), and this was despite the fact that in Dakar, there was compensation given to those who donated blood. His explanation, like that of the British in East Africa, was as telling of European prejudices as of African attitudes. The psychology against giving blood had a number of causes, according to Ouary.

> First the habitual indifference of natives to the suffering of others; then the physical fear, the fear of being weakened by the loss of blood; the mystical

fear because transfusion is a way of trafficking bloods; and more than a few believe in contracting the disease of someone lying next to them receiving their blood. These, more than religious reasons, are the true causes of the lack of donors.

(Ouary 1944)

Ouary went to Algiers to learn about the latest transfusion techniques as part of Benhamou's plan to collect and process blood at the Pasteur Institute of Dakar for shipment to Algiers and then to use the blood at the front (Benhamou 1966). Ouary not only learned the latest medical procedures but he also witnessed the success of Benhamou in obtaining blood from local donors. Ouary attributed this to a combination of effort, including daily propaganda by the press; the offer of supplementary ration coupons for meat, sugar, and oil; and the leadership of the Army, businesses, and government ministries, all of whom urged their subordinates to donate and set examples themselves by donating their own blood. Most important, Ouary noted, were religious leaders:

As for North African natives, they also donate their blood. This was not without difficulty raised at first by religious problems. But they were smoothed out when the Grand Mufti of Algiers approved transfusion and encouraged Moslems to give their blood. The manner in which the peasants of Medjerda and Kabylie have responded to the requests of the mobile teams from the Center has been particularly remarkable. It is they who furnish the major part of blood collected by these teams.

(Ouary 1944)

When Ouary returned to Dakar, the authorities immediately began to implement Benhamou's plan, but because this only began at the end of February 1945, it never achieved the scale that was planned by the time the War ended. Still, in 1945, there were 1,236 donors, from whom 142 litres of plasma were shipped to Algiers. More significant in the long run was that 56 litres of plasma and 25 litres of whole blood were kept for use by hospitals in Dakar (Institut Pasteur 1945). As was indicated by the Minister of Colonies and Ouary before he left for Algiers in 1944, the colonial administration was eager to expand transfusion in the African colonies. As a result, the Pasteur Institute in Dakar continued to function as a blood collection centre after the war, albeit on a lesser scale. In 1948, there were 901 donors (of whom 790 were Africans), who gave 71 litres combined of plasma and whole blood (Institut Pasteur 1948).

In 1950, the French colonial administration decided to create a modern blood transfusion centre to serve not only Dakar and Senegal but all of the French West African colonies and Cameroon. To encourage the great increase in donation that was necessary, especially from Africans, a decree provided for 500 francs for each donation of 300 to 350 cc of blood, plus 100 francs' worth of provisions. Whether motivated by these provisions or not, the new *Centre Fédéral de Transfusion Sanguine*, built on the outskirts of Dakar, registered a dramatic increase in blood donation. The partial year of operation in 1950 saw 268 litres of plasma and whole blood collected, and 896 litres in 1951 (Linhard 1951). In an article published that same year, Jacques Linhard, who became the first director, described the donors as "voluntary," but added that "they are given compensation ["*gratification*"] and a snack at each drawing of blood." He acknowledged that the donors included some European soldiers, many of whom had already donated in France or Indochina. There were also a few European civilians but virtually no women donors. Linhard explained that the great majority of donors were Africans: 1,484 out of a total of 1,939 for the first six months.

Thus, this first and largest centralized blood collection service in sub-Saharan Africa utilized compensation to assure adequate blood donations. The advantages of centralization included the ability to ensure quality of screening, selection, testing, and accountability in the process. But the system was doomed by high cost and ultimately the independence of other colonies. Even before 1960, hospitals in Togo and the Ivory Coast started collecting blood locally for transfusion to avoid the delay and cost of shipment from Dakar (*Croix Rouge togolaise* 1973; *Assemblée Territoriale de la Côte d'Ivoire* 1957). The Dakar centre continued to serve Senegal after independence on a comparable scale, thus providing a model for other countries as well as large hospitals in urban areas, using both paid and volunteer donors.

Early blood donors: the British Red Cross in Africa

The use of "compensation" followed the custom begun in France during the 1920s, in the era before blood storage was possible, when Parisian hospitals offered a payment for the inconvenience of donors who were on call to give blood when needed (Schneider 2003; Hermitte 1996). In contrast, the British developed the practice of uncompensated, "voluntary" donation that became the hallmark of the worldwide Red Cross blood movement, including in British Africa during colonial rule. This was generally based on the model developed in London following World War I, when the local Red Cross chapters established a list of potential donors who could be called upon to give their blood when needed. The extent of this system in Africa was limited before World War II, and there was great variation depending on locale.

The big change after 1945 in the British African colonies (as elsewhere) was the result of the growth of new hospitals and the staffing of medical personnel who were better trained and more likely to give transfusions, which could only be done with more blood donors. Along with the increased use of transfusion, some of the new hospital facilities had the ability to store blood, and that made the system of donor lists increasingly unnecessary in responding to the growing need. For example, a report for the month of May 1954 from the Lagos and Colony Red Cross branch described several emergency calls. One in early May came at such short notice, unfortunately, that by the time volunteers were found, the patient had died. On the brighter side, the report described another call for a rare blood group that found two men at the Military Hospital who were compatible (Chipp 1954). Later that year at an Enugu (Nigeria) divisional meeting, a blood transfusion leader reported: "a most satisfactory situation, the donors continue to increase in numbers." One example he reported was of a "bush mother" who was given three pints of blood at the hospital, and, when it was explained to her husband, he successfully urged additional donors to volunteer (Burton 1954).

One of the innovations adopted to increase blood donations that could be stored was an appeal to existing organizations with many members. This included business enterprises, but the largest numbers were obtained from three other institutions: the military, prisons, and schools. An example of what soon came to be standard practice was Northern Rhodesia, where a 1952 Red Cross report indicated that the African Blood Bank went through a "rather lean period." In response, efforts were successfully made to recruit "members of the Police Force, the Prisons, students from Munali and volunteers from the compounds" (Northern Rhodesia 1952). A similar appeal was used when a blood bank was organized in Lagos in 1953 for blood collected at the General Hospital. After the initial campaign for donors, over 400 men and women were registered from Ikeja airport, the Nigerian police, and workers at the military hospital, the police college, the Nigerian Railway, the Postal school, and Kingsway stores (Nigerian Branch 1953).

The success in obtaining blood donated from upper-level school students caused concern in some colonies when the numbers threatened to make the hospitals overly dependent on this one source. In 1953, following a visit to the Uganda Blood Transfusion Service, a British Red Cross Society field worker, Teresa Spens, reported: "I was impressed by the large number of African blood donors." She noted, however, that they were mostly the senior students at schools and colleges and thought this not satisfactory, although medical authorities did not seem worried. As they explained, "students in residential institutions are often, owing to good food, better able to give blood than other sections of the community." An effort is being made, she concluded, to obtain donors in older age groups (Spens 1953).

A different concern, namely a simple lack of donors, prompted the new Lagos Island Maternity Hospital to adopt a new approach to ensure adequate blood, according to Lady Limerick of the British Red Cross Society, who visited the hospital on her tour of West Africa in 1961: "They get their supplies by demanding that each patient should produce three relatives as blood donors." She reported that husbands were lining up to give their pints as expectant mothers were preparing to give birth. This early example of the "replacement" policy became more widespread as hospitals made arrangements for adequate blood supplies, using methods beyond the British Red Cross model of altruistic donors on lists or who gave blood anonymously for the good of the whole (West Africa 1961).

One final example of donors in a British colony that portended future developments was the transfusion service established at the new Ibadan University College Hospital in 1957. Its importance in the context of who donated blood was the ability of the hospital to mobilize over 5,000 donations annually, whereas in previous years the numbers had been much smaller. The first head of donor recruitment was Una Maclean, who had a medical degree from Edinburgh and who accompanied her husband, Peter Cockshott, to Ibadan, where he was put in charge of radiology at the new hospital. Maclean had worked while in medical school at the Scottish Blood Transfusion Service, so when those in charge of the hospital realized they needed to set up a transfusion unit, Maclean agreed (Maclean 1983; Fleming 1983).

Ibadan was a large city, estimated at the time to have over half a million inhabitants. According to Maclean, before 1957, the small hospital that served the city had no blood bank, so without the ability to store blood, it required patients to secure a donor from family or friends. The new Ibadan hospital followed the Red Cross model of recruiting voluntary donors to supply a blood bank which stored blood for use as needed. As a result, the hospital produced posters and films, while Maclean organized lectures and mobile blood collections. These were done because the new hospital needed large amounts of blood (100 donations per week) and had the storage facilities to accommodate it. Her description in 1958 of a collection was quite graphic:

> A bus loaded with equipment and staff goes every week now to a pre-arranged place, often a school room, and there the sight of other people giving blood does not repel the numerous onlookers as might be feared, but on the contrary, produces so many eager donors that equipment may run out before the supply of volunteers.
>
> (Maclean 1958)

Despite these efforts, the hospital still relied heavily on patients to provide a significant proportion of donors. As Maclean recalled later in a memoir, there were always two categories of donors: "on the one hand members of captive groups of students, soldiers and senior school pupils, on the other, the relatives of patients who had received a blood transfusion." In 1958, after one year of the new hospital's operation, Mclean reported the collection of 4,637 pints of blood, but the percentage of "voluntary" donors was only a little over half (52%) (Maclean 1958).

Post-independence shift to hospital base and family replacement

Following independence, the adoption of these innovations increased the ability of hospitals to obtain blood donors in sub-Saharan Africa. As the use of transfusion grew along with new hospitals, central coordination, including the monitoring and control of blood supply, became more and more difficult. The newly independent governments of francophone West Africa brought an end to the multi-colony responsibilities of the blood centre at Dakar, and they did not invest the funds for new national systems.

In anglophone Africa and the Belgian Congo, the colonial Red Cross branches were unable to continue blood collection when they became national societies following independence. With only a few exceptions, after the 1960s, the role of the Red Cross in such places as Uganda, Kenya, and Congo/Zaire was soon relegated primarily to encouraging blood donation. Hospitals did the actual drawing of blood, and although the Red Cross donors were unpaid, the hospitals were free to make other arrangements for collecting more blood as needed. In the case of the Kenya Red Cross, even in 1960, four years before independence, the collection of blood in Nairobi was turned over to the Nairobi Coordinating Committee based at King George VI (later Kenyatta National) Hospital (Schneider 2013). Even the best Red Cross blood collection program established in sub-Saharan Africa, the Uganda Red Cross, faced similar limitations. In 1962, the Uganda Blood Transfusion Service was established when the new Mulago Hospital opened on the eve of independence. The Uganda Red Cross then shifted its activity toward the recruitment and supply of some equipment. Hospitals, especially outside Kampala, had even more leeway in obtaining blood by other means than had been the case earlier (Schneider 2013).

The transfusion centres at big hospitals in large urban settings were able to meet their growing needs (sometimes including the supply of blood to other hospitals in the region) because they had the ability to obtain and store more blood, including collection from soldiers, prisoners, and schoolchildren. In the case of the large hospital in Nairobi, it sometimes received surplus blood from outlying district and regional hospitals, and replacement donations from families above and beyond what was needed for their relatives. They also expanded the practice of mobile collection, which required a vehicle to transport personnel and blood collected at remote sites.

Many newly independent countries tried to make blood donation an act of patriotism, but it is difficult to assess their success. One standard publicity event – when blood was in short supply or especially at the opening of new facilities – was the photographing of donations of blood given by Ministers of Health or even presidents. For example, at the opening of the new blood transfusion centre in Bujumburu, Burundi, in 1972, not only did the Health Minister donate blood but also the ambassadors from West Germany and the Soviet Union, who attended the building inauguration (Schindler 1976; *East African Standard* 1969).

The oldest and best-known blood donor event in Africa was established by Daniel Arap Moi, the second President of Kenya: an appeal for blood donation the week before Kenyatta Day each October. Newspapers used the occasion to add human interest stories to the pictures of government officials donating blood. "Girls Lead Blood Drive in Mombasa" was the headline of one story about 12 girls from the government's Coast Secretarial College who donated blood at Coast Province General Hospital, saying, "If the men can do it, so can we." For the 1972 Kenyatta Day, the *Daily Nation* aimed more at education with a headline, "Blood … and Why You Need It" ("Girls lead…" n.d., *Daily Nation* 1973).

In the end, and especially during hard times, hospitals were the institutions of last resort that were responsible for collecting blood in most African countries following independence. Given the life-saving nature of transfusion, they there-fore used all means possible to obtain blood, including voluntary, mobile collec-tion, and indirect pressure from military commanding officers, prison wardens, or teachers. When necessary (and if blood storage was possible), hospitals required replacement of blood by the patient's family members themselves or from "friends" at double or triple the amount needed by the patient. The extreme case of Mulago Hospital in Kampala, Uganda, during the difficult times of Idi Amin and civil war shows what hospitals did in desperate times. In 1977, the Mulago Hospital collected 3,493 units of blood for transfusion from family members, compared to 5,849 which came from the Uganda Blood Transfusion Service at Nakasero. In 1984, when the new League of Red Cross Societies blood program director, Juhani Leikola, visited Kampala, he found that between July and September of that year, only 9.5 percent of blood for transfusion at Mulago came from Nakasero (Nzaro n.d.; Leikola 1984).

The 1970s and after: development of centralized, "voluntary" donation

By the mid-1970s, there was a levelling off and in some places a decline in the use of transfusions in sub-Saharan Africa. Among the reasons were the world economic crisis and political instability, which were followed by the AIDS epi-demic ten years later. The first of these to affect blood donation were the eco-nomic decline brought about by the oil crisis and growing instability in several countries of Africa that limited or cut support for central collection. It thus forced families to become more and more responsible not only for finding donors but often also for obtaining equipment and supplies. Many collection efforts were already strained by the increase of transfusion use, as indicated in the fol-lowing 1970 Ugandan Red Cross report: "Each year more blood is required and more demand of refreshments, cigarettes increases. This is a problem every-where and unless we find means and ways of improving this we are bound to lose our blood donors" (Uganda Red Cross 1970).

The economic downturn was precipitated by the oil crisis of 1973. Transfu-sion services had always competed with other health services for funds in newly independent African countries. Generally, these expanded together during the 1960s, when resources were available from growing economies as well as assist-ance from countries of the developed world. The recession that followed the oil crisis of 1973 hit most African countries hard, even though they were not large consumers of oil. It decreased opportunities for foreign aid from countries more immediately affected, and eventually hurt African commodity sales as the world's markets shrank (Nelson 1990). When government budgets flattened or decreased, transfusion services were unable to maintain the level of service they had achieved, let alone continue to expand.

When added to the increased number of coups and civil wars and growing political unrest, the effects were felt in all areas, including African transfusion services. For example, in Uganda, after Idi Amin came to power in 1971, he faced resistance within the country and condemnation by most external powers. In 1975, the Uganda Red Cross complained,

> Blood transfusion service all over the country has experienced two major problems which made it not [*sic*] to collect much blood as it was last year compared to the list given here below showing 1974 collection and 1975 [a decline from 33,855 to 24,227]. There has been [a] transport problem which is a countrywide cry in almost all hospitals where they could not provide vehicles to go and organize blood sessions. Some hospitals fail to find drinks and cigarettes for the blood donors so they fail to hold any sessions.
>
> (Uganda Red Cross 1975)

Ten years later, the AIDS epidemic affected the donation of blood in additional ways. In the short run, it resulted in further reducing the availability of blood donors who were frightened by the possibility of contagion. It was an unwarranted fear but one that was difficult to dispel. According to Didier Fassin, at the CHU hospital in Brazzaville, there was an "abrupt" drop in blood donation due in part to confusion about the risk of contracting the disease by donating blood (Fassin 1994).

To a certain extent, this decrease in donors was mitigated by a decrease in the use of transfusions because of the risk of contaminated blood (Vos *et al.* 1993). Initial tests of blood banks when the AIDS epidemic was first confirmed in Africa provided overwhelming and breath-taking evidence of an 8 to 18 percent infection rate among blood donors in Uganda, Rwanda, and Zaire (Van de Perre *et al.* 1984; Mann *et al.* 1986). An example of the resulting decline in transfusion may be seen in the Nairobi Blood Donor Service, which reported a dramatic drop in donations, from 14,216 in 1988 to 8,163 in 1989. (The peak was over 26,000 in 1981.) For the first time, this annual report mentioned fear of being tested for HIV as a reason for the decline but insisted that the lack of resources that had begun the previous decade was the more important cause of the long-term drop (Nairobi Blood Donor Services 1990).

A more direct impact of the AIDS epidemic on transfusion was the decision to terminate blood collection from military units and prisons because of high sero-prevalence. This reduced available blood even faster than the fear of contagion or decline in use. In fact, the decision by transfusion services to make this change in collecting practice was delayed and came in a manner that was not highly publi-cized because of fears that it would exacerbate shortages. In its annual report for 1990, the Nairobi Blood Donor Services stressed the importance of donations from students at schools and mentioned it had stopped collecting from prisons and the Army due to a high percentage of those testing positive for HIV: "This decision was verbally and quietly communicated to all provincial Laboratory Technologists. It was done so in order not to arouse the suspicion of the press and politicians" (Nairobi Blood Donor Services 1990). The report also cited lack of available trans-portation and refreshments as reasons for a general decline in donations.

In the long run, an unexpected but important change in transfusion that resulted from the AIDS epidemic was the attention drawn to the blood supply and the need for outside support to make it safer. Thus, for example, the AIDS crisis was the main reason for rebuilding the Uganda blood transfusion service at the end of the 1980s with outside assistance. This outside support for African countries was not only bilateral but was also reinforced by the interest of the World Health Organization in encouraging voluntary blood donation and the new policy of the League of Red Cross Societies to assist blood services in less developed countries that began in the mid-1970s. Two early examples were Ethiopia and Burundi, where transfusion services were significantly improved, including recruitment of blood donors. These changes were not, however, sustained because the new institutions and practices did not receive continuing government support (Levene 1984; Schindler 1976). Similarly, in Zaire during the 1970s, two American doctors helped establish a blood bank with voluntary donors at Mama Yemo Hospital in Kinshasa, only to have it disappear soon after their departure in 1978 (La situation actuelle 1983). The Ugandan case was an exception that proves the rule because of the amount and long-term commitment of support from the European Union. This lasted from 1987 through 2000, and after a short break, the U.S. President's Emergency Plan for Aids Relief began providing support for safe blood in 2004 (Winsbury 1995).

Kenya was typical of a country without a centralized system as late as the end of the twentieth century. Historically, the Kenya Red Cross started blood collection for transfusion in the late 1940s using volunteer donors. The Ministry of Health appointed a coordinating committee as early as 1960, thus demonstrating an early government attempt at coordinating blood collection. Yet, figures from 1999 show that the overwhelming majority of donors in Nairobi comes from family/replacement (Nairobi Blood Donor Services 1999). A study done from April 1999 to April 2000 of over 10,000 donors at the two biggest hospitals in Nairobi (including Kenyatta National Hospital) confirms this source of donors. Over 97 percent were "call responsive," the Kenyan phrase for family or replacement donors (Abdalla *et al.* 2005). The U.S. Embassy bombing in Nairobi brought renewed outside attention to the national blood policy and collections system in Kenya, which has since 2004 received US PEPFAR support to install a national system.

Conclusion

Historically, Africans recruited blood donors in a variety of ways in order to meet the growing demand and ability to give blood transfusions. With some significant exceptions, the most important institutions in determining the process, until recently, have been hospitals. From the beginning, with few exceptions, donors were found as needed, from family, friends, and those willing to be on call. Most important in this process was not whether donors were "voluntary" or paid, since in Africa, notions of obligation and compensation were more complicated than in Europe or North America. Rather it was the size and facilities of hospitals or collection centres that dictated whether blood was used immediately, stored for later use, or distributed to other hospitals.

In the national (or regional) transfusion centers like Nakasero in Uganda, or the Dakar center in Senegal, and the new, large, urban hospitals such as Ibadan, Nigeria, there was electricity and refrigeration for storage. These accommodated the collection of a large amount of blood, which required systems of donor recruitment that had a number of features that were different from hospitals where blood was used immediately. When blood was stored in large quantities and not immediately used for a specific patient, the donors were unknown to the patients. Hence, these donors may be characterized as "anonymous," an important distinction in motivation. Even in some situations where donors had to be found by the patient to satisfy the requirement of the hospital that the patient's use of blood from its "bank" was repaid, this was not a direct "debt" in the sense that the patient did not know whose blood was in their body.

More importantly, storage allowed for the collection of more blood for transfusion, and the need to establish a system that used a variety of means to secure donors. This might involve compensation, as was the case in Dakar up until the 1980s, but everywhere, mobile units were eventually used to collect blood off-site. These soon became regular sources of donors at institutions such as army barracks, prisons, and schools. Hospitals, both large and small, still needed to secure immediate donors when conditions or supplies of stored blood were low. The solution was the use of the so-called walk-in, family, and replacement practices. This was reported in all countries, as smaller hospitals found their supplies from larger centres disrupted, or the urban hospitals saw declining donations due to budget cuts or civil strife.

The AIDS epidemic is best characterized as another, albeit extreme, reason for the decline in donors, especially for stored blood collection, because two of the largest sources of donors with high risk of infection were eliminated: prisoners and soldiers. That same crisis, however, brought more careful scrutiny in deciding to use transfusion and renewed outside assistance for organizing national systems of stored blood donated for the general good rather than for a specific patient. These have the advantages of additional flexibility in assuring supplies and maintaining standards of testing, plus the ability to keep records for assessing practices and planning future needs. Time will tell whether governments will provide ongoing and sustainable support.

The best way overall to characterize the historical response to the need for blood donation in Africa was that it was very flexible. Most notably, hospitals were innovative in how they adapted to their circumstances, and the resulting amount of blood secured generally met the ability to give transfusions. This lack of resistance by Africans was not expected and defied predictions of irrational opposition. One way to interpret this was that blood was one medicine that Africans possessed in the same amount and with the same control as anywhere else in the world. There were no drug companies or expensive chemical manufacturing or rare materials involved. As far as donors were concerned, the history of blood transfusion offers a good example of Africans' ability to organize well and adapt their healthcare to other needs when the materials were available to them.

Notes

1 Much of the material for this chapter is drawn from Schneider (2013).
2 See Chapter 11.

References

Abdalla, F., Mwanda, O.W., and Rana, F. 2005. "Comparing walk-in and call-responsive donors in a national and a private hospital in Nairobi." *East African Medical Journal* 82: 531–535.

Allain, J.-P. 2010. "Volunteer safer than replacement donor blood: a myth revealed by evidence." *ISBT Science Series* 5: 169–175.

Assemblée Territoriale de la Cote d'Ivoire. 1957. "Projet de délibération tendant à la création en Côte d'Ivoire d'un Centre de Transfusion Sanguine, 13 Sept 1957." Box 294, Institut de médecine tropicale du Service de santé des armées, Marseille, France.

Bates, I. and Hassall, O. 2010. "Should we neglect or nurture replacement blood donors in sub-Saharan Africa?" *Biologicals* 38(1): 65–67.

Benhamou, E. 1966. "Notes pour servir à l'histoire de la transfusion sanguine dans l'armée française de 1942 à 1945 à partir de l'Afrique du Nord." *Revue des Corps de Santé des Armées Terre, Mer, Air* 7: 859–862.

Burton, C. 1954. "Eastern region report – May 1st, 1954 to June 4th, 1954," June 16, 1954. Acc 0076/36(4) Nigeria, Eastern Region, British Red Cross Society Museum and Archives, London (hereafter cited as BRCS archives).

Chipp, A. 1954. "Organiser's report for the months of March and April 1954." Acc 0076/36(5) Nigeria, Lagos and Colony, BRCS Archives.

Croix Rouge togolaise. 1973. "Rapport d'activité 1973." AO917, Archives of International Federation of Red Cross and Red Crescent Societies, Geneva, Switzerland (hereafter cited as IFRC archives).

Daily Nation (Nairobi, Kenya). 1973. "Blood … and why you need it." October 22.

Dewhurst, K.S. 1945. "Observations on East African Blood Donors." *East African Medical Journal* 22: 276–278.

East African Standard. 1969. "Minister donates blood." October 15.

Fassin, D. 1994. "Le domaine privé de la santé publique: Pouvoir politique et sida au Congo." *Annales. Histoire, Sciences Sociales* 49: 763–764.

Fleming, A. 1983. "Memoir on University College Hospital, Ibadan, and the University of Ibadan, December 1962–July 1966." Alan F. Fleming (dated October 3, 1983), Mss Afr s 1872, no. 52, Oxford Rhodes Library, Oxford (hereafter cited as Oxford Rhodes).

"Girls lead blood drive in Mombasa." 1969. Unlabelled newspaper clipping (presumably 1969) from Kenya National Blood Transfusion Service, Nairobi, Kenya (hereafter cited as KNBTS archives).

Hermitte, M-A. 1996. *Le Sang et le Droit: Essai sur la Transfusion sanguine.* Paris: Editions du Seuil.

Institut Pasteur de Dakar, Annual Report. 1945, 23–24.

Institut Pasteur de Dakar, Annual Report. 1948, 22–23.

Lambillon, J. and Denisoff, N. 1940. "Étude de l'organisation d'un service de transfusions sanguines dans un centre hospitalier d'Afrique." *Annales de la Société Belge de Médecine Tropicale* 20: 279–285.

Leikola, J. 1984. "Report of a Mission to Uganda," November 10–14. Juhani Leikola personal papers, Finnish Red Cross Archives, Helsinki, Finland.

Lejeune, E. 1921. "Transfusion sanguine après hémoglobinurie grave." *Annales de la Société Belge de la Médecine Tropicale* 1: 299–300.

Levene, C. 1984. "Brief history of the development of the transfusion service," *How to Recruit Voluntary Donors in the Third World?* Geneva: League of Red Cross Societies, 22–28.

Linhard, J. 1951. "Le Centre fédéral de transfusion de l'A.O.F." *Médecine tropicale* 11: 957.

Maclean, U. 1958. "Blood donor recruitment in Ibadan: the record of one year's experience." *Journal of Tropical Medicine and Hygiene* 61: 311–312.

Maclean, U. 1983."Nigeria 1956–65." 44pp. of typescript ms, May 10, 1983, Mss Afr s 1872, no. 99, Oxford Rhodes Library.

Mann, J.M., Francis, H., Quinn, T., Asila, P.K., Bosenge, N., Nzilambi, N., Bila, K., Tamfum, M., Ruti, K., Piot, P., McCormick, J., and Curran, J.W. 1986. "Surveillance for AIDS in a central African city. Kinshasa, Zaire." *Journal of the American Medical Association* 255: 3255–3259.

Musambachime, M.C. 1988. "The impact of rumor: the case of the Banyama (Vampire Men) scare in Northern Rhodesia, 1930–1964." *International Journal of African Historical Studies* 21: 201–215.

Nairobi Blood Donor Services. 1989. *Annual Report – Blood Donation 1989*. March 28, 1990. KNBTS Archives.

Nairobi Blood Donor Services. 1999. *Monthly Reports*. January to December, KNBTS Archives.

Nelson, J.M. (ed.). 1990. *Economic Crisis and Policy Choice: The Politics of Adjustment in the Third World*. Princeton, NJ: Princeton University Press.

Nigerian Branch News Sheet. 1953. (No. 5), October. Acc 0076/36(1). Nigeria: BRCS Archives.

Northern Rhodesia Branch. 1952. *Director's and Treasurer's Report to Annual Meeting.* October 22. Acc 0076/38(1) Northern Rhodesia, BRCS Archives.

Nzaro, Dr. Esau. n.d. Private papers. Kampala, Uganda.

Ouary, G. 1944. "Compte-rendu de la Mission effectuée par le Médecin Commandant Ouary au Centre de Transfusion d'Alger (15 Juillet–15 Octobre 1944)." Serie H, 1H1 (1), Senegal National Archives, Dakar, Senegal.

Schindler, E.-B. 1976. *Le Centre de Transfusion sanguine de la Croix Rouge de Burundi, Son organisation et ses activités*. Berne: Croix rouge Suisse.

Schneider, W.H. 2003. "Blood transfusion between the wars." *Journal of the History of Medical and Allied Sciences* 58: 187–224.

Schneider, W.H. 2013. *The History of Blood Transfusion in Sub-Saharan Africa*. Athens: Ohio University Press.

Situation actuelle de la Transfusion dans Notre Pays, La. 1983. *Hôpital africain* 15: 18.

Spedener, D. 1924. "Le traitement des pneumonies des noirs par transfusion de sang des convalescents." *Bulletin Médical du Katanga* 1: 234–238.

Spens, T. 1953. "Notes on a visit to East African branches, Sept. to November 1953." Acc 0076/2(1), BRCS Archives.

Uganda Red Cross Annual Report. 1970. 2, Box 16723, IFRC.

Uganda Red Cross Annual Report. 1975. 5, Box 16723, IFRC.

Van de Perre, P., Rouvroy, D., Lepage, P., Bogaerts, J., Kestelyn, P., Kayihigi, J., Hekker, A.C., Butzler, J.P., and Clumeck, N. 1984. "Acquired immunodeficiency syndrome in Rwanda." *Lancet* 2: 62–65.

Vos, J., Gumodoka, B., Ng'weshemi, J.Z., Kigadye, F.C., Dolmans, W.M., and Borgdorff, M.W. 1993. "Are some blood transfusions avoidable? A hospital record analysis in Mwanza Region, Tanzania." *Tropical and Geographical Medicine* 45: 301–303.

"West Africa: Lady Limerick's tour, January 23 to February 19, 1961." 24, Acc0076/59(2), BRCS Archives.

White, L. 2000. *Speaking with Vampires: Rumor and History in Colonial Africa.* Berkeley, CA: University of California Press.

Winsbury, R. (ed.) 1995. *Safe Blood in Developing Countries: The Lessons from Uganda.* Luxembourg: Office for Official Publications of the European Community.

3 Public health works

Blood donation in urban China[1]

Vincanne Adams, Kathleen Erwin, and Phuoc Le

Introduction

The emergence in recent years of the "Global Health Sciences" field (or various versions thereof) in lieu of "International Public Health" has entailed a concomitant shift in focus of health interventions that potentially diminishes the strength and visibility of national public health programs. Although some have argued that this change in nomenclature reflects no more than old wine in new bottles (Brown *et al.* 2006), globalization itself (reflected in this redefinition of the field) has spurred at least three structural changes in health delivery systems that marginalize, or minimally overlook, national public health programs (Adams *et al.* 2008; Novotny 2007). One of these trends is the globalization of pharmaceutical and biomedical research, which augments local participation in clinical trials research but diverts resources from national public health programs (and, in the worst case, enrollment in clinical trials becomes the only way for the poorest to gain access to health resources) (Petryna 2006). Another trend is the growth of small- and large-scale NGO-based health and development organizations, which cumulatively pose a risk to the role played by large multilateral and bilateral aid organizations in helping countries design and deploy effective policy and practice through public health measures (McNeil 2008). A third trend is the rise of biosecurity programs in the guise of health interventions, which run the risk of undermining integrated health development programs by diverting resources to proposed (or imagined) biological threats response preparedness (King 2002; Lakoff 2008).

With these trends in mind,[2] it becomes increasingly important to consider the value and effectiveness of national public health programs in particular instances, especially in under-resourced nations. We focus on the case of China's national health campaign to promote safe donation that grew out of the contaminated blood crisis which fuelled the spread of HIV in the countryside. Although China is not under-resourced compared to some nations, in its control of infectious diseases and its challenges in restructuring its blood donation and collection practices, China still looks very much like many other developing nations. With the economy and society undergoing massive reform, the nation must develop a modern health infrastructure to meet the needs of its population of 1.3

billion, the majority of whom are poor and rural. Thus, China's experience is instructive for examining how international public health standards and practices can shape national programs, and how national health programs transform such practices to successfully meet local needs.

This chapter focuses on the effectiveness of China's public health system through the lens of the blood donation infrastructure. We recognize that China's public health programs have been widely scrutinized, not infrequently with political overtones. Widely divergent reports have ranged from initially positive reviews of the barefoot doctor movement of the 1970s to more recent and much less laudatory coverage of the national response to SARS and control of avian flu. Our exploration of China's donation system is haunted in particular by the public health crisis that emerged from China's initial inattention to HIV/AIDS prevention, and the mushrooming of HIV transmission from contaminated blood in the early 1990s. Kick-started by this crisis, China's public health infrastructure now actively undertakes HIV prevention efforts. We do not explore the larger HIV/AIDS epidemic and response here, and we recognize that blood collection practices, and ensuring a safe blood supply, are only one dimension of the national epidemic. We focus on this component precisely because it highlights the role of a national health program in managing the conflicting problems of unsafe donation on the one hand and the nation's need for safe blood on the other.

The success of the campaign arises in part from strategies used in China to publicize the need for blood and the marketing of blood donation as a public good in ways that make cultural sense to Chinese donors. Relying on local knowledge to augment participation in public health efforts is not new, and China's example is a good one. Other reasons for the success of the blood donation campaign are particular to China's public health infrastructure and are surely peculiar to China alone. The story of that effort merits more widespread attention than it has received to date.

The data on which this analysis is made come from two years of interview and participant observation research in Shanghai, China, between 2006 and 2008. One hundred and ten adults were interviewed, primarily individually ($n=60$), but also some in focus groups ($n=50$), about their history of blood donation and about their attitudes on donating blood. Data were collected by a team of researchers, and questionnaires were designed in a collaborative process with Chinese and US researchers. Working together, a team of Chinese interviewers was selected representing a range of age, socio-economic status, and occupational interests. The team worked to achieve a representative cohort along lines of gender, age, and socio-economic status of the individuals and groups interviewed. They conducted interviews using snowball methods and focus groups. Interviews were conducted in homes, with IRB approved consent of informants. IRB approval for the research was gained from both US and Chinese collaborating institutions. Data analysis involved each investigator's reading the interviews (in Chinese or in English, with translation). The investigators then discussed findings and analyzed them together over a period of several months.

Results were agreed upon and formed the basis for publications that were written independently by American and Chinese authors, by request of the Chinese investigators.[3] The results are specific to data that come from Shanghai, but we believe many of the insights are true for urban China in general and are informative with regard to China's national public health response.

The problem of HIV and blood donation in China

The HIV/AIDS crisis in relation to blood donation in China has been well documented (Erwin 2006; Jing 2006; Shan *et al.* 2002; Zaller *et al.* 2005, 2006). Briefly, in the early 1990s, following accelerated post-socialist market reforms, China witnessed rapid growth in the commercial procurement of blood (Erwin 2006). Provincial health centres hoping to augment income, as well as private businesses, established numerous blood and plasma donation centres where donors were paid for their donations. In some rural areas, blood sellers returned as often as twice a week. The blood was not tested for HIV, conditions for drawing blood often entailed the reuse of needles, and in the case of plasma, donations were pooled by type, separated by plasmapheresis, and donors were re-injected with pooled blood. By the mid-1990s, it had become apparent that blood donation and transfusion had become a major source of the spread of HIV, with some reports indicating that up to 60 to 80 percent of the adult population of some villages had been infected in this way. Official statistics place the proportion of HIV infections attributable to contaminated blood at 8 to 17 percent, but the actual number is unknown, and some experts have suggested that the spread of HIV in China by way of blood donation and transfusion is much higher (see Erwin 2006). UNAIDS reports that of 75,000 living with AIDS in China in 2005, 22,000 were infected by contaminated blood (UNAIDS: China at a Glance). As disturbing as these figures are, they pale in comparison to the infection rates of Hepatitis B (and C) that – although less noted in the media – have accompanied this crisis. Indeed, Hepatitis B virus (HBV) is endemic in China, with a prevalence of about 10 percent in the general population (HIV prevalence is about 0.05 percent nationwide), and for many Chinese, HBV infection from contaminated blood poses a much more present danger.

Starting in 1996, the central government closed down many of the state-run commercial centers, and in 1998, it outlawed commercial blood procurement. Since then, it has invested more than 200 million Yuan in the construction of new blood centres, and the implementation of more stringent screening and collection procedures. More importantly, it has deployed effective propaganda campaigns to both promote voluntary blood donation, particularly in urban areas, and minimize public fears of the risk of contamination (Wang 2004; Qu 2006). It is important to note that "propaganda" in China is understood as a form of mass public education and does not have the negative political connotations with which it is attributed in the USA and many other Western countries.

Operating on the internationally accepted assumption that eliminating "blood selling" would eliminate a source of contamination, China made this the linchpin of its campaign. It utilized a combination of educational and compulsory strategies to increase donation at legitimate blood centres – particularly in urban areas where demand is greatest – but donation has been historically low. Relying on the existing social structures of the universities and work units with which the large majority of healthy adult Chinese are affiliated, the Ministry implemented a "planned" (*jihua*) donation system, in which a quota was established for the work unit, and not the individual. In China, the work unit, or *danwei*, refers to state-owned or state-run enterprises where most urban Chinese continue to work. Although a growing number of Chinese are now self-employed or work in private enterprises, the work unit remains a fundamental social and economic structure in China, and a primary reference point for Chinese. Simultaneously, mobile vans were deployed to make blood donation both more visible and more convenient. In its campaign, the Public Health Bureau took advantage of the media, the established relationships that people had with their work unit, and the knowledge that in order for citizens to trust in the state's demands for blood donation, they would have to be convinced of not only its safety but its worthiness, as a contribution to the national good. We describe these techniques, and the intersection and synergy of the structural and educational strategies, below.

Suffice to say that Chinese public health officials and researchers note that this campaign has resulted in dramatically decreasing the proportion of blood supplied by paid donors and increasing the blood supply from voluntary donors. Shan et al. report that in one city, the number of voluntary whole blood donors increased between 1993 and 2001, from 55 to 96,320 donors. Wang (2004) reported similar increases in voluntary donations, such that by 2004, 58.6 percent of blood came from voluntary donors, 29.9 percent from employer-organized donors, and 11.5 percent from paid donors. Statistics from the Shanghai Blood Centre estimate that 30 percent of blood for clinical use is purchased from other provinces, and voluntary donations comprise another 21 percent. The remaining 50 percent comes from work units and universities fulfilling their quotas under the planned donation system (*China Daily*, October 19, 2004 (eastday.com)). Shanghai's continuing reliance on commercial sources is in part due to the high demand for blood in the megalopolis, where numerous hospitals and clinics and the medical infrastructure engage in advanced medical and surgical procedures that may require more blood.

Whole blood donations represented by these statistics account for a large proportion of China's overall procurement infrastructure, and are certainly the thrust of the public health campaign. But they do not account for all donated blood. In China, whole blood donation, primarily used in clinical settings, is regulated by the Ministry of Health and is thus integrated into the public health system. Plasma donation, used in the blood products/derivatives industry, is regulated by the National Institute for the Control of Pharmaceutical and Biological Products. While we do not have statistics on the latter, we suspect that "commercial" donation remains a primary source of blood for these commercial plasma centres.

Nevertheless, the concerted effort which China has directed toward transforming its public health donation system has proven overall effective in attending to two national health needs: reducing the spread of transfusion transmissible infections (TTI) while increasing its supply of safe and clean blood. We note that some evidence shows that voluntary donors at mobile units have a slightly lower rate of TTIs than at blood donation centres (which are often used by work units), and this number decreases for donors who give more than once (Zaller *et al.* 2006). Still, donations by way of the work unit remain the most plentiful source of what is considered on the whole to be a means to ensure a safe blood supply. The details of how this broad-reaching transformation was achieved are instructive and point to the critical importance of the public health campaign in accomplishing these dual goals.

Addressing the cultural and social impediments to blood donation

In addressing the challenge of eradicating unsafe donation while ensuring an adequate, safe blood supply, Chinese public health officials had to address several issues at once. These were both cultural and sociological in the sense that one pertains to cultural notions derived from classical Chinese medicine and gender ideologies about blood and blood loss, while the other pertains to social evidence concerning the effects, and risks, of blood donation.

Cultural beliefs about blood

Cultural beliefs about blood, and the health effects of its depletion, predispose many Chinese against blood donation (Erwin *et al.* 2006; Shan *et al.* 2002). In classical Chinese medicine (also called TCM), blood is understood as a vital bodily essence (similar to *qi*), and loss of this essence can lead to long-term decline in health and vitality. Although educated urban Chinese are familiar with biomedical understandings of blood as a regenerative tissue, many nevertheless retain some intrinsic fear of lost health and vitality associated with blood donation. In many cases, this fear was enacted through overt resistance to donation, such as young women who would deliberately lose weight at the time their work unit was called upon to donate in order to fall below the 45kg minimum weight requirement. We found that Shanghainese were forthcoming about their fears of donating:

> Sometimes my friends would say impulsively "I'm going to donate blood." But they never put their words into action. I heard a colleague in her forties by then had donated blood and slept for a whole day after donation. Later when her son's work unit called employees to donate blood, she desperately stopped him from donating, afraid that he would feel dizzy. Her son finally skipped it. About six or seven years ago when I was in school, people felt frightened upon hearing about blood donation. Girls stopped eating to lower their body weight so that they would be able to avoid donation.
>
> (#29 F24)

[Wife]: At first I believed that giving blood was scary and believed that taking blood out was harmful to the body.... From my own experience, I felt fatigue no matter how much rest I took after donating. As I went out under the sun, I had a shock and sudden blindness that made me have to crouch to recover. I'm not sure if it was caused by blood donation or the extremely high temperature that Uganda Red Cross Annual Report day.

[Husband]: Actually there is a seasonal choice for blood donation. It's suitable to donate in spring and autumn instead of summer and winter. The neighbors said my wife shouldn't have donated on such a hot day. The *qi* could be harmed without proper rest and as much nutrition intake as possible.... Male donors would feel tired and listless after donation. Laborers' work had to stop because of their inner deficiency of blood. It would be ok after two to three days' rest.... Women would feel sore in the waist after donation.

(#24 F46 (wife), M49 (husband))

Sentiments about loss of vitality were sometimes expressed in relation to semen, which is known as another vital essence influenced by the strength of the blood (see also Kleinman 1981):

We have a saying, that "one drop of semen equals ten drops of blood." It refers to the relationship of blood and spirit. *Jing* (semen) may refer to the spirit of a person and link with blood, as we usually say "A flourishing *qi* and blood makes a person fit." A healthy person means he or she has healthy blood, which leads to good spirit. Thus, taking blood out of the body may affect human spirit. This is my understanding.

(#11 F50)

Semen is the essence of man, so is blood. Both are too precious to lose much. If you do, your health is impaired. Most emperors died at early ages. They had many concubines besides an official wife. This [early death] may be due to high frequency for their sex life, which affects health and longevity. This is told and passed from generation to generation. I'm not sure if it's scientifically correct, but it is widely accepted among Chinese. Now blood donation is encouraged. A normal and appropriate frequency for sex life is fine. Excessively high or low is harmful to health. This is why we say that ten drops of blood equals one drop of *jing*.

(#14 F34)

Many feared that even a small amount of blood loss (200 to 400 cc) would not only compromise one's health temporarily – for example, requiring a rest of a few hours and a nutritious meal to recuperate – but could also risk one's long-term health, requiring up to several weeks' rest and the consumption of a special diet for several days. Thus, many Shanghainese described the ways in which one could restore one's health after blood loss through special nutritious foods (red dates, red beans, hen soup) as well as through traditional Chinese medicines and albumin supplements. Most believed that three to five days was the minimum required for a small donation (200 cc) and that two weeks or more of rest was needed to recuperate from a donation of 400 cc. While many younger people believed that these practices were sufficient to recuperate, others felt that even these remedies were not enough to undo the potential harm brought about by blood loss.

The value placed on blood as a vital essence, and the concomitant fears about blood loss, framed the perception that it was only people who were desperate for money who would willingly part with their blood. "Blood selling" in particular was seen as compelled by poverty – a troubling act of desperation, or even "backwardness" (*luohou*) (Erwin 2006). Only someone who was in extremely dire straits already would consider selling his or her blood for money and suffering the ill-health effects (to self, family, and lineage) thereafter. Indeed, reframing the motivation, or conditions under which one would willingly donate blood, was one of the key challenges facing the public health program that hoped to both eliminate paid and augment voluntary donation. We explain how this challenge was met below.

Social fears of contamination

Even before widespread public disclosure of the contaminated blood crisis in 2001, many urban Chinese already knew about blood selling practices in the countryside and associated it with the desperate poverty of the rural population (Erwin 2006). Even those unaware of the threat of HIV already feared HBV contamination from blood donation, and it was not uncommon for Chinese to know someone who had contracted hepatitis from blood donation. These extant fears were, to some extent, reinforced by the disclosure of the contaminated blood crisis and reports of high rates of HIV infection and AIDS in the countryside. Zaller *et al.* (2005, 2006) reported that in 2002 in one region of Western China, up to 69 percent of 1,280 interviewed respondents (Han and Uyghurs) said that the fear of becoming infected with TTI (hepatitis or HIV) from donating blood was an inhibitory factor when considering donation.

For public health officials, the escalating rates of HIV-contaminated blood surely sparked concerns over how to set national policy for eliminating vectors of transmission while avoiding a sharp decline in the blood supply. Following standard recommendations of international blood banking first laid out by Titmuss in 1970 (Titmuss 1987) and promulgated by the International Red Cross, the Public Health Bureau implemented more rigorous screening and testing to identify TTIs, required the purchase and use of new and sterilized equipment (rather than reusing needles), and, importantly, advocated that donations should come only from voluntary, unpaid donors rather than from paid ones.

Perhaps the most challenging aspect of China's campaign was eliminating paid blood donations without severely reducing the blood supply in an environment in which contemplation of blood donation instilled both fear of contamination and fear of depletion of vitality from blood loss. Resolving this quandary was the key-stone to restoring a safe and adequate blood supply in China. The strategy relied on outlawing the practice of blood selling while encouraging voluntary donations through the familiar infrastructure of the work unit. The resolution produced an interesting "fiction" in China's public health culture.

China's adoption of internationally accepted blood donation practices that rely on voluntary, unpaid donations to ensure a safe blood supply was taken up as a public health cause celebre. Commercial blood selling was outlawed and illegal donation centres shut down. At the same time, campaigns to increase vol-untary donations were widely promoted. The logic of this two-pronged approach rests on the assumption that offering compensation for blood is more likely to attract unhealthy donors (injection drug users, the poor) who will lie about their risk status and their likelihood of having contaminated blood. In the absence of foolproof screening techniques, deciphering the underlying blood health of donors becomes critical. Social measures, including evidence of drug abuse and poverty, end up standing in for biological measures of exposure. Although some critics have argued that blood donation systems could also entail various forms of compensation and still produce safe blood, the idea that blood donations should be unpaid still circulates as the best practices standard for ensuring safe blood. Although promulgated as the linchpin of China's strategy, we will see that such measures were nevertheless shaped by local social and institutional norms, producing the interesting fiction to which we alluded.

It is worth remembering that the contaminated blood crisis in China was less a direct result of rural populations being more "at risk" because of their poverty or drug use than a result of unhygienic practices at the collection centres themselves: the use of unclean needles, failure to screen and test blood, and the pooling of blood and re-injecting of donors. These practices were allowed because commer-cial blood donation flourished in an environment of rural poverty and virtually non-existent government regulation. Indeed, Jing (2006) cogently argues that the sweeping market reforms authorizing the commercial selling of blood were part of a larger trend toward exploitation of the rural poor in post-Mao China. This phe-nomenon offers a sad case of unregulated and unscrupulous commercialism that, as we will see below, was exactly how it was portrayed by the Health Bureau in a campaign to "clean up" practices of blood donation in the long run.

While it took political will, financial resources, and technical training to outlaw the commercial blood centres, to create the infrastructure to support vol-untary donation, particularly in urban areas where demand is highest, and to implement hygienic clinical practices and stringent screening and testing proced-ures, these steps represent only one component of the transformation that needed to occur to ensure a safe and adequate blood supply. The deeper challenge, perhaps, was transforming the cultural and social framework in and through which people decided to willingly donate blood. Effectively deploying local knowledge and institutional structures facilitated this transformation of public perception and practice. The data we collected from Shanghai illustrate this larger story about how public health "works."

Public health works

In looking at the outcomes of China's policies and strategies to eliminate the spread of HIV and hepatitis through blood donation, we do not intend to suggest that these effects were always deliberate on the part of officials within the health bureaus. Nevertheless, the public health outcomes were effective. We explore several here.

The effort to increase voluntary donation and eliminate blood selling as a way of stemming transmission of TTIs effectively convinced many Shanghainese that the element of risk in blood donation was swiftly contained. Public health campaigns used television commercials, movies, billboard advertisements, and leaflets within the work unit to explain how donating blood was "glorious." Celebrities were depicted donating blood to show the public not only how safe it was but how good it made one feel to be part of a national movement.

The more important technique used by the Health Bureau in its media campaign, however, was its subtle shift in identifying who and what was "risky" about blood donation. By acknowledging the experience of the desperately poor and rural "blood sellers" at the hands of unscrupulous, illegal commercial buyers – as opposed to the unhygienic practices – the government was able to deflect popular concerns about whether the state apparatus was in fact what should be feared. Urban Chinese already viewed rural inhabitants as uneducated, backward, and culturally unlike them. That the blood sellers were from rural areas made the problem seem a distant one that was unlikely to touch them. Moreover, criminalizing blood selling allowed for a popular understanding that giving blood in other ways (i.e., through voluntary donations) would *not* be risky because it was regulated and a public service (not for private monetary gain). Along the way, blood selling came to be portrayed as an occurrence that was confined in time and place. Television coverage of the contaminated blood crisis was effective in creating a popular understanding that the spread of HIV through blood donation was limited to rural poor communities and to a very small region of China. Listen to this 42-year-old woman from Shanghai talk about the scope and boundaries of the emerging epidemic caused by blood donation:

> I know [about AIDS and blood donation] from TV about the AIDS village in Henan province, where they are poor and short of medical facilities. Some people organized villagers to sell blood for money. I saw it on TV, and the village is dirty as hell. They are so ignorant and irresponsible for their own lives. People are dying everyday according to the TV report, though recently we have heard less about it. This rarely happens in big cities like Shanghai where it is safer and has proper protections.
>
> (#5 F24)

In some cases the emerging epidemic was not seen as national in scope but rather seen as limited to a single village, or even to a single individual:

I heard on TV about AIDS [and blood donation]. It happened in a village. A villager was infected with AIDS and demeaned by other residents because it is hard to tell if he had done something bad or was infected through the blood he received. According to the TV coverage, he was given vigilant scrutiny by local residents. The disease is not easily transmitted, but AIDS infection was found in him after he donated blood.

(#27 M34)

By containing media coverage from the outset, and framing the disclosure limited in time and place, the impact of the crisis on public perception about the safety of blood donation was effectively controlled. By 2006, we found that Shanghainese were largely convinced that the epidemic had been contained and in any case was limited from the outset. Although a few expressed concern about receiving transfusions, for the most part, they reported that they were not afraid of contamination from donating blood – an idea that was for them coupled with the assumption that urban hospitals and donation centres would be cleaner, safer, and more modern than those in rural areas.

I have seen that from TV and newspapers. These events are more often in backward areas, I have not heard that happened in Shanghai.

(#43 M 57)

There is a village in Henan where most residents sold blood for a living at unofficial places and were all infected with AIDS. In TV news, a pregnant woman received blood transfusion when she delivered and her baby was infected. There are quite a few similar cases.... They gave blood through unofficial channels. I believe such incidents would not happen in official hospitals.

(#31 F34)

Despite successfully minimizing public concern for the risk of infection from donation, public health campaigns still had to overcome widespread popular sentiment that donating blood was in and of itself deleterious to one's health. This cultural assumption was in place long before HIV, or even blood donation, existed in China. Hence, it is important to put blood donation in the historical context of China's efforts to augment donations in general, and then to recognize what the effort to outlaw "selling blood" accomplished with regard to overcoming this more deeply held fear.

Worldwide, demand for blood for transfusion and other surgical or medical procedures grew after World War II. As medical techniques became more advanced, the need for blood also grew, and at an increasing pace over time. China experienced a similar increase in demand, which grew slowly at first and then increased more rapidly in the 1970s, spiking more dramatically in the 1980s with the combination of economic expansion and a growing population. Thus, for most of the Maoist era (1949–1976), China was able to meet its demand for blood by relying on a mandatory donation system managed by the state-run communes, work units, and universities. Each unit was assigned its quota, and donations were minimally compensated. Since quotas were an integral part of the planned economy – in this case "planned donations" – they were very much a part of the everyday landscape of Chinese socialism.

> During the Cultural Revolution, my work unit was organized to give blood regularly. The work unit was Food Shop of North Station. We got 50 Yuan annually, donating blood once every two or three months. We donated quite frequently over a period of a year. We were organized to go traveling afterward for four to six days. The money was for compensation but the holiday was to replenish health … I managed the manufacturing, and I was the assistant of the workshop director. The workers went to donate blood based on the job number, but we could not tell them just to donate blood. We went first, [but] I was not qualified…. The factory prepared the tonics and money to pay the workers. We Ningbo people steam red dates, red beans, and walnuts [to replenish]. We cook soybean curd with a little steamed food [nutritional tonics]. The blood station gave a bottle of milk and two cakes. At the time nothing was compensated. Honestly, we had high morality.
>
> (#1 M57)

Nevertheless this same 57-year-old man goes on to say:

> Nothing was compensated for us except for 300 RMB. We went to donate blood voluntarily, and we did not care about the money … [but] even if you gave 300 RMB, people would not donate blood. But 300 RMB was not a little amount in the 1980s. Workers from textile mills were rich then. They did not think much of 300 RMB, but they thought 200 cc of blood was more valuable. [He also took three days' rest paid vacation.]
>
> (#1 M57)

This reference to compensation provides an interesting foreshadowing to practices under the current planned donation system. They point not so much to a break with the past, or creation of an entirely new means of encouraging donation today, but rather to the continuity and familiar infrastructure onto which current practices have been laid. What is perhaps "new" therefore, is the fiction around unpaid donation that has arisen as a result of adopting international standards of blood collection and banking to make public health work in China.

Since the 1980s, with China's burgeoning economic growth, both the capacity and the demand for more advanced medical treatments – and the blood they require – grew. The system of compulsory donation through state-run units continued during this era, but supply no longer met growing demand. It was in this context that commercial blood donation began to flourish. The dismantling of the communes and centrally planned economy, and the underdeveloped private enterprise taxation system, meant that the central government no longer had the resources to fully fund public health. Provincial health bureaus and other public and private entities saw an opportunity to raise capital by purchasing blood locally (and cheaply) and selling it to urban hospitals (or pharmaceutical companies) where demand was high. While uncompensated donation at the work units grew only slowly, purchased blood (from the countryside) escalated.

This system continued into the 1990s, until the crisis of contaminated blood – first discovered in 1995 – forced the government to reorganize blood donation and compensation systems, specifically re-emphasizing "planned giving" as its primary public health strategy for ensuring an adequate blood supply. Recognizing the need to respond to new economic realities, work units began increasing remuneration to those workers who agreed to donate on behalf of the work unit. Compensation from the work unit was not seen as the same as blood selling for two reasons: (1) workers were asked to voluntarily participate to meet the quota, and compensation was offered as an expression of caring and appreciation for the willing donation of one's valuable essence; and (2) the "profit" motive associated with selling blood to the urban public hospitals was removed. Although hospitals still had to pay for blood, the payment was to cover legitimate costs of screening, testing, and storage of blood, not for profit. Likewise, compensation to the donor was not motivated by personal profit (as in selling one's blood) but by the willingness to contribute to the public good. Thus, by the mid- to late 1990s, receiving compensation for one's donation was not only a legitimate practice, but one that was seen as furthering the adoption of modern blood procurement practices.

Compensation provided by work units to those who donated could be quite generous. Some work units gave donors up to 20 percent or 50 percent of their monthly salary in pay and a week or two of paid vacation, or a trip to a resort. In other work units, the standard was for money and a few days off, but no paid vacations.

As in other work units, donors at our *danwei* were given subsidy and a few days off. The subsidy was 1,500 yuan [US$200] and one week vacation.

(#21 F23)

The vacation was kind of incentive. It was given and allowed by the work unit and had nothing to do with the blood center. It was not payment. It was a kind of encouragement. It is usually referred to as a fund for nutrition because in the first day or two, donors need to take some supplements.
[*INTERVIEWER:* Is the economic compensation standard high? I have heard that some work units give 2000 to 3000 RMB.]
SECOND WOMAN: So much? Our work unit only gives us 1000.
FIRST WOMAN: No work unit can give 2000 to 3000 RMB.
THIRD WOMAN: The economic compensation is different in different units.
FIRST WOMAN: It is different, for the work unit has different profit. The country should unify this economic compensation, and it shouldn't be given by the work unit. Work unit with good income, with abundant source, and work unit with poor income, the country should consider this.

SECOND WOMAN: After blood donation, the work unit will send people to visit you, and they can not accompany you for long. This is the fact.

[*INTERVIEWER:* Then should the country set the compensation standard? And according to the standard, how much do you think is proper for Shanghai?]

FIRST WOMAN: For Shanghai, I think it should be 2000 to 3000.

SECOND WOMAN: It should be 2000 to 3000.

[Note: the average annual salary for this group was 46,000 Yuan].

(#49 F40)

As noted above, the outlawing of commercial blood donation centres did not eliminate the practice of compensating donors for their blood. Rather, it occurred in the context of a set of social structures and cultural practices already in place, and was made possible by the clever distinction made between compensation from the work unit and "blood selling." Blood selling had become identified as a public health disaster, while providing compensation via the work unit was perceived as underpinning a voluntary and safe procurement system – quite antithetical to the coercion of poverty that compelled blood selling by rural peasants.

We found that Shanghai donors were clear on the distinction between blood selling and work unit compensation, even though both amounted to monetary compensation for donating one's blood.

I don't think it is payment [when asked about work unit compensations]. It is a humane way of showing care and friendship from leaders and colleagues. The kindness, which is more important than the gifts [or money], makes people happy to realize blood donation is glorious.

(#5 F24)

Similar sentiments were expressed by a 46-year-old woman and her 49-year-old husband:

HUSBAND: Blood donation is public interest oriented and a kind of contribution, totally different from selling blood. Unpaid blood donation reflects a person's high morality. Selling blood for money is to survive poor living conditions.

WIFE: Selling blood is the last choice for poor people.

HUSBAND: It is an obligation for those employees in work units, who are allocated with a quota for blood donors who are compensated. We donated blood as a social contribution, not for money or fame.

(#24 F46 M49)

A 42-year-old woman who worked as a household cleaner told us:

It is not payment. It is encouragement for this highly conscientious deed. A woman, who had the same cleaning job as me, once asked if donors were paid. I said "No. They would not do it then. If not for the certificate [showing it was not paid], it would be misunderstood as selling blood." In my hometown, blood donation refers to selling blood. They don't have the notion of blood donation not for payment. The payment from work units is more symbolic. It is not money oriented as is blood selling.

(#26 F42)

Part of the reason the public was able to distinguish between "bad" kinds of paid donation and "good" compensated donation was that the public health campaign created a media discourse which used celebrities to endorse the idea that giving blood was to be celebrated:

I had seen some ads on TV. Chen Rong [a popular star] donated blood, and there was the slogan, "A drop of blood may ignite hope."

(#41 M 20)

Q: Did you hear about blood donation through media?
THIRD MAN: Yes; in broadcast and TV.
FOURTH MAN: On internet. There are advertisements with famous stars, like Yao Ming, Sun Li, and Xu Rongzhen, and all of them participate in these advertisements.
THIRD MAN: Chen Rong also did. She donated blood herself, and told people the benefits, so it was convincing.
FOURTH MAN: Public advertisements advocate for all people to help, because the blood bank is in need, all types of blood are needed.

(#60 64M, 33M)

Our interviewees repeated the sentiments they had garnered from public health campaign slogans which portrayed voluntary donation as glorious and patriotic:

Donors should take the opportunity to "spread love."

(#9 F48)

It is glorious to give blood as we donated blood to save lives.

(# 22 F22)

Voluntary blood donation began to be seen as a "glorious" and "patriotic" gesture that was safe for the body, despite deep-seated sentiments that it could harm one's health. In the end, we found many donors who were compelled to give, and did so, sometimes simply as an act of individual patriotism rather than as a response to a work unit demand. However, in many of these cases, we found that donors still worried about the possibility that their donation would have residual ill-health effects. That is, the idea of donating blood became embedded in a larger set of sentiments about personal sacrifice to the larger society, to the nation, even at the expense of one's own personal health. In a response to a question regarding where she had learned about blood donation, a 24-year-old woman told us:

From TV commercials and news reports of insufficient blood supply of certain types of blood. The public was called to donate.... Many people think it harms health, but if it harms the body, there shouldn't be so many blood donors. Some of them even donate annually. Giving blood was a taboo for my mother's generation. I am influenced by TV and commercials, which are successful in promoting [it]. Actually blood donation is so simple to finish at once. It is far less complicated than marrow donation, which requires many steps and procedures. All we need is an incentive or compulsive measure. No extra compensation is necessary except a favorable policy for usage after donation.

(#29 F24)

In another vein, a 31-year-old man reported:

Previously, I thought blood donation was harmful to health. There are many negative opinions about this, such as that it is harmful to *yuan qi*. I felt confused and that it was irrelevant to me. The public had no contact with information about it. Seniors usually think blood donation affects health in the long run. According to them, the side effects include dizziness, tiredness which influences daily work. Especially it causes male sterility, which I feared the most. Later more information has been made available on the media. More friends and colleagues devoted themselves to this public deed. The notions changed gradually. Blood donation became acceptable to more and more people, including the fact that it is harmless to health and even good. Also, understanding the fact that the human body can restore itself after proper rest, made it appropriate to think that blood donation is absolutely good to your health and harmless. *As for my own understanding, I don't believe blood donation has no influence on health. But it is recoverable, controllable, and temporary* [emphasis added].

(#16 M31)

Interestingly, this donor went on to explain how he was so motivated to give blood for the sake of his society that he donated on his own at a blood mobile unit one day while walking past a department store with a friend. He explained that he was "caught by the 'patriotism bug' and wanted to make a donation to feel 'glorious'." He then explained that his work unit organized blood drives and paid large compensation: two weeks' vacation and 2,000 to 3,000 yuan. He did not donate when this was offered because he felt that the health risk must be high if the reward was so great. He felt the payment to donors should enable them to buy nutritious tonics after donating. At the mobile van, he was only given cookies, mineral water, and an umbrella.

Continuing, we found that this donor exemplified some of the ambivalence surrounding compensation versus no compensation for blood donation, and it points to a delicate balance the work units must strike: offering enough compensation to express appreciation for the individual's sacrifice and contribution, without instilling either a sense of coercion or of fear among potential donors. Although this man begins by noting that uncompensated donation is the best kind of donation, he reveals that, in the end, he would have wanted compensation in order to ensure his long-term health. He said that he donated without any need for compensation, and when he went home, he "didn't dare tell his parents." In fact, he played badminton with a friend and went swimming, but on the third day, he had a fever of over 38°C. The febricide he took for his fever did not work. He was scared. He had to tell his parents under their questioning before going into hospital (for an infusion). After three days of fluid infusions, his fever abated. He felt confused and was unsure whether the fever had been caused by the blood donation or whether it was because he was overexcited and did not rest properly after donating. He would be more conservative next time, he said, making sure to rest for three to four days after donating.

The idea of packaging donation as rewarding in and of itself caught on to some degree. A few donors considered voluntary uncompensated donation to be the ideal for contemporary China. And indeed, the public media and blood centres continue to emphasize that this is the ideal type, which should eventually replace even compensated donation through the work unit. But among donors, the ideal donation remains one that is compensated by the work unit. The idea that the donor has made a sacrifice for the social good was accompanied by the idea that society, by way of the work unit, should care for the donor. Compensated blood donation is thus distinguished from "blood selling" and is understood as the best, most productive, and most effective way to ensure donations among the public. It also attended to cultural fears about the potential harm to one's health from donating. It did not eliminate such fears so much as answer them by rewarding the donor with ample resources to replenish his or her health and, more importantly, to be acknowledged as a person who sacrificed their health for their nation.

Making compensation a reward for glorious service to one's country distinguishes it from blood selling. Blood selling was represented as a societal failure, in the sense that it made visible the desperately poor citizens for whom the state had failed to adequately care. In contrast, compensated donations represented the success of both socialist and post-socialist reforms: they reinforced the idea that the social system worked to take care of its patriotic citizens. Remuneration by the work unit was seen as a way for the work unit to reward the donor, take care of him or her, and acknowledge the large sacrifice made on behalf of the donor for the good of society.

Conclusion

For blood donation, propaganda has not many effects. People all have a caring heart, and their qualities are improved. If a hospital needs blood, and show a line of words on the TV, many people would go to donate blood, and they don't ask for compensation. We had a case before. In 1995 or 1996, we had a person with negative Rh blood [rhesus factor], and she bled much when delivering the baby. There was no such blood in blood bank, neither in the blood bank from the city, and we called the TV station. After the information was sent out, many people with negative Rh blood came and packed in the examination room. They came just to save a mother and a baby, and they went to visit the mother after blood donation.

(#46 F54)

The story of how a nation, which had a long-standing cultural objection to voluntary blood donations, as well as an emerging epidemic tied directly to blood donation practices, was able to produce a group of willing donors is a compelling one. It is compelling not simply for what it can tell us about China's peculiar blood donation practices in relation to epidemics but also for what it can tell us about effective public health programs.

The story begins for us with several important turns in China's public health campaigns. Minimizing the fear of contamination through unsafe blood donation practices was accomplished by depicting the problem of blood donation risk as one associated with an isolated time, place, and set of economic circumstances in which poverty served to coerce blood selling. Outlawing blood selling meant that legal blood donation centres could be identified as "safe" centres for donors to willingly contribute to a public good. Very quickly, much of the urban public came to think of contamination risk as limited to a single remote region where poor, rural blood sellers – people who were quite different from them – lived.

At the same time, long-standing cultural objections to blood donation because of its potentially deleterious effects on vitality and *qi* had already set in motion a slightly different set of fears. These too were in some sense addressed by the public health campaign to criminalize blood selling. Voluntary donation was depicted as glorious and patriotic, reminding audiences of a higher moral calling. Celebrities endorsed this in media campaigns that called upon ordinary citizens to give "freely" and out of "love" for one's countrymen.

Still, the idea that one might suffer ill-health effects from blood loss, even for a glorious cause, was deeply embedded in a cultural system of reciprocity that pre-dated socialism but was nevertheless sustained and remade over time from the early days of collectivization through the contemporary years of post-socialist market reform (Yang 1994; Anagnost 1997; Greenhalgh 2008). The idea that donors would sacrifice their blood, and potentially their health, for the work unit, for the larger society, or for the nation, was met with an expectation that such sacrifice would be compensated. Work units compensated donors with money, vacations, and food. Despite that fact that compensation is an openly recognized part of an "incentive" system, it was still clearly distinguishable from blood selling. Compensation by way of work units is a symbolic reward for the sacrifice of the patriotic citizen rather than as payment, since blood purchasing is not only illegal but also operates externally to and separately from regulated, state-run enterprises.

In the end, the factors which probably made the most difference in China's ability to limit the spread of HIV by way of blood donation had little to do with the actual elimination of financially remunerated blood and much to do with

improving upon screening systems and hygienic withdrawal and pooling practices at donation centres. However, given that the early health crisis could have
led to egregious declines in blood donation and in the national blood supply, it is
remarkable how swiftly things turned around and how rapidly China was able to
build its own blood banking systems based largely on local voluntary donations
(keeping in mind that China contributes greatly to the international supply of
plasma products but purchases no blood from outside for internal use). We
suggest that it accomplished this, at least in urban areas, by being able to endorse
types of donation that were already part of the culturally accepted repertoire of
what was considered appropriate exchange between citizens and larger institutions of social welfare (namely the work units). Donation was not only done
willingly (and, in that sense, was voluntary) but was also a contribution to the
work unit's (and by extension, society's) success only when the donor was suffi-
ciently "taken care of" through compensation. Even though this type of donation
represents a twist on (if not a break with) international standards for ensuring
safe procurement, it works well in China.

One of the important lessons from China's experiences with blood donation
is that it suggests the need for flexibility in defining international standards and
strategies for public health when it comes to the safety of blood. Although international strategies for producing safe blood generally insist on voluntary, unpaid
donations, the case of China suggests that cultural specificity may require that
different techniques of blood collection and compensation be used to ensure a
safe blood supply. There is some debate in the international community
regarding the ethics of compensation for whole blood (see Daar 1992; Marshall
and Daar 1998), China's example suggests that this debate should remain open.

The importance of national public health programs is not that they can simply
be a conduit for larger international agendas in health development, whether in
the rise of pharmaceutical industries and research, in the decentralized practices
of local NGO work, or in their ability to deploy risk-oriented security regimes.
Rather, the importance of national public health programs is in their ability to
tailor their methods, resources, and strategies in ways that are locally informed,
and that make sense in a cultural context. Responsiveness to local health scen-
arios is best accomplished by working through national public health infrastructures that already have an understanding of what makes cultural sense and what
is logistically possible. Public debates about the structure of blood donation – or
other public health or health promotion efforts – need to be less about imposing
a "universal" notion of ethics and more about ensuring the implementation of
effective strategies and the delivery of successful outcomes.

In some ways, the story of China's response to the blood donation-related
HIV epidemic is very specific to China, both in the sense of its large capacity for
generating propaganda that penetrates to even the most rural villages and in the
sense of its being able to criminalize activities and authorize others with an executive swiftness that is unfamiliar to most modern nations. At the same time, the
example that China presents us with of a public health program that was able to
attend to local crises in specific ways and to respond to the emerging epidemic

of both HIV and potential decline of blood supply is one that reveals the importance of having strong local public health programs anywhere.

Acknowledgments

Funding for this research was provided by the NIH R21 MHO73415. This grant was originally procured by Kathleen Erwin, who was PI on the project. Vincanne Adams took over as PI on the project in 2006 and has been working collaboratively with Kathleen Erwin on the project since then. Phuoc V. Le (MD, MPH, Global Health Equity Resident at Brigham and Women's Hospital in Boston) has worked on the project as co-investigator since 2006. The authors would also like to thank and acknowledge the support and intellectual engagement of colleagues at the Shanghai Academy of Social Sciences.

Notes

1 This chapter has been previously published in Adams, A., Erwin, K., and Le, Phuoc V. 2009. "Public health works: blood donation in urban China." *Social Sciences and Medicine* 68(3): 410–418.
2 While recognizing that it is impossible to generalize these trends to all countries, and while also recognizing that some of these trends may contribute indirectly to strengthening public health programs in some instances, we begin with this scenario to make the point that we should be worried. So, for example, some will note that pharmaceuticals and bioscience research projects that are conducted collaboratively in under-resourced nations can help build local infrastructures for scientific research and potentially stem the net outflow of qualified biomedical researchers from poor to wealthy nations. In addition, in some regions, NGO programs are required to work through national ministries or bureaus of health, enabling national public health programs to coordinate efforts to build a strong national public health system. Finally, we note that biosecurity programs can also augment local national public health infrastructures when they focus on the eradication of vectors of transmission, even if they may undermine other programs, such as small business loans for chicken farmers and other livestock businesses (which are eradicated in programs to eliminate vectors) (see work by Benjamin Hickler, Graduate Program in Medical Anthropology (UCF)).
3 The collaboration with Chinese researchers was initiated by Kathleen Erwin, who has a history of conducting research in urban China.

References

Adams, V., Novotny, T., and Leslie, H. 2008. "Global Health Diplomacy." *Editorial Medical Anthropology* 27(4): 315–323.
Anagnost, A. 1997. *National Past-Times: Narrative, Representation and Power in Modern China*. Durham, NC: Duke University Press.
Archard, D. 2002. "Selling Yourself: Titmuss's Argument Against a Market in Blood." *The Journal of Ethics* 6: 87–103.
Brown, T., Marcos Cueto, M., and Fee, E. 2006. "The World Health Organization and the Transition from International to Global Public Health." *American Journal of Public Health* 96(1): 62–72.
Daar, A.S. 1992. "Rewarded Giving." *Transplantation Proceedings* 24: 2207–2211.

Erwin, K. 2006. "The Circulatory System: Blood Procurement, AIDS, and the Social Body in China." *Medical Anthropology Quarterly* 20(2): 139–159.

Greenhalgh, S. 2008. *Just One Child: Science and Policy in Deng's China.* Berkeley: University of California Press.

Jing, S. 2006. "Fluid Labor and Blood Money: The Economy of HIV/AIDS in Rural Central China." *Cultural Anthropology* 21(4): 535–569.

King, N.K. 2002. "Security, Disease, Commerce: Ideologies of Post-colonial Global Health." *SSS* 32(5/60): 763–789.

Kleinman, A. 1981. *Patients and Healers in the Context of Culture.* New York: Campus Books.

Lakoff, A. 2008. "The Generic Biothreat, or, How We Become Unprepared." *Cultural Anthropology* 23(3): 399–428.

Marshall, P.A. and Daar, A.S. 1998. "Cultural and Psychological Dimensions of Organ Transplantation." *Annals of Transplantation* 3(2): 7–11.

Mastro, T.D. and Yip, R. 2006. "The Legacy of Unhygienic Plasma Collection in China." *AIDS* 20(10): 1451–1452.

McNeil, D.G. Jr. 2008. "Gates Foundation Influence Criticized." *New York Times*, February 16.

Novotny, T. 2007. "Global Governance and Public Health Security in the 21st Century." *California Western International Law Journal* 38: 101–122.

Petryna, A. 2006. "Globalizing Human Subjects Research," in *Global Pharmaceuticals: Ethics, Markets, Practices*, ed. A. Petryna, A. Lakoff, and A. Kleinman (33–60). Durham, NC: Duke University Press.

Qu, L. 2006. World Blood Donation Day. People's Republic of China, Shanghai. www.who.int/worldblooddonorday/archives/2006/wbdd_prchina/en/index.html (last accessed December 16, 2014).

Shan, H., Wang, J.-X., Ren, F.-R., Zhang, Y.-Z., Zhao, H.-Y., Gao, G.-J., Ji, Y., and Ness, P.M. 2002. "Blood Banking in China." *The Lancet* 360: 1770–1775.

Titmuss, R.M. 1987. *The Gift Relationship, From Human Blood to Social Policy*, ed. A. Oakley and J. Ashton. New York: The Free Press.

UNAIDS: *China At a Glance.* www.unaids.org.cn/en/index/page.asp?id=197&class=2&classname=China+Epidemic+%26+Response (last accessed December 16, 2014).

Wang, Y. 2004. "Encouraging Volunteers to Give Blood." *China Daily* (online edition).

Whyte, G. 2003. "Ethical Aspects of Blood and Organ Donation." *Internal Medical Journal* 33: 362–264.

Yang, Mayfair Mei-Hui. 1994. *Gifts, Favors and Banquets: The Art of Social Relationships in China.* Ithaca, NY: Cornell University Press.

Zaller, N., Nelso, K.E., Ness, P., Wen, G., Bai, X., and Shan, H. 2005. "Knowledge, Attitude and Practice Survey Regarding Blood Donation in a Northwestern Chinese City." *Transfusion Medicine* 15: 277–286.

Zaller, N., Kenrad, E., Nelson, P.N., Wen, G., Dewir, T., Bai, X., and Shan, H. 2006. "Demographic Characteristics and Risks for Transfusion-transmissible Infection Among Blood Donors in Xinjiang Autonomous Region, People's Republic of China." *Transfusion* 46: 265–271.

4 The contaminated blood affair in France

A turning point in blood donation[1]

Sophie Chauveau

Introduction

Starting in the early 1980s, France saw a large number of transfusion patients become infected by blood transfusions contaminated by the human immunodeficiency virus (HIV) and the hepatitis C virus (HCV). The country sustained one of the highest rates of contaminated transfusion recipients and hemophiliacs in Europe. This high contamination rate may be largely explained by the organization of blood collection in France at the time and the particularities of its blood derivative industry. However, these institutions cannot be held solely responsible for the crisis; politicians and French health administrators also played an important role. Indeed, intensive media coverage of the crisis, as well as the indictment of a number of doctors and high-ranking officials, helped transform this issue into a scandal at the dawn of the 1990s. In the public's mind, the contaminated blood affair became the country's first health crisis (Chauveau 2011). It also significantly altered the way politicians and public authorities manage health safety concerns.

The affair has had several consequences. The organization of blood transfusion underwent several reforms over the 1990s that resulted in the introduction of new regulations for blood donation and the manufacture of blood derivatives. These transformations were justified by the need to improve the safety of blood products offered to patients, as well as to adapt blood transfusion establishments to the requirements of industrially producing blood-derived medicinal products. Although the principle of voluntary, anonymous, and non-remunerated blood donation was never called into question, these changes transformed the very moral economy of blood transfusion. If blood donation is still valued as an altruistic gesture in blood-drive campaigns, it is also an increasingly regulated and codified practice subject to health, industry, and commercial standards.

Blood transfusion in France now coexists as both a gift economy, which oversees the obtaining of blood as a raw material, and as a market economy, which involves the preparation and distribution of blood-derived products.[2] This coexistence was not instituted with the contaminated blood affair but appeared at the beginning of the 1970s, when the preparation of blood-derived products became more systematic in many blood establishments. Until the contaminated blood affair broke out, however, neither public authorities, nor transfusion specialists, nor donors, nor patients accepted the ambivalence of this economy of blood transfusion. Since then, the reorganization of blood transfusion in France has sanctioned this activity as a component of the bio-industry.

Today, the *Établissement Français du Sang* (EFS), which reports to the Health Ministry, is the organization responsible for collecting blood from voluntary, anonymous, non-remunerated donors.[3] The EFS was founded in 2000, following legislation passed on July 1, 1998, which strengthened the state's supervision of all products destined for human consumption. In replacing the *Agence Française du Sang* (AFS), the EFS was given a twofold mandate: (1) to meet the blood needs of the French population; and (2) to ensure conformity of transfusion practices to accepted medical, scientific, and technological standards, while respecting ethical principles. The EFS was also tasked with supplying the *Laboratoire Français du Fractionnement et des Biotechnologies* (LFB) with the raw plasma necessary to meet national needs for stable blood products and blood-derived medicinal products. These products are considered medicinal because they are subjected to the same safety and commercial standards as pharmaceutical medications. The 1993 designation of blood-derived products as medicinal complied with a related European directive dated June 14, 1989, itself modeled after legislation passed in the United States two decades earlier. Designating blood products as medicinal facilitated their circulation throughout Europe and led to safety improvements in their production (Directive 89/381 du *Conseil des Communautés Européennes*).

Yet, how has voluntary, anonymous, and non-remunerated blood donation been preserved in France, even when it seemed doubly condemned by the implementation of stricter safety requirements and by growing industrial and commercial constraints? The implementation of stricter screening procedures resulted in the identification of a growing number of threats to the blood supply and widening exclusion of some segments of the population from donating. These changes challenged an entrenched culture of donation whereby donors were often conferred the status of hero. Tensions were also introduced by the need to meet an ever-growing demand for blood-derived products. These tensions trace to the contradiction of having blood, which is freely and voluntarily donated, transformed into commercial products on an industrial scale. These combined pressures outraged many blood donor associations, which resented that much of the blood donated was being transformed into therapeutic products mostly consumed, at the time, by a minority of patients, primarily hemophiliacs. Many blood donor associations resisted the industrialization of blood transfusion at the end of the 1970s and the beginning of the 1980s.

This chapter argues that key changes in the moral economy of blood transfusion eventually eased the tensions between the gift and market economies of blood-derived products. Specifically, France retained a blood system entirely based on voluntary and non-remunerated donation, in part because of the influence of a strong public service sector and the presence of a strong moral economy of blood transfusion. This chapter also draws attention to the motivations of key stakeholders who preserved France's blood system as a voluntary system, including doctors, donors, patients, and public authorities.

In the first section, this chapter examines the measures put in place to manage the contamination risks posed by the HIV and HCV viruses; the second section offers an analysis of the discourse on blood donation during the contaminated blood affair. This analysis reveals that while the principle of voluntary, anonymous, non-remunerated blood donation was never challenged in France, questions were nonetheless raised about the usefulness of this principle in the wake of the contaminated blood affair. Finally, the third section situates the principle of voluntary, anonymous, non-remunerated donation in relation to the commodification of blood transfusion. A powerful rhetoric was deployed to defend this principle, partly to maintain the trust of donors and the sufficiency of the blood supply (Healy 2006). However, this rhetoric also served to hide growing tensions within the French blood transfusion system between market rules (e.g., the pricing of blood transfers) and a gift economy.

The following analysis is based mainly on data about blood transfusion activities obtained from a study of archival collections released by the French *Ministère de la Santé*. Among these archives, files addressing problems with transfusion safety, as well as the meeting minutes of the *Commission Consultative de Transfusion Sanguine* (CCTS),[4] provide the most important information. The contaminated blood affair led to several inquiries ordered by the *Ministère de la Santé* and undertaken by the *Inspection générale des affaires sociales*.[5] Chief among these was a report by Michel Lucas, *Transfusion sanguine et sida en 1985: Chronologie des faits et décisions pour ce qui concerne les hémophiles*. The report was the main source used by journalist Anne-Marie Casteret, who played a key role in breaking the scandal (Casteret 1992). Members of the French Parliament also investigated the contaminated blood affair and the measures taken in connection with the acquired immunodeficiency syndrome (AIDS) epidemic (Sourdille and Huriet 1992; *Rapport de la commission d'enquête sur l'état des connaissances scientifiques et les actions menées à l'égard de la transmission du sida* 1993). Finally, the author conducted interviews with key players from this period, including high-ranking officials, transfusion specialists, and the leaders of blood donation associations.

The contaminated blood affair and its aftermath have been the subject of numerous analyses by social science researchers. Inspired by the pioneering work of Ulrich Beck (2001[1986]), some researchers have examined this health crisis in relation to issues of risk management.[6] Others have focused on the legal and judicial dimensions of the crisis and, more generally, on the legal ramifications of blood transfusion and the use of the human body (Hermitte 1996). Still others have investigated the contaminated blood affair from specific angles: the question of screening, the situation of hemophiliacs, information management in public health, and the role of the media.[7]

Unlike these previous analyses, this chapter focuses on the organizational aspects of blood donation. It argues that the principle of voluntary, anonymous, non-remunerated donation in France was preserved through important transformations in the moral economy of blood transfusion. This economy rests on a combination of values about the status of blood, the practices associated with collecting blood and manufacturing blood-derived products, and the social meanings attributed to blood collection and the delivery of blood products. This moral economy also brings together key players (donors, physicians, patients, managers, and politicians) involved in the organization of blood transfusion (Fassin 2009).

The end of universal donation: exclusions from blood donation

In 1983, before the HIV virus was positively identified as the cause of AIDS, most virology and immunology specialists were almost certain that "gay cancer," as it was referred to at the time, was transmitted both sexually and by blood (Epstein 2001; Lestrade and Pialoux 2012). This understanding of AIDS transmission explains why restrictions on blood donation were among the first preventive measures adopted by countries confronting this emergent risk.

Although blood donation was considered to be a universal practice in principle, meaning that any individual could give blood, in reality, there were already several restrictions placed on donation. For example, in France, the frequency of donations was limited over time and women were not permitted to give as often as men. Children and the elderly were also prohibited from donating. Donors were required to be in good health and free of blood-borne illnesses. Donors who wanted to donate frequently were required to submit the results of their syphilis screens or Bordet–Wassermann tests on a regular basis. In the 1960s, the risk of hepatitis B transmission led to the exclusion of hepatitis carriers, and hepatitis screens became mandatory for all blood donations in 1971. Exclusion was done via biological screening: blood was collected from donors as usual, but if testing of their blood packs detected hepatitis antibodies, their blood would be removed from the pool. Biological screening also became the established method for managing the risk posed by the HIV virus. However, the introduction of HIV screening was delayed, first by the challenges involved in identifying the virus, and later by the difficulties involved in developing a reliable screening test.

At the start of the HIV crisis, numerous uncertainties thus confronted doctors, donors, patients, and public authorities. The clinical profile of AIDS only became clear over a period of months: the first victims, reported in 1981, did not die from the same disease; rather, they suffered from a number of opportunistic illnesses which they acquired following the collapse of their immune defenses. A hypothesis emerged that a virus provoked these immune deficiencies, but the transmission modes of the virus were still being debated. Nonetheless, well before HIV was proven to be blood-borne, the first exclusionary measures for blood donation were put in place, based on clinical signs and observation of at-risk behaviors.[8]

A circular letter dated June 20, 1983, recommended the implementation of screening for the clinical signs of disease and for at-risk behaviors that would increase the likelihood of a donor carrying a blood-borne pathogen.[9] The circular recommended the exclusion of prospective blood donors on the basis of sexual orientation, state of health, intravenous drug use, and travel to Haiti or Africa (CCTS minutes, meeting of June 9, 1983).

Transfusion specialists initially resisted the use of this screening. Some feared that homosexuals would refuse to answer questions regarding their private lives, while others were afraid of being accused of racism if they turned away donors of African origin (CCTS minutes, meeting of June 9, 1983). Although any prospective blood donor was expected to submit to a brief clinical examination, many doctors were bothered by the invasive nature of the screening and feared angering donors. Furthermore, doctors did not understand why a biological test could not be used instead, as was the case for hepatitis B. In 1983, the virus had only just been identified and no screening test was available; a few doctors nevertheless suggested that an individual found to be a carrier of hepatitis B antibodies might be a carrier of HIV, as opposed to an individual in good health.

A 1984 investigation by the director of the Brest transfusion centre revealed that directives contained in the 1983 circular were improperly and inconsistently applied in many blood transfusion establishments (Saleun 1984a, 1984b). The circular called for the handing out of a note to prospective donors, requesting that they identify themselves if they belonged to at-risk groups (based on clinical signs indicative of AIDS, sexual behavior, drug consumption, and trips to Haiti or Africa) (*Circulaire Direction Générale de la Santé* 3B no. 569). In some establishments, donors were not always asked about their at-risk behaviors in pre-donation interviews (Chauveau 2011, 62–71), while other establishments relied instead on alternate preventive measures such as forgoing blood collection in prisons due to the higher prevalence of AIDS-specific risk factors in prison populations.

In the end, the world of transfusion – doctors and donors alike – responded ambivalently to the threat of AIDS. Transfusion specialists were generally quite uncomfortable bringing up the risk of AIDS with donors. It was as if the selfless nature of donors forbade the view that they could pose a threat to the health of blood recipients. This view was perhaps reinforced by the muted reaction of blood donor associations to the risk of HIV contamination. These organizations reproduced in their newsletters information from the 1983 circular but abstained from commenting on it.[10] The prevailing view at the time was that blood contamination was more likely to come from remunerated donations, which were not permitted in France, or from the use of imported commercial products.[11]

The failure to adequately implement screening as outlined in the June 20, 1983, circular was harmful in light of the fact that such pre-donation interviews would have excluded at-risk populations and significantly reduced the number of HIV-contaminated transfusions.[12] Only after a steep increase in the number of contamination cases and the confirmation of HIV as a blood-borne virus did French doctors implement more rigorous screening procedures. In January 1985, a new circular was released that restated most of the information contained in the 1983 circular. But it also warned the directors of blood transfusion establishments that they would be held accountable if they did not follow the circular's directives (Chauveau 2011, 70).

By April 1985, two screening kits became available in France: one manufactured by the American firm Abbott, the other by a subsidiary of Pasteur Production, Diagnostics-Pasteur. In June 1985, French Prime Minister Laurent Fabius made HIV screening mandatory for all blood donations. But the government contracted the French supplier of screening kits, Diagnostics-Pasteur, even though the company was still struggling to mass produce a reliable test. (Abbott, its American competitor, was already doing so.) The *Ministère de l'Industrie* even exerted pressure to delay making screening mandatory until the French firm was in a position to supply the test kits. Indecision over the selection of the test and over what information to give HIV-positive donors served to justify this delay.[13]

Mandatory screening of all blood for the HIV and HCV viruses became a logical extension of practices already in place to manage the risk of hepatitis B. This solution was easier to implement and, in a sense, preserved the principle of universality, as any exclusions that occurred took place after the donation, when blood packs were tested. However, the fact that contaminated blood came from voluntary, anonymous, non-remunerated donors raised some questions about the effectiveness of non-remuneration in protecting the safety of the blood supply – particularly since tests were now available to screen all donated blood. The next section explores this debate.

Non-remunerated blood donation: myths and realities

As the public authorities struggled to implement measures to prevent HIV contamination of the blood supply, voices were raised to defend the value of non-remunerated blood donation as a precautionary measure. In the early 1980s, French blood donor associations, in particular the *Fédération Française des Donneurs de Sang Bénévoles* (Marty 1985), took up arguments already made in the late 1960s and early 1970s by Titmuss, who championed voluntary and unpaid donation as a principle of solidarity that organizes social relationships (Titmuss 1971; Fontaine 2002). These arguments followed a familiar line: without a policy enforcing non-remunerated donation, poor and marginalized individuals would be tempted to sell their blood, while their ill health would make it more likely for unsafe blood to be collected from them. Reports of mercenary blood transfusion practices in developing countries further reinforced this view and entrenched the idea that blood or plasma from remunerated donors was more likely to carry viruses and contagious diseases than blood obtained from non-remunerated donors (Anderson and Snow 1994; Drake *et al.* 1982; Hagen 1982).

These condemnations of remunerated donation and the fact that such donation was closely linked with the acquisition of hazardous products led to a portrayal of AIDS as an external threat; however, the discovery of contamination among young hemophiliacs who had used products from France nullified the argument.

Even so, non-remunerated blood donation continued to be viewed as superior, and it was thought that "voluntary" blood could not be contaminated by HIV, since it was pure blood, not tainted by commercial transaction, as the leaders of blood donation associations continued to reiterate. Paradoxically, even though the contaminated blood affair revealed that voluntary donation itself could be a vehicle for contamination, the principle of voluntary, anonymous, and non-remunerated donation emerged strengthened from the crisis. In the end, however, this principle was undermined less by the AIDS contamination crisis than by the shift toward a blood economy centred on the industrial production of blood-derived products.

The practice of non-remunerated donation in France has a rich history. The practice was mandated by law in France only in 1993. Article 2 of a bill dated January 4, 1993, states that "Blood transfusion is performed in the interest of the recipient and is governed by the ethical principles of voluntary and anonymous donation, as well as the absence of profit" (JO 1993; my translation). Yet, unpaid donation did not always prevail in France: only in the 1950s did voluntary, anonymous, and non-remunerated donation become the rule. During the inter-war period and World War II, donor remuneration was justified by the urgency of the gesture. Indeed, because blood could not be conserved, donors were called upon when the need for donations arose, often in emergency situations. Beginning in the 1930s, the first efforts to conserve blood led some doctors to question the compensation of donors.

During the Liberation of France, opposition between voluntary and paid donors intensified. Remunerated donors were equated with Nazi collaborators, while volunteers were seen as embodying the spirit of the Resistance. Resistance networks, and especially armed resisters, had equipped themselves with underground transfusion teams whose donors were volunteers and did not ask for compensation, even for emergency transfusions. Volunteer donation was practiced in a spirit of solidarity that characterized the ideals of the Resistance. The *Code du Donneur de Sang* (blood donor's code) written in 1944 by donor associations specified that donors should commit to answering any call, including emergencies, whether compensated or not.[14] Paid donation was quickly side-lined, and compensation increasingly took on the form of fixed sums intended to compensate donors for the inconvenience of having to answer an urgent call for donation. Even then, paid donors almost always remitted their compensation to solidarity funds such as the *Mutuelle du sang*, which assisted the families of donors in need (*Archives Charles Mérieux* 1943–1945, 1950; *Fédération Française des Donneurs de Sang Bénévoles Assemblée Générale* [1949]).

The rule of voluntary and non-remunerated donation was instituted in July 1952 with the adoption of the July 21, 1952, bill concerning the therapeutic use of human blood and plasma, as well as their derived products. The bill stipulated that no profit could be made from the transfer of blood products and that their preparation and distribution fell under the exclusive preserve of the medical establishment. This non-profit rule was interpreted in different ways by blood donor associations in the early 1950s. Indeed, these associations considered that an absence of profit implied that blood was acquired freely; in other words, it was given by volunteers and hence should be distributed free of charge (1954: *Compte-rendu du Congrès national de la fédération des donneurs de sang bénévoles:* 42; Chauveau 2007, 194–199). However, in the view of the *Administration de la Santé*, this free model of blood donation could not become the established norm. Preparing blood bottles and blood-derived products requires expensive handling (grouping of blood, addition of preservatives, etc.). Consequently, blood products were distributed upon payment of a transfer price corresponding to the cost of preparation, with no provision for profit. This principle has endured up until today: transfer fees still provide the financial resources for blood establishments.

Such debates on donor remuneration and the price of blood left a deep and abiding mark on the world of blood transfusion in France. The generosity and altruism of blood donors in a sense made them heroes, rewarded with medals and diplomas in accordance with how much blood they gave. The existence of such bonuses produced reservations; certain doctors in charge of transfusion establishments preferred to emphasize fraternal solidarity (Raoul-Duval 1956; Trambouze 1957). Conversely, those who promoted such rewards maintained that they made it possible to hold up blood donation as a model of altruistic behavior.

The promotion of non-remunerated donation in France was by no means limited to donor associations. Transfusion specialists, and especially those in charge of transfusion establishments, were very much attached to unpaid donation. Starting at the end of the 1940s, as the first blood transfusion establishments were opened and blood collection was organized at the national level, such specialists defended this model. For these doctors, non-remunerated donation reflected a respect for human dignity (1949: Etienne Aujaleu, minutes; 1952: *Documents parlementaires, Assemblée Nationale*, March 14, 1952). Yet, the reality is that after World War II, there was never a plan to develop transfusion activities based on paid donation, as was the case in the USA. This is why the controversies sparked by the writings of Richard Titmuss found little resonance in France in the 1960s and early 1970s. Indeed, blood donors as well as transfusion specialists at this time still perceived transfusion as a matter of organizing blood collection and distribution, and refused to take into account emergent constraints resulting from the industrialization of certain activities in line with the transformation of blood products.

Starting in the second half of the 1970s, the organization of blood transfusion in France grew in complexity alongside the introduction of new fractioning technologies and the manufacture of a large variety of blood-derived products, such as albumin or anti-hemophilia fraction. Prices for these products continued to be fixed by public authorities: stable products, derived from plasma, were transferred to transfusion establishments at very high prices, while labile products, such as red blood cell concentrates, were transferred at very low cost. To compensate for the costs associated with these products' manufacture, some blood establishments started to collect large quantities of blood for fractioning. As a result, larger establishments with large donor pools were favoured, although blood was also commonly wasted (Chauveau 2007).

Unsurprisingly, during this period, the relationships among blood donors, those in charge of major blood establishments, and hemophilia representatives deteriorated (Bastin 1978). Hemophiliacs had come to use treatments that required very large quantities of plasma, which meant a high number of donations. These treatments enabled them to live virtually normal lives. Donor associations were fairly critical of these practices, unlike certain transfusion specialists who encouraged plasma drives that only served the interests of a small number of patients. The spirit of solidarity that had reigned over blood donation was, in a sense, flouted.

Blood donors also proved very critical of an organizational structure that seemed interested only in profit and patient satisfaction. They felt that the altruism and solidarity of their act was no longer respected. At the same time, it was fairly difficult for them to take a clear-cut position: they would then be criticized for not being as generous as they claimed to be and for being too concerned about obtaining rewards for their actions in the form of decorations.

Up until the contaminated blood affair, non-remunerated donation in France was not questioned. No voices were therefore raised to defend the recourse to payment in order to obtain more plasma. To meet the growing demand for certain blood-derived products, the public authorities preferred to authorize imports, without being able to verify whether these products originated from unpaid donations. These products were imported very discreetly: they were a stopgap solution for hemophilia doctors who normally preferred to use products supplied by French establishments (Soulier 1978). However, the French transfusion system appears to have been substantially weakened by internal tensions. Indeed, blood transfusion partly became an industry exhibiting certain traits shared with the drug industry (*Rapport de la Cour des comptes* 2005). Blood itself had become a commodity, a product from which various other derived products could be extracted for therapeutic use: blood bags were given a value, and this economic logic ran counter to the ideal of non-remunerated donation. The contaminated blood affair compelled a profound reorganization of blood transfusion in France which saw the adoption of new safety rules and some level of reconciliation between the logic of the gift and the logic of the market.

The gift and the market

From its beginnings, blood transfusion in France was organized in the context of a market economy. Blood products were subject to commercial transfer: the payment of a sum corresponding to a transfer rate established by the *Ministère de la Santé* was needed to finance the running of blood transfusion establishments and, in particular, the activities of analyzing and testing blood bottles, as well as preparing blood-derived products. This transfusion economy relied on a freely obtained resource – blood – which may be described as a "thing outside commerce" (Moine 1997). A given object escapes commerce by virtue of its inalienable nature, or because it is hazardous, or because it belongs to the public domain. An object's commercial nature is based on an ability to circulate between different subjects, between different estates, and the number of these transfers is unlimited. Blood, like organs taken from the human body, cannot be an object of such exchange. This characteristic of being "outside commerce" is not a mere quality of blood but rather a fundamental feature of its exchange between human beings. Blood cannot be acquired or transmitted. Nor is blood donation a hand-to-hand gift, since the donor must submit to a medical examination before giving blood and the collected blood undergoes numerous transformations before being used for therapeutic purposes.

The organization of blood donation in France has all the attributes of a public service, and the donor's gesture constitutes an occasional collaboration to ensure the proper functioning of this public service. Indeed, until the end of the 1980s, transfusion activities were entrusted to non-profit associations. Associations were disinterested organizations that fulfilled their administrative mission without concern for profit. Blood was given to the community, and a moral commitment was made to the donor concerning the use of the blood: given that the donation was free, it could not be a source of profit. In this manner, blood remained a "thing outside commerce": a "thing so closely associated with human beings by rights that they could not, even voluntarily, relinquish ownership of it without denying their humanity" (Moine 1997, 222; our translation).

Keeping blood "outside of commerce" became increasingly difficult as pressures to commercialize blood packs mounted, especially for labile and stable blood products. Beginning in the 1970s, as collected blood entered commercial preparation and production, it became subject to transactions whose rates were fixed by public authorities. Private businesses were not permitted to manufacture blood products until the 1980s and 1990s. Finally, and most importantly, blood donor associations were very hostile to any form of commodification of blood, including blood-derived products. Yet, by the early 1990s, the reorganization of blood transfusion in France, together with safety requirements, required a greater integration of blood products in a market economy and clarification of the ambiguities surrounding their commercialization for therapeutic use. In the wake of reforms begun in the 1990s, the principle of non-remunerated donation was reinforced, while the integration of blood collection into a new economy of transfusion gradually came to be more accepted.

A substantial drop in the number of blood donations following the contaminated blood affair accelerated the introduction of new practices to reduce the need for blood transfusion and the development of blood substitutes, notably for treating hemophiliacs.[15] Blood donations did indeed decrease significantly starting in the 1990s: in 1980, four million blood units were collected in France, but in 1992, when the contaminated blood affair became a public scandal, it dropped to 2.9 million units (Chauveau 2007). These shortages also prompted blood establishments to improve donor recruitment practices and public communication about the need for blood (Malet 2004).

Since 1998, the EFS has been the only French operator of blood drives. This institution must meet the needs of hospitals as well as of the *Laboratoire Français du Fractionnement*. The use of some of the blood donated by volunteer donors to prepare blood-derived medicinal products has met with much reluctance and criticism from blood donors. The contaminated blood affair also resulted in profound changes in the relationships among donors, donor associations, and blood establishments. Blood donor associations, which had been involved in the running of blood transfusion establishments, were now excluded by the reforms initiated in 1992. Association members had been regular participants in blood drives, organized recruitment campaigns, and assisted in blood collection. The introduction of stricter safety guidelines meant that association members could no longer take part in these activities.

Blood transfusion organizations also altered their blood donor screening practices. The need for conducting a pre-donation screening had not always been well understood, particularly since blood packs were systematically tested afterwards. Donors were made more aware of their responsibilities and were required to sign a sheet acknowledging that they had been informed about the donation process (Bastard 2006).

Blood donor associations were initially very hostile to the designation of plasma products as "medication derived from blood." Many donors feared becoming "suppliers" to an industry profiting from blood-derived products (1991: *Compte-rendu des travaux du colloque de Cognac*, December 14–15, FFDSB). However, by the 1990s, there was greater acceptance of this market economy as reflected by the French government's decision to align the prices of its blood products with international prices.

Over time, and with dialogue between public authorities, transfusion specialists, and donor associations, these reforms have gradually gained acceptance. The European Parliament's support of the principle of voluntary, anonymous, non-remunerated donation also played a role in this development. Specifically, the European Parliament's directive of September 14, 1993, recommended that blood donation be voluntary, that the origin of all blood be known, that no profit be made on unpaid donation, and that the commercialization of blood and its products be progressively abandoned (1993: *JO des Communautés Européennes*). Blood donor associations eventually appointed themselves as the guardians of voluntary donation within this new economy of blood transfusion.

However, there is no doubt that the principle of voluntary, anonymous, non-remunerated donation was harmed by the contaminated blood affair. It brought to light the contrasting features of the French blood transfusion system: on the one hand, it has a relatively rudimentary organizational structure for collecting blood, and, on the other hand, it maintains large, complex, quasi-industrial establishments involved in preparing blood-derived products. A gift economy characterizes blood collection, while a market economy characterizes the preparation of blood-derived products. These two logics have been preserved by the reforms begun at the start of the 1990s and aiming to improve the safety of blood products. At the same time, existing market mechanisms have been taken into account, as demonstrated by the alignment of blood product prices in France with international prices.

Overall, the principle of voluntary, anonymous, non-remunerated donation has been preserved in France despite the introduction of stringent safety standards, mandatory testing of all blood, and rigorous pre-donation interviews. The French government has publicly committed itself to defending and promoting the principle of voluntary, anonymous, non-remunerated donation among other European states. The survival of this principle traces to cultural factors – it would be impossible to neglect the fact that voluntary donation finds more advocates in countries with a Catholic tradition than elsewhere – and also to political factors. The mobilization of blood donors remains an ongoing challenge, and the support of donor associations is crucial in achieving this task: the government understands it cannot alienate these organizations with policies or practices that undermine a principle which they cherish. The transformation of the French blood transfusion system is thus embedded in the very logic of the technical transformations that blood transfusion has undergone over more than 50 years.

Concluding remarks

The coexistence of the gift economy with a market economy is not a recent abnormality, nor is it difficult to accept; rather, it is an extension of the way blood transfusion had always been organized in France. The contaminated blood affair helped resolve existing ambiguities in this relationship. Striking a balance between market forces and the promotion of voluntary donation has been made possible by adherence to values based on the respect and protection of all human beings from exploitation.

The current consensus over the value of voluntary, anonymous, non-remunerated blood donation traces back to the late 1940s and early 1950s, when transfusion establishments promoted blood donation as serving the interests of the nation. The contaminated blood affair may have temporarily weakened the resolve of French donors, but it also spurred changes that made blood transfusions safer and reaffirmed voluntary, anonymous, non-remunerated blood donation as a fundamental aspect of a renewed moral economy of blood – one that now includes blood donor associations, patients, physicians in the hospital, general practitioners, public officers in health administration, and the manufacturers of blood derivatives.

Notes

1 A previous version of this chapter has been published in Johanne Charbonneau and Nathalie Tran (eds). 2012. *Les Enjeux du Don de Sang dans le Monde*. Rennes: Presses de l'EHESP. However, this chapter, originally published in French, has been updated, and additional ideas have been included in the analyses and conclusions.
2 On the gift, see Mauss 1950; Godelier 1997; Godbout and Caillé 1992; Caillé 2005; Bourdieu 2000; Boltanski 1990. On the blood economy, see Cooper and Culyer 1968;

Alchian 1973; Titmuss 1970. On the commodification of life, see Scheper-Hughes and Wacquant (eds) 2002; Waldby and Mitchell 2006. On the coexistence of the gift economy and the market economy, see Callon (ed.) 1998; Chauveau 2009; Steiner 2010; Wailoo *et al.* (eds) 2006; Healy 2006.

3 At a national level, the EFS organizes blood collection activities, the biological quali-fication of LBP, and their distribution to health establishments. It is endowed with a monopoly over these activities. The EFS has national headquarters and 17 regional and inter-regional blood transfusion establishments. (ETS is short for *Établissements de Transfusion Sanguine*.) These establishments are under the management and responsibility of a doctor or pharmacist acting on behalf of the EFS president, who determines the geographical and technical activity sectors of the ETS in compliance with the provisions of territorial plans for blood transfusion. All ETS centres must be certified by the national agency for drug and health products safety (ANSM: *Agence Nationale de Sécurité du Médicament et des Produits de Santé*).

4 The CCTS was established in 1946 and brings together directors of blood transfusion establishments and plasma fractionation centres, as well as representatives of the *Dir-ection Générale de la Santé*, the *Direction des Hôpitaux* (for the *Ministère de la Santé*), and the *Direction de la Sécurité Sociale*. The commission deals with all transfusion-related matters: the opening of transfusion establishments, the definition and standardization of blood products, the fixing of transfer prices, the establishment of collection practices, etc.

5 The *Inspection Générale des Affaires Sociales* (IGAS) is an inspection unit whose mission is to verify and investigate administrations and public services in matters of health, labour, and employment. The unit comprises high-ranking officials, often from the *École Nationale d'Administration* (ENA), as well as doctors. In France, most administrations have their own inspection units (*Finances, Éducation nationale, Police nationale*, etc.).

6 See Callon *et al.* (eds) 1998; Chateauraynaud and Torny 1999; Noiville 2003; Chau-veau 2004; Borraz 2008.

7 See Setbon 1993; Bastin *et al.* (eds) 1993; Carricaburu 2000; Fillion 2009; Grémy 2000; Marchetti 2010.

8 These first clinical screening tests were implemented starting in May 1983 in France at the collection points of the *Centre National de la Transfusion Sanguine*, at the request of Jean-Pierre Soulier, the institution's director. *Procès-Verbal de la CCTS, Séance du 9 juin 1983, Sécurité transfusionnelle* (1956 1993), *ministère de la Santé, Direction générale de la Santé*, 19960402/14.

9 These risks are as follows: operations and transfusions undergone by the donor, acu-puncture treatment, tattoos, hepatitis, trips outside France, episodes of malaria, intrave-nous drug use, relations with multiple homosexual partners, weight loss, unexplained fever, and the appearance of nodes. Questionnaire cited in Soulier (1992).

10 For example, Genetet 1983: *Informations UNAADSBPTT*).

11 On the subject of plasma from remunerated donations, Cagnard, a medical advisor, wrote that "at-risk donors such as drug addicts would sell their blood to acquire drugs, which is not the case in France, where donation is on a volunteer basis" (1983: *Le donneur de sang bénévole*, 429).

12 Four out of 1,000 donors were turned away from giving blood subsequent to an inter-view in 1983 (Soulier 1983). This proportion is comparable to that of donors who were turned away following a test (Nguyen *et al.* 1985).

13 Minutes of the inter-ministry meeting on May 9, 1985, chaired by Mr. Gros (Lucas 1991, 38–39; Soulier 1992, 55–57).

14 "I pledge on my honour … to remain worthy of being a Blood Donor, to respect rules of morality, proper conduct and human solidarity … to answer any need for transfu-sion (whether entailing compensation or not)" (*Code du Donneur de Sang* 1951; my translation).

15 The use of biotechnologies, and especially advances in recombinant products, provided some relief from plasma supply problems. Simultaneously, advances in immunopurification procedures reduced risks of sensitization to circulating anticoagulants, a factor that had limited the effectiveness of treatments (Bugnard 2002).

References

Primary sources

1944. *Lettre de G. Lafontaine, président de la Mutuelle du Sang pour Lyon au maire de Lyon*, Archives Charles Mérieux, Transfusion Sanguine, 1943–1945.

1961. *Compte-rendu des travaux du colloque de Cognac, 14–15 décembre 1991, Fédération Française des Donneurs de Sang Bénévoles*, 1961–1994, Associations de donneurs, ADTS et Gamma TS, Ministère de la Santé, Direction Générale de la Santé, CAC 19960402/46.

1983. *Circulaire DGS 3B no. 569 relative à l'éventuelle transmission du sida par la transfusion sanguine*, June 20, 1983, non parue au JO, *Bulletin Officiel du ministère de la Santé Publique*.

1983. Informations UNAADSBPTT.

1989. Directive 89/381 du Conseil du 14 juin 1989, JO des Communautés européennes.

1991. *Compte-rendu de la réunion interministérielle tenue le 9 mai 1985 sous la présidence de M. Gros, M. Lucas*, "Transfusion sanguine et sida en 1985. Chronologie des faits et décisions pour ce qui concerne les hémophiles." Paris: IGAS, annexe 17.

1993. *La souffrance à distance: morale humanitaire, médias et politique*. Paris: Métailié.

1993. *Loi du 4 janvier 1993 relative à la sécurité en matière de transfusion sanguine et de médicament*, JO (January 5, 1993), article 2.

1993. *Résolution du Parlement européen du 14 septembre 1993 sur l'autosuffisance et la sécurité de l'approvisionnement dans la communauté européenne* (October 4, 1993), JO des Communautés, C 268.

1993. *Rapport de la Commission d'enquête sur l'état des connaissances scientifiques et les actions menées à l'égard de la transmission du sida*. Paris: Union Générale d'Éditions, collection 10/18.

2004. JO des Communautés (March 30, 2004), L 91.25.

2005. "Les transformations du service public de la transfusion sanguine" dans *Rapport de la Cour des Comptes pour l'année 2004*. Paris: Cour des comptes.

2007. "Du don au marché. Politiques du sang en France (années 1940–années 2000)." Habilitation dissertation. Paris: École des Hautes Études en Sciences Sociales.

2009. "Between Gift and Commodity: Blood Products in France." *Economic Sociology. The European Electronic Newsletter* 11(1): 24–28.

2011. *L'affaire du sang contaminé (1983–2003)*. Paris: Les Belles Lettres.

Secondary sources

Alchian, A. 1973. *Economics of Charity: Essays on the Comparative Economics and Ethics of Giving and Selling with Application to Blood*. London: Institute of Economic Affairs.

Anderson, L. and Snow, D.A. 1994. "L'industrie du plasma." *Actes de la recherche en sciences sociales* 104: 25–33.

Assemblée Générale. 1950 [1949]. *Le Donneur de Sang*, 1, séance du 20 novembre.

Assemblée Nationale. 1952. *Documents parlementaires*, séance du 14 mars.

Bastard, B. 2006. "Donner son sang: un droit individual ou l'exercice d'une responsabilité sociale? Débat sur la place du donneur dans la transfusion." *Transfusion clinique et biologique* 13: 215–255.

Bastin, N. 1978. "Les hémophiles et le réseau transfusionnel." *La Gazette de la transfusion* 15.

Bastin, N., Cresson, G., and Tyberghien, J. 1993. *Approche sociologique de la demande en réparation du préjudice thérapeutique: le cas du sida*. Lille: ANRS-Clersé.

Bastin-Vieillard, N. 1977. "L'Organisation transfusionnelle française. Une contribution à l'étude du système de santé." Ph.D. diss. Lille: Institut de préparation aux affaires et IAE.

Beck, U. 2001 [1986]. *La société du risque*. Paris: Aubier.

Boltanski, L. 1990. *L'amour et la justice comme compétences: trois essais de sociologie de l'action*. Paris: Métailié.

Borraz, O. 2008. *Les politiques du risque*. Paris: Presses de Sciences Po.

Bourdieu, P. 2000 [1972]. *Esquisse d'une théorie de la pratique*. Paris: Le Seuil.

Bugnard, S. 2002. "Sécurité virale des médicaments dérivés du sang au Laboratoire français du fractionnement et des biotechnologies." Ph.D. diss. Paris: University of Paris 5.

Cagnard, J.-P. 1983. "Réflexions sur le SIDA." *Le Donneur de Sang Bénévole* 429.

Caillé, A. 2005. *Don, intérêt et désintéressement: Bourdieu, Mauss, Platon et quelques autres*. Paris: La découverte.

Callon, M. 1998. "The Embeddedness of Economics Markets in Economics." In Callon, M. (ed.), *The Laws of the Markets*. Oxford: Blackwell.

Carricaburu, D. 2000. *L'Hémophilie au risque de la maladie: de la maladie individuelle à la contamination collective par le sida*. Paris: Anthropos.

Casteret, A-M. 1992. *L'affaire du sang*. Paris: La découverte.

Chateauraynaud, F. and Torny, D. 1999. *Les sombres précurseurs. Une sociologie pragmatique de l'alerte et du risque*. Paris: Editions de l'EHESS.

Chauveau, S. 2004. "Genèse de la sécurité sanitaire. Les produits pharmaceutiques en France aux XIXe et XXe siècles." *Revue d'histoire moderne et contemporaine* 51–52: 88–117.

Chauveau, S. 2007. *Du don au marché. Politiques du sang en France (années 1940–années 2000)*, mémoire de recherche inédit pour l'HDR. Paris: EHESS.

Chauveau, S. 2009. "Between Gift and Commodity: Blood Products in France." *Economic Sociology – The European Electronic Newsletter* 11(1): 24–28.

Chauveau, S. 2011. *L'affaire du sang contaminé (1983–2003)*. Paris: Les Belles Lettres.

Code du Donneur de Sang. 1951. *Le Donneur de Sang*.

Compte-rendu du Congrès National de la Fédération. 1954. *Le Donneur de Sang*.

Cooper, M.H. and Culyer, A.J. 1968. "The Price of Blood: An Economic Study of the Charitable and Commercial Principle." *Hobart Paper 41*. London: Institute of Economic Affairs.

Direction Générale de la Santé. 1983. *Procès-verbal de la CCTS, Séance du 9 juin 1983, Sécurité transfusionnelle (1956–1993), Ministère de la Santé*, 19960402/14.

Drake, A.W., Finkelstein, S.N., and Sapolsky, H.M. 1982. *The American Blood Supply*. Cambridge, MA: MIT Press.

Epstein, H. 2001. "AIDS: The Lesson of Uganda." *The New York Review of Books* 48(11): 18–23.

Fassin, D. 2009. "Les économies morales revisitées." *Annales HSS* 64–66: 1237–1266.

Fillion, E. 2009. *À l'épreuve du sang contaminé. Pour une sociologie des affaires médicales.* Paris: Éditions de l'EHESS.

Fontaine, P. 2002. "Blood, Politics and Social Science. Richard Titmuss and the Institute of Economic Affairs, 1957–1973." *Isis* 93: 401–434.

Genetet, B. 1983. "Le SIDA. Flash d'information à l'intention des donneurs et donneuses de sang." *Le Donneur de Sang Bénévole* 427.

Godbout, J. and Caillé, A. 1992. *L'esprit du don.* Paris: La découverte.

Godelier, M. 1997. *L'énigme du don.* Paris: Fayard.

Grémy, F. 2000. "Savoir, connaissance et communication en santé publique: réflexions à propos de l'affaire du sang contaminé." *Santé Publique* 12(1): 91–108 and 12(2): 229–244.

Hagen, P.J. 1982. *Blood, Gift or Merchandise: Towards an International Blood Policy.* New York: Alan R. Liss.

Healy, K. 2006. *Last Best Gift: Altruism and the Market for Human Blood and Organs.* Chicago, IL: University of Chicago Press.

Hermitte, M-A. 1996. *Le Sang et le droit: essai sur la transfusion sanguine.* Paris: Le Seuil.

JO des Communautés. 2004. L 91.25, March 30.

Leroux, A. 1980. *Exposé de A. Leroux, Séance officielle du samedi 3 mai 1980, XXIIe congrès de la FFDSB à Lisieux*, May 1, *Le Donneur de Sang Bénévole* 397.

Lestrade, D. and Pialoux, G. 2012. *SIDA 2.0. Regards croisés sur 30 ans de pandémie.* Paris: Fleuve Éditions.

Malet, J. 2004. "Donner son sang en France." Paris: CERPHI et EFS.

Marchetti, D. 2010. *Quand la santé devient médiatique. Les logiques de production de l'information dans la presse.* Grenoble: Presses Universitaires de Grenoble.

Marty, A. 1985. "Le respect du donneur." *Le Donneur de Sang Bénévole* 444: 1.

Mauss, M. 1950. "Essai sur le don. Forme et raison de l'échange dans les sociétés archaïques." *Sociologie et anthropologie.* Paris: Presses Universitaires de France, 143–279.

Ministère de la Santé, Direction Générale de la Santé. 1949. "Affaires générales et rapports sur la transfusion sanguine." *Notes d'Eugène Aujaleu sur le projet de loi sur l'utilisation du sang humain et de ses dérivés en vue de transfusion sanguine*, 1949–1989, CAC 19960402/1.

Moine, I. 1997. *Les choses hors-commerce: une approche de la personne humaine juridique.* Paris: LGDJ.

Morelle, A. 1996. *La Défaite de la santé publique.* Paris: Flammarion.

Nguyen, M., Mathez, D., Leibowitch, J., and Pinon, F. 1985. "Donneurs de sang volontaires de la région parisienne et anticorps anti-HTLV-III/LAV." *Gazette de la Transfusion* 37–38.

Noiville, C. 2003. *Du bon gouvernement des risques: le droit et la question du risque "acceptable."* Paris: Presses Universitaires de France.

Raoul-Duval, P. 1956. *Allocution du docteur Raoul-Duval à l'occasion du 50 000e diplôme de donneur. Le Donneur de Sang* 60.

Resnik, S. 1999. *Blood Saga. Hemophilia, AIDS and the Survival of a Community.* Berkeley: University of California Press.

Saleun J.-P. 1984a. "Impact pratique des instructions concernant le Sida." *Revue Française de Transfusion et Immuno-hématologie* 27(4): 513–520.

Saleun J.-P. 1984b. "Le SIDA à la manière de…" *Gazette de la transfusion* 33.

Scheper-Hughes, N. and Wacquant, L. (eds) 2002. *Commodifying Bodies.* London: Sage.

Setbon, M. 1993. *Pouvoirs contre sida. De la transfusion sanguine au dépistage: décisions et pratiques en France, Grande-Bretagne et Suède.* Paris: Le Seuil.

Soulier, J.-P. 1978. "Ressources actuelles pour les hémophiles." *L'Hémophile* 78.

Soulier, J.-P. 1983. "Le SIDA." *Revue française de Transfusion et d'Immuno-hématologie* 26(4): 437–445.

Soulier, J.-P. 1992. *Transfusion et sida. Le droit à la vérité.* Paris: Frison-Roche.

Sourdille, J. and Huriet, C. 1992. *La crise du système transfusionnel français. Rapport de la commission d'enquête du Sénat.* Paris: Economica.

Steiner, P. 2010. *La transplantation d'organes. Un commerce nouveau entre les êtres humains.* Paris: Gallimard.

Titmuss, R. 1971. *The Gift Relationship: From Human Blood to Social Policy.* London: Allen & Unwin.

Trambouze, M. 1957. *Allocution de M. Trambouze au IXe Congrès de la Fédération* (June). Pau: Le Donneur de Sang, 71.

Wailoo, K., Livingston, J., and Guarnaccia, P. (eds). 2006. *A Death Retold: Jesica Santillan, the Bungled Transplant and Paradoxes of Medical Citizenship.* Chapel Hill: University of North Carolina Press.

Waldby, C. and Mitchell, R. 2006. *Tissue Economies: Blood, Organs and Cell Lines in Late Capitalism.* Durham, NC: Duke University Press.

Part II

The institutional politics of donor recruitment

5 The marketing of blood donation in Canada

Organizational discourse, practice, and symbolic tension in a blood donation clinic

André Smith

Introduction

Finding effective ways to recruit blood donors is vitally important in the context of a rising demand for blood due to an aging population, strict donor deferral criteria, and the limited shelf life of blood products (Drackley *et al.* 2012; Riley *et al.* 2007). Researchers addressing this issue have overwhelmingly focused on the behavioural and psychological characteristics of donors in their efforts to determine what motivates some individuals and not others to donate (Crawford *et al.* 2008; Piliavin and Callero 1991; Reich *et al.* 2006; Shaz *et al.* 2009). Much less attention has been devoted to the influence of social contexts, although we know from epidemiological research that blood donation rates vary significantly by community; ethnic groups have different donation rates; and there is a relationship between age, gender, education, social class, occupation, religion, and blood donation (Alessandrini 2007; Zou *et al.* 2008). We know even less about the organizational factors that influence blood donation, including the role of blood collection agencies in leveraging social resources to recruit and retain donors.

In his comparative analysis of donor recruitment practices across three blood collection regimes in the European Union (state-run, Red Cross, and blood banks), however, Kieran Healy (2000) alludes to such factors' importance when he states that "blood can be seen not as something that individuals donate but as something that organizations collect" (71). Indeed, his investigation reveals that blood collection agencies produce different donor rates and donor bases depending on the social meanings they impart to blood donation during efforts to recruit donors. For example, in state-run systems, donor recruitment results in donor bases that are representative of their countries' social compositions, whereas the Red Cross attracts donors with religious affiliations and community service values. Healy (2006) contends that donors across all types of blood systems tend to view themselves as motivated by altruism because that is the message that blood collection agencies emphasize in their donor recruitment campaigns. Because Healy's research is epidemiological in nature, however, it does not provide a finer-grained understanding of the interplay between donors' motives and the activities of blood collection agencies. Many questions about this interplay persist, including those about the organizational dynamics involved in donor recruitment activities, how local recruitment efforts integrate with national policies and guidelines, and how the blood donation experience intersects with donor recruitment activities.

To advance understanding on this issue, research was undertaken of donor recruitment and blood collection activities at the Canadian Blood Services (CBS), the agency responsible for overseeing blood collection in Canada (with the exception of the province of Québec), in four communities with substantially different donation rates. This chapter specifically reports on a case study of one clinic in a community with substantially higher rates of donation. This case study seeks to illustrate how clinic practices, which are guided by national policies, professional standards, and regulations, also reflect unique local beliefs, ideologies, and organizational cultures (Geertz 1973; Lee 2000; Powell and DiMaggio 1991).

Theoretical approach

The blood donation clinic is conceptualized as an environment where employees construct and legitimate their activities in the context of shifting structural contingencies (Meyer and Rowan 1977), and where "social relations [are] deliberately created, with the explicit intention of continuously accomplishing some specific goals or purposes" (Stinchcombe 1965, 142). In this case study, the aim is to understand how employees operated under the numerous constraints impinging upon donor recruitment and blood collection, such as the varying demand for blood, the complex safety procedures involved in the collection and handling of blood, the changing characteristics of the donor base, and the restrictions associated with national policies and guidelines.

Central to the investigation is the concept of organizational culture, which is defined as:

> pattern[s] of basic assumptions – invented, discovered, or developed by a given group as it learns to cope with its problems of external adaptation and internal integration – that [have] worked well enough to be considered valid and, therefore, to be taught to new members as the correct way to perceive, think, and feel in relation to those problems.
>
> (Schein 1985, 9)

As a key aspect of institutions, organizational culture is reflected in members' beliefs, values, and rationalizations. It also serves as a powerful mechanism for coordinating actions and decisions, including those involving practices that address service recipients' needs (Alvesson 2002; Bowker 1982).

Also relevant to the analysis is Michel Foucault's view "that discourses constitute social phenomena, that they are practices, and operate as fields of fluid power/knowledge, where power and knowledge directly imply one another"

(Harding 1997, 137). This case study shows how the practices at the clinic drew from knowledge that intersected the fields of medicine (how blood can save a life), marketing (how to appeal to donors), and social psychology (how to enhance the donor experience). One signal feature of this knowledge is its involvement in constituting donors as subjects of interventions (in recruitment and blood collection, for example) and the comparison of donors against established norms (as in the terminology of "lapsed" donors and "repeat" donors).

In this theoretical context, this chapter identifies the practices employed by clinic employees to recruit donors and enhance donors' experiences. It also offers insights into clinic employees' tacit knowledge of donor motivation and how this knowledge informs the development of local strategies, as well as strategies that reflect national policies and guidelines set by the CBS.

Methods

This case study forms part of a larger research project that compares blood collection and donor recruitment in four cities with substantially different blood donation rates. In this chapter, the focus is on the activities of one donor clinic operating in a city surrounded by a large, dispersed catchment area. The clinic operates out of a permanent site but also runs a mobile clinic to serve its catchment area. At the time of the investigation, this clinic consistently reported blood donation rates that were higher than those of the other cities in the overall study sample.

The findings originate from a combination of ethnographic observations of donor recruitment and blood collection activities at the blood clinic along with in-depth interviews with 14 CBS employees (nurses, administrative personnel, and donor recruitment staff), eight repeat donors, two first-time donors, and two non-donors in ten organizations participating in Life Link, a donor recruitment program that supports organizations to educate employees about the benefits of blood donation. The interviews lasted between 30 minutes and one hour. Life Link interviews were conducted at participants' workplaces and the interviews with CBS employees were held at the clinic.

Observations were conducted of a range of donor recruitment activities in businesses and in not-for-profit and public sector organizations using rapid ethnography, a method for speeding up data collection without sacrificing complexity and depth of investigation (Baines and Cunningham 2011; Millen 2000). By following the same procedures as traditional ethnography (e.g., field notes, thick descriptions) but restricting observation lengths to shorter time periods, researchers were able to carefully document clinic activities while remaining unobtrusive. At the clinic, data were obtained from spending two two-hour periods (morning and afternoon) each day observing employees as they collected blood and interacted with donors. Further data were collected by shadowing the coordinator responsible for donor recruitment for periods of one to two hours over the same three days. All these ethnographic observations were recorded in field notes using a semi-structured observation guide.

All interviews were audio-recorded and transcribed verbatim, field notes were typed, and the data were entered into Atlas.ti, a software program for qualitative data analysis (Smit 2002). The transcripts were line-numbered and coded using the principles of thematic analysis. The documents were systematically scrutinized using an iterative process based on the procedures of grounded theory as interpreted by Juliet Corbin and Anselm Strauss (1990). In a first step, using open coding and the constant comparison method (Thorne 2000), the author and one research associate independently read the transcripts and field notes for important passages and keywords denoting a theme, and gradually clustered these themes into higher order categories based on recurrence and relevance. This iterative process of interpretation continued until the themes seemed repetitive or saturated (Patton 2001).

Qualitative methodology involves unavoidable compromises about reliability and generalizability in order to enhance interpretive validity (Morse and Mitcham 2002). To verify interpretive validity, "emic" and "etic" validity checks (Guba 1981; Harris 1976) were performed. The former involved returning to participants with a request that they review the meanings that were attributed to their statements and observations of their practices. Interpretive validity was assessed by determining the position and significance of each theme in relation to the objectives of the study. For the "etic" validity check, the study triangulates data from multiple sources and thus corroborates findings from different perspectives. Generalizability is not a criterion that applies in qualitative research because of the use of purposive sampling and naturalistic methods. Instead, internal validity was maintained by remaining vigilant for rival explanations over the course of data collection and analysis.

The following section provides an overview of the Canadian blood system and its regulatory history in an effort to contextualize the way clinic activities reflect: (1) locally situated conceptualizations of donors and their motivations, as well as broader discourses in the blood system; (2) strategies for diffusing ideas about blood donation and its importance within the community; and (3) tensions between local initiatives and national guidelines for donor recruitment and blood collection. The section concludes with a discussion of how donor recruitment and blood collection practices are rooted in local and specific circumstances, and how they at times emulate but also subvert national guidelines designed to standardize such practices as part of the CBS's corporate governance mandate.

The Canadian blood system

Canada's blood system developed from a partnership between the Canadian Red Cross (CRC) and Connaught Laboratories, a company that, in the 1940s, developed a process for manufacturing freeze-dried human serum for use during World War II (Picard 1998). As Richard Titmuss (1972) notes, issues of demand and supply, and debates about the ethics of commercializing blood, arose soon after blood became widely available for transfusion. Canada adopted a donor program that relied on voluntary donation; by the 1950s, this program had expanded to supply blood to hospitals across the country. Soon afterwards, the federal and provincial governments granted the CRC an exclusive mandate to be the sole operator of Canada's blood system (Krever 1997, 43–46). By the late 1980s, the CRC was operating 17 blood centres and several mobile clinics supporting blood drives in rural areas, community centres, churches, schools, legion halls, and factories (Krever 1997).

This situation changed drastically when blood supplies in Canada and around the world were contaminated with the human immunodeficiency virus (HIV); approximately 1,100 Canadians became infected with the HIV through contaminated blood transfusions (Canadian Hemophilia Society 2010). The contamination of the Canadian blood supply seriously undermined public trust in the Canadian blood system and resulted in a dramatic decrease in rates of blood donation, thus raising concern about the sufficiency of the blood supply (Gilmore and Sommerville 1999).

In an effort to identify factors that had resulted in the blood supply's contamination, the federal government established the Royal Commission of Inquiry on the Blood System in Canada, led by Justice Horace Krever. After reviewing all Canadian blood system activities that took place between 1993 and 1997, Krever singled out the "ineffective and half-hearted" (Krever 1997, 293–294) risk-reduction strategies of the CRC and found that the organization had not responded to the HIV crisis quickly enough by excluding populations that posed a contamination risk to the blood supply, such as men who have sex with men (Weinberg *et al.* 2002).

On November 26, 1997, Krever tabled a report in the House of Commons that contained several recommendations for overhauling the collection, processing, and management of blood in Canada. Underlying these recommendations was a desire to restore Canadians' trust in their blood system in order to improve the blood system's ability to recruit and retain new donors. Krever recommended that the Canadian blood system adopt a precautionary approach to risk decision-making, addressing a key criticism of the CRC: namely, that it could have prevented many cases of infection had it deferred high-risk donors on a precautionary basis instead of waiting for scientific confirmation of the HIV threat. This recommendation stipulated that consideration be given to actual as well as theoretical risks in the event that "a potential disease-causing agent is or may be blood borne, even when there is no evidence that recipients have been affected" (Krever 1997, 1049). Krever (1997, 1047) also proposed several other guiding principles: that blood should remain a public resource; that donors of blood and plasma should not be paid for their donations, except in rare circumstances; that whole blood, plasma, and platelets must be collected in sufficient quantities in Canada to meet domestic needs for blood components and blood products; and that Canadians should have free and universal access to blood components and blood products.

On September 10, 1996, federal, provincial, and territorial health ministers agreed to create a new national blood authority that would operate independently from government and be responsible for managing all aspects of a voluntary blood system. In 1998, two new not-for-profit organizations, Canadian Blood Services (CBS) and Héma-Québec (HQ), took over responsibility for managing the blood system from the CRC: CBS took over responsibility for English Canada's blood supply, whereas HQ was incorporated as a non-profit organization on March 27, 1998, with responsibility for the province of Québec's blood supply. Although these organizations differ on some of their policies and procedures, they are both regulated by Health Canada and must meet the same national regulatory standards (Wilson *et al.* 2003, 2004).

Under the Food and Drugs Act (1985), Health Canada regulates both CBS and HQ through its Biologic and Genetic Therapies Directorate, which considers blood and blood products to be pharmaceutical products (Health Canada 2006). This agency is responsible for disease surveillance, including the surveillance of known blood-borne pathogens (e.g., HIV) and emergent pathogens that could threaten the blood system's safety. It issues binding recommendations to the blood operators about the collecting, processing, testing, and transfusing of blood and the exclusion of pathogens from the blood supply (Health Canada 2006). The blood operators are thus bound by federal regulations: they may exceed existing safety standards, but new safety measures must be approved by Health Canada (Wilson *et al.* 2004a). As was the case with the CRC, the CBS and HQ collect blood from volunteer donors, believing such donors to be inherently safer than paid donors, who may have "a financial motive for giving blood even if they were not healthy enough to do so" (Krever 1997, 211).

Overall, as Violaine Roussel (2003, 124) remarks, the period surrounding the tainted blood scandal marked the emergence of a blood safety culture in which public decision-makers were increasingly being denounced and held criminally responsible for their lack of foresight in managing new risks to public health. Roussel suggests that the public outcry and scrutiny associated with the tainted blood scandal have made it necessary for blood experts to look for more thorough and efficient ways of anticipating and responding to emergent risks in order to retain their legitimacy and, ultimately, to rebuild public trust. Earlier in this book (Chapter 4), Sophie Chauveau argues, in a parallel vein, that the tainted blood scandal in France transformed that country's blood system into an increasingly bureaucratized organization in which blood products were subjected to a wide range of health, industry, and commercial regulations. The author concludes that the tainted blood scandal produced an intriguing juxtaposition of a moral economy of voluntarily, non-remunerated donation and a market economy driven by the pharmaceutical production of commercial blood products. While both Roussel and Chauveau focus on the circumstances surrounding the tainted blood scandal in France, their comments apply equally to the Canadian situation, particularly in light of the criminal charges laid against the former head of the CRC, other health officials, and an American pharmaceutical company (Canadian Broadcasting Corporation 2006). In addition, the designation of blood and blood products as pharmaceutical products under the

Food and Drugs Act (1985) has allowed the Canadian federal government to play a dominant role in overseeing the safety of the blood supply (Smith *et al.* 2011).

The implementation of strict regulatory regimes also paradoxically created new challenges in terms of ensuring the sufficiency of blood supplies. Stringent deferral criteria led to the exclusion of an increasingly large segment of the population from donating, while the inconvenience and invasiveness of donor screening procedures undermined the donor experience, thus making first-time donors less likely to return (Halperin *et al.* 1998; Hillgrove *et al.* 2012). Under these circumstances, donor recruitment acquired heightened importance as blood agencies sought to avoid a new risk to the blood supply: insufficiency. The importance of this issue for CBS is evidenced by the fact that in each annual report, sections on blood safety discuss the safety of blood and blood products, the technologies available to test known and emerging pathogens, and "Security of Supply" (with a focus on donor recruitment and blood sufficiency). For example, CBS's 2003–2004 *Report to Canadians* states that "ensuring a secure supply is a constant challenge for Canadian Blood Services. It … requires increasingly sophisticated programs to recruit and continually attract committed blood donors" (27).

To address these issues of safety and sufficiency, the CBS operates in accordance with a corporate structure: decision-making is centralized within a publicly accountable administrative structure whereby its CEO is the focal point of accountability, reporting to a "13-member board of directors whose members have been appointed to represent various regions and constituencies" and which is "responsible to the members of the corporation, who are the provincial/territorial ministers" (Rock 2000, 35). The CBS also has several vice-presidents who oversee finance, regulatory and quality assurance, operations, and medical and human resources. It has also equipped itself with a substantial marketing department, which has adopted the language and techniques of social marketing in strategizing to improve donor recruitment and the donor experience (Carter *et al.* 2011; Healy 2006). Under this administrative structure, the CBS oversees the operation of blood centres that operate in the nine provinces, excluding Québec, and the three territories. Each provincial centre is managed by a director who reports to the national office and oversees blood collection that is carried out in fixed and mobile clinics.

Donor recruitment and symbolic tension

A central feature of donor recruitment at the time of the investigation was the Life Link program, a CBS-wide initiative aiming to encourage employees from participating organizations to consider donating blood. As part of this program, the clinic employed a full-time Community Development Coordinator (CDC) whose primary responsibility was to visit businesses and not-for-profit and public sector agencies to generate support for blood donation. Donor recruitment in this case involved selecting local employees (typically, experienced blood donors) and tasking them to motivate non-donating employees to become first-time donors.

The CDC viewed his role more broadly as that of an "ambassador" of blood donation in his community. He emphasized the importance of participating in parades and fundraising events to raise the profile of the clinic, as indicated by this comment:

> You don't necessarily have to have a media personality with the CDCs but get involved in your community. Get out there, plant trees, walk grandma across the street, help be a cub leader, be scout leader, be a Girl Guide leader, volunteer as a chairperson of something. Because the more your face is in there, the face then is associated like mine is to Canadian Blood Services. They don't look at me, they see a community guy who represents Canadian Blood Services. They say: "You're the blood guy!"

The CDC noted the challenges posed by the negative reputation that blood donation still retained in some circles. Specifically, he pointed to the reluctance of some charitable organizations to lend their support to blood drives:

> They don't, they don't come forward. I can see why, 'cos I was here when the blood program was on the front page every day for killing people with tainted products. So, if I was another organization, would I want to partner up with a group that has to deal with West Nile Virus, Mad Cow, SARS? That's just what we have right at this moment. Probably not. [They'd say:] "I've enough headaches, thanks."

The clinic also used donor recruitment strategies that were imbued with a strong business and marketing ethos. Although the CBS employees described blood collection as distinct from any sort of business, they nonetheless often relied on the language of business in describing their involvement in donor recruitment. For example, they described recruitment initiatives using terms such as "project marketing" and referred to the CBS as a "manufacturing plant." As the CDC put it:

> It's a unique organization. They tell us to run it like a manufactured business but yet we're dealing with people's lives. You know? All that said and done, I understand both worlds. I understand the business world, I also understand the touchy feely warm customer service and we just haven't as a nation reached that medium. And I would like to think that in my community we have. I do some questionable practices, but nothing that I feel is offensive to anyone or any group.

One administrator echoed this comment by reflecting on the paradox which Chauveau described in the previous chapter: having to care for donors as human beings while at the same time working in an environment where the meaning of blood is reduced to that of a healthcare product.

We take a product from a human being and we process it and we ship it off. So really in basic terms, we are like a manufacturing plant. We try to be as understanding and as compassionate and empathetic as we possibly can because we know what we're taking from someone should be the most pleasant experience for them to go through. I mean, it's not like it's a completely painless procedure. So we recognize that, but at the end of the day we're a manufacturing plant.

Another administrator felt that donor recruitment practices had been heavily influenced by the corporate shift of the CBS in managing the blood system. He said, "A lot of the people at head office worked in the corporate world as well and while the principles of marketing are the same in the corporate world versus the non-profit world, we use slightly different language." One nurse nostalgically commented, "I think with the Red Cross, there was more that sense of it being a humanitarian organization."

The discourse of business and marketing was reflected in several practices the clinic used to leverage blood donation from the organizations that participated in the Life Link program. For example, the clinic sought to foster friendly competition among organizations through a reward system: organizations whose employees donated the most blood were publicly recognized in a newsletter and with a plaque handed out in an informal ceremony hosted at the clinic. Through personal connections, the CDC also arranged for the winning organizations to be acknowledged in the local community newspaper. This unique practice was justified on the basis that it gave the winning organizations welcomed publicity, instilled pride in their employees, and increased staff morale. This donor's comment from a participating business validates this view:

I think it's a good opportunity because of corporate image. Especially for us, but for any corporation, I don't think anyone can negatively put a spin on it no matter what they do. So I would hope it would spread to other communities. I'm not quite sure how it could spread but I would say any corporation, if they're looking for some solid corporate citizen-type stuff, it's a really great opportunity.

The clinic employees viewed this strategy as an effective means of generating first-time donors whom they felt were more likely to become repeat donors at a later stage because of their commitment to their workplace.

The discourse of marketing is also reflected in the following comment from one CDC about how to manage media interviews during blood drives:

You've got a short period of time to make your case, and all it takes is that person. The attention span of a radio listener in a car is very short and then they always catch the first beginning, the middle, forget it, and the last ten seconds. And that's where you really gotta sell it. Really gotta sell it.

Blood collection employees also described donor recruitment as an aspect of their engagement with the community and felt they played an active role in enhancing the visibility of the clinic among local businesses. As one employee remarked, "We all intertwine. We're all focused on the same thing, and that is the need for blood ... and I don't even like that: for the need for blood. How about we change it: for getting blood!" Some of the strategies they employed were low key but apparently effective. For example, since nearly all the employees shopped in the catchment area of the blood clinic, they reminded other customers about the importance of blood donation whenever they were out running errands. In one example, a nurse spoke about how she and several of her co-workers who had purchased a new car at a dealership lobbied its employees to donate blood in appreciation of their patronage. In this practice, employees capitalized on their reputation as valued consumers and respected members of their community (e.g., many attended churches, volunteered in various charitable organizations, and coached little league clubs). As one clinic nurse explains:

> Well again we're in a unique position, because we are all from this community, have all been here for years and we all have connections to the community as does our community development coordinator. And so that brings local knowledge and connection to the people that walk in the door.

Employees considered these informal recruitment practices to be one sign of their commitment to the cause of blood donation. But they also spoke of their clinic as a type of business and of blood donation as the service they promoted.

Managing the donor experience

Another prominent theme pertained to how clinic employees viewed the donor experience as an extension of donor recruitment, particularly when it came to first-time donors. Employees' aim was to produce a "satisfied customer," a process that involved engineering the clinic as a social space and engaging donors in a personalized manner. Clinic employees adopted several strategies, as reflected in this comment from one clinic nurse:

> I think a lot of us make the rewards come out of the contact with the donors. That's the part where we remember people's names, we remember their birthdays, you know, have a chat with them when they come in, so they're, they're almost like family members when they come back.

Personalizing the donor experience also involved engaging volunteers from the community, many of whom became familiar faces to the repeat donors and to the occasional first-time donor who recognized a volunteer from a previous encounter in the community. Here is how the CDC described the value of volunteers:

That's right, especially people who recognize other people, because a lot of times, the volunteers are our spokespeople and our flag people and, I don't know if you witnessed this … that today at K–, but you saw them say, "Oh, Hi Stanley! Hi Ethel! Hi Bev! Hi Margaret! Hi!" And they talk to the donors.

Blood collection employees also identified several barriers to the donor experience, including the use of deferral criteria to identify and exclude individuals posing a contamination risk to the blood supply. While employees saw such deferrals as an effective and necessary safety measure, they nonetheless expressed concern about the impact of the deferral process on donor satisfaction, particularly when newly introduced criteria result in the deferral of long-term donors who derived a sense of self-worth from donating blood. As the CDC explained, "There are so many people that are absolutely terrified, knowing that they have many sexual partners in their past, or may have done something way in the past…. We're talking people in their forties, late thirties, fifties, even sixties, that are just terrified of knowing." Using the language of marketing, the CDC also described the consequences of how deferrals were handled by CBS in terms of the negative publicity this engendered for the blood clinic:

> [People] are getting harassed everywhere to come and donate blood, and when they do come out and donate blood, then they're deferred or for whatever reason, and they're handled very, very roughly. They walk out, and then they take that negative message, and spill it out of their mouth, all over the world. If you ease them down with good customer service, and good customer care, they're less likely to spill out anything negative. In actual fact, they won't even talk about their deferral experience at all.

Nurses also identified the use of complex medical procedures to collect blood (e.g., vena-puncture, labelling blood bags) as another potential barrier to "customer satisfaction." Although these procedures were an unavoidable aspect of their practice, nurses felt that such procedures' increased complexity distracted them from their ability to relate to and interact with donors. As one nurse noted, "There's so much regulation…. It's just so highly regulated, but that is a challenge getting all that in order, and understood." Another nurse commented, "the donors and the volunteers, they go, 'I don't want any part of that…. It's like going into a hospital.' " The CDC also expressed concerns about the impact of these procedures on the donor experience:

> I mean, we've removed ourselves to be so sterile, because safety is such an issue, which it is! But it shouldn't be so overpowering of an issue that we remove ourselves, or disconnect from the general community, or the general public, so the public feels like, "Well, hold on…" Again that goes back to that hierarchy of Ottawa looking down upon you, you know, and I mean, we

can't make the clinics, or the environment, or the staff too sterile. We still need that touchy feely ... that sense of humor, that sense of realness, a sense of same-level communication.

Clinic staff also implemented several unique initiatives to improve the donor experience, including exhibiting art by local artists that became the focal point of animated discussions and holding spontaneous games of *Trivial Pursuit*.

Resistance to corporate governance

Clinic employees expressed significant frustration with what they saw as a disconnection between local donor recruitment initiatives and the policies and guidelines imposed on them by the CBS's head office in Ottawa. This disconnection is reflected in this comment from an administrator: "We have national campaigns that are being layered on, which in some cases are more of a pain in the neck than anything else." These campaigns were often centred on televised advertisements, which several employees critiqued as discouraging people from donating, as suggested by this comment from a nurse:

They have all the commercials you see on TV. Where they have that poor person "by my baby's first birthday I will be having leukemia" and those commercials make me mad. I don't like those commercials. They are "guilting" me into giving blood. I said those are depressing, they guilt me, and it puts my back up and I'm just like "who the hell are you to tell me that?" I say, I would respond myself and I know other people would too. [But] people aren't stupid. Give them some facts out there of reality, you know? Because when I see this "it's in you to give" and "I'm gonna have leukemia and I have to go through all this and if the blood's not there," well, the first thing that pops in my head is "what? I'm never gonna have leukemia and this is never gonna happen to me" you know.

Clinic employees' frustration about the centralized management of donor recruitment also appeared evident in their discussion of a recently cancelled program targeting first-time donors. This initiative had involved giving every new donor a "first-time donor kit," which employees felt helped these donors entice other people to give blood. As one CDC described it:

The volunteers were saying how positive the response was about that, and the first-timers were taking that information back and putting it on their fridge, or wearing that pin, and then becoming an advocate of ours. And not only coming back and turning that first-timer and having a positive experience to coming back to be potentially a third- or fourth-time donor throughout the year, but also the fact that they would tell their friends, "Hey come on and donate blood. Look what you get."

After CBS discontinued this program, new donors were only giving a pin and a "thanks," which the CDC saw as reducing not only the incentive to donate, but also the incentive to act as an advocate on behalf of the CBS. He further commented:

> Yeah, they decided to remove that after two years of great success. The volunteers were very disappointed, and so were the donors. Now, we give you a pin, one pin. Yeah, yeah, one pin. No letter, no dispenser, no rah-rah, no little plastic bag, nothing.

Clinic employees had come to conceptualize this program as a mechanism for reaching out to new donors and its cancellation as exemplifying head office's ineptitude and lack of foresight. As one employee remarked, "it should be a national, really sexy program, that's … that's um, bring a friend and … and a partnership … uh, call it … there's lots of names for it."

Several clinic employees felt alienated by what they perceived to be unnecessary interference by head office in reprimanding local initiatives they saw as successful but that in some way contravened national guidelines – only to reintroduce them later as national initiatives. Here is how the CDC conveyed his sense of alienation:

> The big giant head interferes way too much. They're learning their lesson now … and it's finally starting to come around, and starting to realize that they have spoiled years of wonderful marketing ideas across this great country.

He added that such interference over time undermined the morale of clinic employees, impacting their willingness to engage fully with the task of recruiting donors and enhancing the donor experience:

> The staff, they're tired of being burnt by head office. Because, the thing is, it's one thing to be frustrated about the big giant head … the big giant head always frustrated with you. But then to add on the workload, more and more of a workload, and then with all that negative stress on you, and then compounded by not being rewarded.

Discussion and conclusion

This investigation is inspired by Healy's (2000, 2006) work, which compares the donor recruitment practices of state-run systems and those of Red Cross blood systems in the European Union. Healy found that state-run systems attract diversified donor bases that tend to represent the overall demographic composition of their countries; by contrast, Red Cross systems are more likely to attract donors with religious affiliations and strong community service values. Healy's later research on the market and non-market exchanges of whole blood, plasma, and organs further draws attention to the organizational dynamics that generate altruistic donors. Healy problematizes altruism as an organizational construct rather than as an inherent personality characteristic. He argues that the act of donating blood is thus "structured, promoted, and made logistically possible by organizations and institutions with a strong interest in producing it" (Healy 2004, 387).

In the wake of Healy's arguments, this case study problematizes the organizational dynamics of blood donation in one community where CBS operates a combination of a permanent and a mobile clinic. The focus is on how clinic employees constructed blood donation at the intersection of two sets of contingencies. On the one hand, there were the contingencies that arose from the need to constantly recruit new donors in order to maintain the blood supply and meet local quotas for donation rates; on the other hand, clinic employees operated in the context of centralized policies and guidelines that restricted the type of donor recruitment strategies they could employ in their community. Despite these limitations, clinic employees' unique knowledge of their community permitted them to develop donor recruitment strategies that uniquely blended marketing tactics with efforts to promote blood donation as an altruistic behaviour.

Blood collection employees also employed a marketing narrative in describing their efforts to enhance the donor experience, invoking the importance of personalizing contact with donors, "demedicalizing" the donor experience, and equally valuing first-time and repeat donors. Several studies validate how strengthening the positive aspects of blood donation can lead to an increase in the rate of repeat donors (e.g., Devine *et al.* 2007; Masser *et al.* 2008; Ringwald *et al.* 2010). As Dana Devine and colleagues (2007) remark, the experience of blood donation has been undermined by the use of "guilt messages to recruit donors and poorly executed aspects of the donation experience such as excessive wait times, poor needle insertion, insufficient communication and lack of appreciation throughout the donation experience" (254).

This chapter describes how the new regulatory arrangements of blood systems have transformed the "gift of life" into a scarce commodity that constantly raises concerns over safety and supply. In this context, donor recruitment has acquired a heightened importance, which has arguably resulted in the commodification of donors through an expanded use of social marketing technologies. As Margaret Lock (2002) remarks, "all forms of commodification involve a complex interaction of temporal, cultural, social, and political factors" (46). The findings underline the interplay of these technologies in the context of a clinic with a high donor rate and unique donor recruitment practices. This process unfolded within localized systems of meaning (Appadurai 1986) that accommodated but also adapted national policies and guidelines. Clinic employees thus enacted a discourse that represented donors as subjects to be appealed to and ultimately manipulated into donating their blood, but paradoxically, they did so in a way that seemed to reflect genuine engagement and concern. They also viewed what they did as unique and different from other clinics' work, a perception that speaks to their knowledge as "specific and local, grounded in the exigencies of a particular set of constraints and possibilities" (Rhodes 1991, 174). As Lorna A.

Rhodes (1991) notes, this kind of knowledge represents what Foucault (1980) calls "subjugated knowledge." Rooted in the local circumstances of the clinic, this knowledge permitted the strategic use of practices in a manner that suggested the existence of resistance to power, "for power inevitably creates and works through resistance" (Lupton 1997, 102).

Overall, the practices of blood clinic employees were shaped by specific organizational dynamics and local belief systems about how best to recruit blood donors and enhance their donation experience. These practices also evolved in the context of an ever-growing demand for blood and enormous social pressures to ensure its safety and sufficiency. The success of this particular clinic in generating much higher donor rates than comparable clinics richly suggests the value and efficiencies of situated knowledge and practices in meeting the challenges of blood sufficiency.

Acknowledgments

This study was made possible by a grant from the Bayer Canada-Canadian Blood Services-Héma Québec, Canadian Institutes for Health Research Partnership Fund.

References

Alessandrini, M. 2007. "Community Volunteerism and Blood Donation: Altruism as a Lifestyle Choice." *Transfusion Medicine Reviews* 21: 307–316.

Alvesson, M. 2002. *Understanding Organizational Culture*. Thousand Oaks, CA: Sage.

Appadurai, A. 1986. "Introduction: Commodities and the Politics of Value." In *The Social Life of Things: Commodities in Cultural Perspective*, edited by A. Appadurai, 3–63. Cambridge: Cambridge University Press.

Baines, D. and Cunningham, I. 2011. "Using Comparative Perspective Rapid Ethnography in International Case Studies: Strengths and Challenges." *Qualitative Social Work* 12: 73 88.

Bowker, L.E. 1982. *Humanizing Institutions for the Aged*. Lexington, MA: Lexington Books.

Canadian Blood Services. 2005. A Report to Canadians, 2004/2005. www.bloodservices.ca/centreapps/Internet/UW_V502_MainEngine.nsf/9749ca80b75a038585256aa20060d703/aaf1aa83a2ebfeb685256f31006c968f?OpenDocument (last accessed December 16, 2014).

Canadian Broadcasting Corporation. "Tainted-blood Trial Will Go Ahead: Crown." February 21, 2006. www.cbc.ca/canada/story/2006/02/21/tainted-blood060221.html (last accessed December 7, 2013).

Canadian Hemophilia Society. 2010. "Case of Freeman vs. CBS & Attorney-General of Canada Ends: Decision Expected in Summer." www.hemophilia.ca/files/Freeman%2002%20-%20EN.pdf (last accessed December 16, 2014).

Carter, M.C., Wilson, J., Redpath, G.S., Hayes, P., and Mitchell, C. 2011. "Donor Recruitment in the 21st Century: Challenges and Lessons Learned in the First Decade." *Transfusion and Apheresis Science* 45: 31–43.

Corbin, J. and Strauss, A. 1990. "Grounded Theory Research: Procedures, Canons, and Evaluative Criteria." *Qualitative Sociology* 13: 3–21.

Crawford, S.O., Reich, N.G., An, M.W., Brookmeyer, R., Louis T.A., Nelson, K.E., Notari E.P., Trouern-Trend, J., and Zou, S. 2008. "Regional and Temporal Variation in American Red Cross Blood Donations, 1995 to 2005." *Transfusion* 48: 1576–1583.

Devine, D.V., Goldman, M., Englefriet, P., Reesink, H., Heatherington, C., Hall, S., Steed, A., Harding, S., Westman, P., Gogarty, J., Katz, L.M., and Bryant, M. 2007. "International Forum: Donor Recruitment Research." *Vox Sanguinius* 93: 250–259.

Drackley, A., Newbold, K.B., Paez, A., and Heddle, N. 2012. "Forecasting Ontario's Blood Supply and Demand." *Transfusion* 52: 366–374.

Food and Drugs Act (R.S. 1985, c. F-27).

Foucault, M. 1980. "Power-Knowledge: Selected Interviews and Other Writings, 1972–1977" (translated by Gordon, C., Marshall, L., Mepham, J., and Soper, K.), edited by Gordon, C. Hassocks: Harvester Press.

Geertz, C. 1973. *Interpretation of Cultures*. New York: Basic Books.

Gilmore, N. and Sommerville, M. 1999. "From Trust to Tragedy: HIV/AIDS and the Canadian Blood System." In *Blood Feuds: AIDS, Blood, and the Politics of Medical Disaster*, edited by Feldman, E., 128–159. Oxford: Oxford University Press.

Guba, E.G. 1981. "Criteria for Assessing the Trustworthiness of Naturalistic Inquiries." *Educational Communications and Technology Journal* 29(2): 75–91.

Halperin, D., Baetens, J., and Newman, B. 1998. "The Effect of Short-term, Temporary Deferral on Future Blood Donations." *Transfusion* 38: 181–183.

Harding, J. 1997. "Bodies at Risk: Sex, Surveillance and Hormone Replacement Therapy." In *Foucault, Health and Medicine*, edited by Petersen, A. and Bunton, R., 134–150. London: Routledge.

Harris, M. 1976. "History and Significance of the Emic/Etic Distinction." *Annual Review of Anthropology* 5: 329–350.

Healy, K. 2000. "Embedded Altruism: Blood Collection Regimes and the European Union's Donor Population." *American Journal of Sociology* 105: 1633–1657.

Healy, K. 2004. "Altruism as an Organizational Problem: The Case of Organ Procurement." *American Sociological Review* 69: 387–404.

Healy, K. 2006. *Last Best Gifts: Altruism and The Market for Human Blood And Organs*. Chicago, IL: University of Chicago Press.

Hillgrove, T.L., Doherty, K.V., and Moore, V.M. 2012. "Understanding Non-return After a Temporary Deferral From Giving Blood: A Qualitative Study." *BMC Public Health* 12: 1063. doi:10.1186/1471-2458-12-1063. www.biomedcentral.com/1471-2458/12/1063 (last accessed December 8, 2013).

Krever, H. 1997. *Commission of Inquiry On The Blood System In Canada*, Volumes 1, 2, and 3. Ottawa: Canadian Government Publishing.

Kriebel, D. and Tickner, J. 2001. "Reenergizing Public Health through Precaution." *American Journal of Public Health* 91(9): 1351–1355.

Lee, O. 2000. "The Constitution of Meaning: On the Practical Conditions of Social Understanding." *Current Perspectives in Sociological Theory* 20: 27–64.

Lock, M. 2002. *Twice Dead*. Berkeley: University of California Press.

Lupton, D. 1997. "Foucault and The Medicalisation Critique." In *Foucault: Health and Medicine*, edited by Petersen, A. and Bunton, R., 94–112. London: Routledge.

Masser, B.M., White, K.M., Hyde, M.K., Terry, D.J., and Robinson, N.G. 2008. "Predicting Blood Donation Intentions and Behavior among Australian Blood Donors: Testing an Extended Theory of Planned Behavior Model." *Transfusion* 49: 320–329.

Meyer, J.W. and Rowan, B. 1977. "Institutionalized Organizations: Formal Structure as Myth and Ceremony." *American Journal of Sociology* 83: 340–363.

Millen, D. 2000. "Rapid Ethnography: Time Deepening Strategies for HCI Field Research." portal.acm.org/citation.cfm?id¼347763, 2000 (last accessed December 8, 2013).

Morse, J.M. and Mitcham, C. 2002. "Exploring Qualitatively-Derived Concepts: Inductive-Deductive Pitfalls." *International Journal of Qualitative Methods* 1(4): Article 3. www.ualberta.ca/~ijqm (last accessed December 8, 2013).

Patton, M.Q. 2001. *Qualitative Research and Evaluation Methods.* Thousand Oaks, CA: Sage.

Picard, A. 1998. *The Gift of Death: Confronting Canada's Tainted Blood Tragedy.* Toronto: Harper Perennial.

Piliavin, J.A. and Callero, P.L. 1991. *Giving Blood: The Development of an Altruistic Identity.* Baltimore, MD: Johns Hopkins University Press.

Powell, W.W. and DiMaggio, P.J. 1991. *The New Institutionalism in Organizational Analysis.* Chicago, IL: The University of Chicago Press.

Reich, P., Roberts, P., Laabs, N., Chinn, A., McEvoy, P., Hirschler, N., and Murphy, E.L. 2006. "A Randomized Trial of Blood Donor Recruitment Strategies." *Transfusion* 46: 1090–1096.

Rhodes, L.A. 1991. *Emptying Beds: The Work of an Emergency Psychiatric Unit.* Berkeley: University of California Press.

Riley, W., Schwei, M., and McCullough, J. 2007. "The United States' Potential Blood Donor Pool: Estimating the Prevalence of Donor-exclusion Factors on the Pool of Potential Donors." *Transfusion* 47: 1180–1188.

Ringwald, J., Zimmermann, R., and Eckstein, R. 2010. "Keys to Open the Door for Blood Donors to Return." *Transfusion Medicine Reviews* 24(4): 295–304.

Rock, G. 2000. "Changes in the Canadian Blood System: The Krever Inquiry, Canadian Blood Services and Héma-Québec." *Transfusion Science* 22(1): 29–37.

Roussel, V. 2003. "New Moralities of Risk and Political Responsibility." In *Risk and Morality,* edited by Ericson, R.V. and Doyle, A., 117–144. Toronto: University of Toronto Press.

Schein, E.H. 1985. *Organizational Culture and Leadership.* San Francisco, CA: Jossey-Bass.

Shaz, B.H., Demmons, D.G., Hillyer, K.L., Jones, R.E., and Hillyer, C.D. 2009. "Racial Differences in Motivators and Barriers to Blood Donation among Blood Donors." *Archives of Pathology and Laboratory Medicine* 133: 1444–1447.

Smit, B. 2002. "Atlas.ti for Qualitative Data Analysis." *Perspective in Education* 20: 65–76.

Smith, A., Fiddler, J., Walby, K., and Hier, S. 2011. "Blood Donation and Institutional Trust: Risk, Policy Rhetoric, and the Men Who Have Sex with Men Lifetime Deferral Policy in Canada." *Canadian Review of Sociology* 48(4): 369–389.

Stinchcombe, A.L. 1965. "Social Structure and Organizations." In *Handbook of Organizations,* edited by March, J.G., 142–193. Chicago, IL: Rand McNally & Company.

Thorne, S. 2000. "Data Analysis in Qualitative Research." *Evidence Based Nursing* 3: 68–70.

Titmuss, R.M. 1972. *The Gift Relationship: From Human Blood to Social Policy.* New York: Vintage Books.

Weinberg, P.D., Hounshell, J., Sherman, L.A., Godwin, J., Ali, S., Tomori, C., and Bennett, C.L. 2002. "Legal, Financial, and Public Health Consequences of HIV Contamination of Blood and Blood Products in the 1980s and 1990s." *Annals of Internal Medicine* 136(4): 312–319.

Wilson, K., Wilson, M., Hébert, P., and Graham, I. 2003. "The Application of the Precautionary Principle to the Blood System: The Canadian Blood System's CJD Donor Deferral Policy." *Transfusion Medicine Reviews* 17: 89–94.

Wilson, K., McCrea-Logie, J., and Lazar, H. 2004. "Understanding the Impact of Intergovernmental Relations on Public Health: Lessons from Reform Initiatives in the Blood System and Health Surveillance." *Canadian Public Policy* 30(2):177–194.

Zou, S., Musavi, F., Notari, E.P., Rios, J.A., Trouern-Trend, J., and Fang, C.T. 2008. "Donor Deferral and Resulting Donor Loss at the American Red Cross Blood Services, 2001 Through 2006." *Transfusion* 48: 2531–2539.

6 The influence of blood collection organizations on blood donation motivations and practices in Québec, Canada

Johanne Charbonneau and Anne Quéniart

Introduction

A long-term blood supply can only be guaranteed on the condition that new donors are continually being generated from within the population. There have been numerous studies in the field of behavioural psychology in recent decades to determine the psychosocial factors that prompt individuals to develop a blood donation practice and maintain it over the long term (Giles and Cairns 1995; Ferguson 1996; Armitage and Conner 2001; Misje *et al.* 2005; Godin *et al.* 2007; France *et al.* 2007; Sojka and Sojka 2008; Lemmens *et al.* 2009; Veldhuizen *et al.* 2011; Bednall and Bove, 2011; Ferguson *et al.* 2012; Masser *et al.* 2012). However, although these studies may have made reference to the potential influence of the social context, researchers have not studied it directly. Instead, such influence has always been perceived through the mediation of individual cognition. According to Healy (2006), one must go beyond psychosocial analyses of individual motivations to gain a better understanding of the cultural and institutional factors that shape blood donation practices. This view of the importance of considering blood donation from a more social standpoint is shared by Piliavin and Callero (1991, 179):

> To understand the wide-ranging power a social structure can have on blood donation, we must first recognize that blood donation is a social act, which means it cannot be completed alone or in private; it requires the cooperation of a larger community. With this premise we make the assumption that sociological factors independent of the psychological decision-making process affect the community pattern of blood donation. This means, for example, that changes in the rate of blood donation by a particular social group or category of donors cannot be fully explained at the level of the individual.

As was noted in the previous chapter, no one can give blood without a blood collection organization having first set up a place for them to do so. Such organizations are also responsible for establishing qualification criteria as well as temporary and permanent deferral guidelines. Future blood recipients do not make direct requests for donations; rather, it is hospitals that assess needs and submit requests to blood product suppliers. Thus, the organizations which serve as intermediaries between blood donors and recipients play a key role in the blood flow process. In a study carried out with plasma and platelet donors, Henrion (2003) observed that this way of proceeding allows donors to forge ties with the staff at blood collection centres but never allows donors and recipients to create direct ties to one another. This may lead donors to think they are giving their blood to the organization itself rather than to future recipients, whom they have difficulty imagining.

The present analysis will draw on the work of Kieran Healy (2006), who encourages researchers to study the institutional context responsible not only for the conditions surrounding the practice of blood donation but also for the rhetoric of altruistic donation.

As Hall and Taylor (1996) have pointed out, institutions such as blood collection agencies provide cultural and moral templates designed to shape individual behaviour within given fields of action. Meyer and Rowan (1977) have also noted that it is vital for such organizations to demonstrate that the myths upon which their structure is based are effective and contribute to the realization of the intended goals. Only in this way will they be able to produce the necessary levels of satisfaction and trust. In the field of blood donation, donor and recipient satisfaction and trust are issues of the utmost importance. Recipients need to be confident that the blood products they are given are safe; donors must also be satisfied and have confidence in the process, as their donations are voluntary and they could stop donating at any time, thereby jeopardizing the entire system.

The aim of this chapter is to identify the processes by which such organizations influence blood donation motivations and practices among blood donors in Québec. Our analysis is based on the results of four complementary research projects conducted between the winter of 2009 and the fall of 2011 by the Research Chair on the Social Aspects of Blood Donation, in collaboration with Héma-Québec. Analyses in this chapter are based on interviews with 185 regular and former donors. Despite having different objectives, all four interview surveys made it possible to obtain a description of participants' blood donation experiences and to explore their reasons for developing and maintaining – or abandoning – the practice over time.

Using a cross-analysis of themes common to all four surveys, we identified five types of factors underlying donor motivations: (1) trust in and familiarity with the blood product supply system; (2) an understanding of the practical value of blood and hence the need for blood products; (3) personal motivations (some of which were associated with the identity-construction process during the transition to adulthood); (4) social motivations (family, community, and civic); and (5) institutional conditions favorable to the practice of donation. This chapter will focus specifically on the influence of blood collection organizations on the practice of blood donation. As we will see, these organizations play a substantial role in connection with each of the types of motivation factors. First, however, we will briefly outline the theoretical concepts that inspired our analysis, as well as the methodological approach used in the surveys.

Kieran Healy's (2006) concept of institutional regimes

Healy's proposition is a critique of lines of reasoning centred on individual and altruistic motivations. Drawing on Wuthnow's (1991) analyses concerning money, selfishness, and altruism, Healy maintains that individuals rarely think in terms of "motivations"; instead, they tend to describe the circumstances surrounding their actions. When giving personal accounts, they relate the series of contingent circumstances that led them to make a specific decision. According to Healy, people who cite altruistic motivations to justify their blood donation practices merely borrow the language produced and refined over the years by blood collection organizations themselves.

> Organizations procuring blood and organs create and sustain their donor pools by providing opportunities to give and by producing and popularizing accounts of what giving means. This means that the structure and practices of these organizations play a larger role in our understanding of blood and organ donation than much of the debate on the relative merits of self-interest and altruism would lead us to believe.... They shape our ideas about altruism and donation by producing accounts of what it means to be a donor.
>
> (Healy 2006, 17–18)

Healy does not deny that individuals have their own personal reasons for donating blood but rather contends that organizations contribute to establishing a set of potential reasons from which donors are able to pick and choose. They do this, for example, by stressing the fact that few people give blood, thus making the donor into someone special, even a hero (who saves lives):

> By analyzing the social basis of exchange in human goods, we can better understand how opportunities to give are successfully created by organizations in the short run. We can also learn how acts like this are culturally sustained and morally valued in the long run. The goal, in other words, has been to see which organizations make gifts best, and how institutions make gifts last.
>
> (Healy 2006, 132)

Following Healy's lead, we will begin by asking whether individuals truly think in terms of motivations. We will primarily attempt to determine how blood collection organizations influence blood donor motivation. In short, how do these organizations contribute to reinforcing the blood donor identity?

A constructivist approach for a better understanding of relationships of trust

According to Barman's (2007) studies on the field of charitable giving, donor behavior may be accounted for by examining personal attributes while focusing on social relations between donors and fundraising organizations, and analyzing the dynamics of the organizational field. Sociological institutionalism (Di Maggio and Powell 1983; Meyer and Rowan 1977; Scott and Meyer 1983) is also centred on analysis of the internal dynamics of organizational change, which it regards as responsible for the definition of strategies of solicitation, i.e., the opportunities and constraints surrounding donation. However, this institutional approach offers few avenues for specifically analyzing how such opportunities or constraints are perceived by donors themselves, other than donors who form associations to defend their views. In the field of blood donation, the donor practice is essentially an individual activity. Donor associations today serve mainly as intermediaries for the dominant organizations in the field (collection agencies) by promoting blood donation practices consistent with the rules governing blood product safety.[1] Other associations tend to represent either citizens who are excluded from blood donation (such as homosexuals) or recipients (such as hemophiliacs) rather than active donors. In our opinion, a study of the views of these various associations would not be sufficient to permit us to truly understand how individual donors perceive opportunities and constraints, or how they react to the rhetorical discourse designed to convince them to donate blood and to develop a long-term practice. A constructivist approach may be used to study the temporality of practices. This perspective, which was adopted by Piliavin and Callero (1991) in their study of blood donor "careers," views blood donation as a constructed social role.

Giddens' (1984) approach offers a promising avenue for thinking about the interaction between the blood collection system and individual donors. According to Giddens, the relationship between institutions and social representations is a dynamic one. Agent and social structure are interdependent, with neither dominating the other. Structures are defined by rules and resources. When engaging in action, agents draw on the traces these rules and resources have left in their memory. Thus, an approach that focuses analysis on agent/social structure relationships offers a way to address both the question of how blood donor identity is constructed, as well as the importance of relationships of trust between donors and blood collection organizations. Giddens' theoretical propositions emphasize agent reflexivity and autonomy, with the question of trust taking on a central role. Trust is what allows individuals to take action in a context of uncertainty, taking into account their actual, memorized experiences on the one hand and the contingency of new possibilities on the other. In a postmodern society, trust acts to reduce complexity (Bachmann 2001). The institutional context itself must ensure agents' ontological security, thereby increasing their sense of trust.

Focusing on the dynamic relationship between agents and social structures and stressing the importance of mutual relationships of trust, this premise is a logical complement to our analysis. In recent decades, especially since the contaminated blood scandal, the questions of trust and health hazard management have had a major influence on blood collection organizations' ability to convince the public to donate blood. As we will see, the establishment of mutual trust between donors and blood collection organizations is one of the chief conditions for blood donation.

A cross-analysis of four surveys' results

We have chosen to use the donor standpoint as the basis for our analysis of motivations. According to the definition of methodological individualism (Weber 1913; Boudon and Filleule 2012), collective phenomena may be analyzed based on individuals' actions, mutual interactions, and representations of the social world. Between the winter of 2009 and the fall of 2011, our research team performed four interview-based surveys in Québec (Table 6.1). All the surveys were supervised by the same team of researchers, and several assistants took part in more than one survey. The interview guides used for each survey were all patterned after one another. They included the same introductory and concluding sections, which provided the analytical results presented here, while each survey also included a distinct portion associated with the specific goals of the individual research project. The interviews were conducted by one or two of the researchers and assistants, and lasted for between one and two hours. All interviews were audio-recorded and transcribed verbatim. The data were analyzed by the same group of researchers and assistants, using the same data classification codes from one survey to the next.

Despite having different goals, all four interview surveys supplied a description of participants' blood donation experiences and explored the motivations and circumstances that led donors to develop and maintain their practice over time (or not).

In all surveys, our primary aim when interviewing regular or former donors was to attempt to determine how they had first become involved. We asked them to try to remember their first blood donation experience and to describe how it unfolded. We were able to discuss with all donors the main changes experienced over the course of their donor career. Our aim was to identify changes in the collection sites frequented, the integration of the practice in their everyday lives, the individual or collective nature of the experience, the way they described their experience at blood drives, and their experiences of deferral or exclusion; as well as changes in their perceived motivations and their reasons for changing the frequency of their donations or, if applicable, for abandoning the practice altogether. They were also invited to reflect more broadly on the role which the cause of blood donation played in their lives, to give their opinions on facilitating factors

Table 6.1 Distribution of interviewed donors by research project

Research project	Project code	% of interviewed donors/ 185 interviews
Ethnic minorities and blood donation in Québec	E1	29
Young people, altruism, and blood donation	E2	24
Family, altruism, and blood donation	E3	17
Blood donation according to living environment	E4	30

Table 6.2 General characteristics of interviewed donors (*n*=185)

Characteristics	Number	%
Men	106	57
Women	79	43
Under 30 years old	63	39
Over 30 years old	99	61
Regular donors	136	74
Former donors	49	26
Urban setting	119	65
Suburbs	30	16
Rural setting	35	19

and obstacles affecting the practice of donating blood, and to talk about their future intentions. They were also asked other questions depending on the goals and target population of the given survey.

Analyses in this chapter are based on interviews with 185 regular and former donors (Table 6.2). Non-donors were also recruited for three of the surveys:[2] youth activists and volunteers (youth survey, *n*=17);[3] parents and young people who had not donated blood, although their children or parents had (family survey, *n*=10),[4] and representatives of ethnic or religious associations (ethnic minorities survey, *n*=23). The non-donors were asked to describe their perceptions of the cause of blood donation, to identify their reasons for not giving blood, to express their opinions on barriers or facilitating factors affecting the practice, and to compare blood donation with other forms of social or political engagement. The contents of these interviews will be explored during our analysis of the factors that act as barriers to the practice of blood donation.[5]

To complement our survey data, we also used the results of annual surveys conducted by Héma-Québec to monitor its public image (SOM 2013).

Results: the essential role of blood collection organizations

As predicted by Healy, some donors did indeed struggle to explain why they donated blood. In fact, when asked why they donated, 28 donors (15%) were unable to give a specific reason.

> I don't know. I have no idea why. I mean, I could give you lots of theories, but I don't think I really know. It's sort of a habit that I got into. I never stopped.... I guess it's part of who I am, one of those things that make me a good person, and people who know me know I'm a good person. It's not something that I feel a need to externalize.
>
> (Man, 27 years old, regular donor, student, E2)

However, all the other donors (i.e., the vast majority) were able to answer the question and explain their commitment to the practice. Healy hypothesized that donors would prefer to discuss the circumstances that had initially led them to start donating blood. In our survey, those who remembered their first donation did indeed cite all the contextual elements that had caused them to donate, while those with extensive donor careers discussed the circumstances that allowed them to continue their practice.

All donors, however, also cited broader *motivations* for donating blood, since while there are indeed always multiple circumstances surrounding a first donation, *there are always multiple motivations as well.* This plurality of motivations has also been observed in other surveys, such as Henrion's (2003). As Caillé (2000) has suggested, this plurality readily encompasses a combination of self-interested reasons (selfishness), selfless reasons (altruism), and social obligations (pressure from people around the donor), but it also always includes institutional aspects as well (direct appeals and easy access to blood drives, for example).

We will examine our results based on the categories of motivations mentioned above.

Familiarity with the system and trust in blood collection organizations

Blood collection organizations have a responsibility to make themselves known to non-donors. They accomplish this, for example, by partnering with primary and secondary schools to raise young people's awareness of the cause before they are even old enough to donate blood (Charbonneau *et al.* 2014). However, few members of the general population can explain how donated blood is processed into blood products or are aware of the volume of blood products used by hospitals. Instead, the public trusts the organizations responsible for supplying blood products to properly assess the amounts required to meet needs. As Alessandrini (2006) has pointed out, the cause of blood donation is viewed positively in our societies and trust in blood organizations has improved greatly since the contaminated blood affair.

Yearly surveys conducted by Héma-Québec confirm that the organization has a good reputation with residents of the province. In the 2013 survey (SOM 2013), 46 percent of respondents spontaneously identified Héma-Québec as the organization responsible for the blood product supply in Québec, while 83 percent stated that they had previously heard Héma-Québec's name, a result that has remained stable over the years. According to the survey, 89 percent of Québec's adults who are familiar with the organization (at least by name) view it positively. In this regard, the 2013 results are similar to those obtained over the previous six years, confirming that most Québecers trust the organization. Fifty-nine percent of respondents stated that they would not be at all worried about developing a disease after having donated blood. In fact, only 15 percent said that they would be moderately or very worried, and many of these were among the respondents who were not at all familiar with the organization. In addition, 83 percent of respondents believed that Héma-Québec was managing blood reserves fairly or very well, an opinion that has remained stable over the years. In addition, 92 percent stated that they were somewhat or completely confident in the blood collection and distribution system in Québec.

When asked directly why they donated blood, donors in our surveys rarely answered spontaneously that it was because they trusted Héma-Québec or because they trusted the organization to use blood wisely. An analysis of non-donors' answers reveals why this question is so important. For example, those who had wanted to donate blood in the past but had been deferred may tend to question the legitimacy of the criteria used to exclude them and express their distrust in the organizations responsible for establishing such criteria.

> As soon as I got back from India, I went to Héma-Québec's offices and started answering the questions. They said, "You were in India? You can't donate." That made me angry. I said, "Yes, but I had blood tests done when I got back" to make sure I didn't have any diseases, even if I wasn't sick over there, to be sure my blood was healthy.... I know I have good blood, but to this day, I still can't donate.
>
> (Woman, 21 years old, no donations, student, E2)

> I can't go, unless I lie.... I'd like to have a long-term relationship, but I don't have one. What can I say? It's one of the criteria now, long-term relationships, but I'd say that for the past five years, I've had a new boyfriend – you wouldn't really call him a boyfriend, we're not living together – still it isn't safe.... It's their criteria, you know.
>
> (Woman, mother of three children, no donations, nurse, E3)

The bond of trust between Héma-Québec and blood donors can also be broken by even temporary deferral. Seventy-four of the donors (40%) had had such an experience.[6] More women (51%) had experienced deferral than men (32%), while more individuals born abroad (82%) said they had experienced deferral than individuals born in Canada (29%). However, 57 percent of respondents who had undergone such an experience continued to be regular donors. Experiencing deferral or anticipating the possibility of it caused donors to question the legitimacy of decisions made by blood collection organizations.

> I was refused because they said my blood hadn't passed the HIV test. They wrote me a letter saying they had "done an initial test that found that I had HIV," but it was like a screening test. It wasn't very precise. Then they said, "We did a confirmatory test, so now we're sure you don't have it, but we would still prefer if you never donated blood again." I found that stupid because I'd given blood just once and now I can never give again for the rest of my life.... Afterwards, I went to see my doctor. I had other blood work done to be sure.... "No, no, everything's fine." But even with a note from the doctor I can't ever give blood again.
>
> (Woman, 19 years old, one donation, student, E2)

I'm not going to change my travel plans because of this, but at some point I will no longer be able to give blood, apparently. It's too bad.... Even if I do travel, that doesn't mean I'm going to inject myself with drugs and things like that. No. It's a bit ridiculous.

(Woman of Senegalese and Guinean origin, 25 years old, regular donor, community organizer, E1)

Similar questions were asked by those who refused to donate blood out of solidarity with people they knew who had been or were still excluded.

Why did I stop donating blood? Because I realized Héma-Québec was often discriminatory. There's a new co-worker who was hired who's Haitian. He explained to me that he and the whole black and Haitian community are systematically discriminated against.... I didn't know about that, but after he explained the situation to me clearly, I followed his example.

(Man, 39 years old, former donor, biomedical engineering technician, E4)

Thus, the population first needs to trust blood collection organizations before its members will take part in blood drives. Blood collection organizations have attempted to foster such trust by tightening donation criteria since the contaminated blood affair in order to reduce fear among potential donors. At the same time, however, they also need to respond to criticism from people who are now disqualified from donating blood for the very same reasons and who, in questioning the legitimacy of exclusion criteria, express a loss of confidence in these organizations. Relationships of trust clearly work in both directions. Individuals' questioning of the criteria used to select donors can lead them to refuse to become involved in the cause and even to convince others to do the same. This situation is, of course, problematic for an organization seeking to convince the population to give blood.

Understanding the practical value of blood and the need for blood products

Of the regular and former donors interviewed, 82 (44%) stated that they donated or had donated blood to meet very concrete societal needs for blood products, or because they considered the gesture "useful." The donors were motivated to give blood because the substance was valuable, rare, and irreplaceable, and because it met the needs of both the sick and accident victims.

Our survey data point to a number of circumstances that may inform this practical view of blood donation. Donors may have needed transfusions themselves or known others who needed them. They may have witnessed accidents or worked in the health sector where people who need blood are a familiar sight. They may have been motivated to donate out of a belief that they themselves, or members of their families, would have access to such products if they needed them one day in the future.

Another source of awareness about blood products is the information disseminated in the media, in public space, and via blood collection organizations, as
seen in the previous chapter. Héma-Québec communication strategies rarely
promote blood donation by encouraging donors to meet the "need" for blood
products. In fact, only six donors mentioned Héma-Québec directly as a source
of awareness of blood product needs. However, it is also important to mention
the people to whom the organization appeals by phone to meet specific needs, as
such direct appeals obviously reinforce a sense of the usefulness of blood donation. A number of donors referred to these direct appeals.

> We often hear about supplies being low, and one day when I'll need it, I
> hope the supply won't be low. That's kind of why I do it. That's pretty
> much the reason.
>
> (Woman, 30 years old, regular donor, nursing student, E2)

> I listen to the news fairly often. I try to keep informed, and sometimes I hear
> that supplies are getting low, that they need more.
>
> (Man, 29 years old, regular donor, officer in the Canadian Army, E2)

> They've called me once or twice before: "Listen, we have a shortage for
> your donor type, can you come make a donation?" … If they call me
> because there's a shortage, it's because it's really important. It's not just
> about showing up and doing my part. In that case it's more out of necessity.
> And when it comes to that, I can't believe that a man out there will die
> because he was short a litre of blood.
>
> (Man, 21 years old, regular donor, student, E2)

The most convincing argument, and also the one used most often to convince the
public that blood is a useful substance which fulfills a fundamental need, is
undoubtedly the argument that it "saves lives."

"Give blood. Give life." For many years, this expression appeared as part
of Héma-Québec's website address. The association between the gift of blood
and the gift of life is the most frequently recurring element in the rhetorical
discourse of blood organizations. It is probably the oldest and most internationally widespread element used to encourage the public to donate blood.
That donors in our surveys borrowed this vocabulary from Héma-Québec's
discourse became evident when they cited advertisements which state that
"one blood donation can save *four* lives."

> I've continued to donate because the first time, one of the nurses [told me],
> "You know, you can save four lives with one blood donation." So I thought,
> "Well, that's cool." It made me feel like a superhero, like I was going to do
> something good for society. That's why I kept donating. When I was able
> to, when they called me, and I wanted to go, well, I went.
>
> (Woman of Senegalese and Guinean origin, 25 years old, regular donor,
> community organizer, E1)

My understanding is that with one blood donation, I think you can save up to four lives. Because they take … it's not just blood. There are platelets, too, or white blood cells. It means saving lives in my mind.

(Woman, 34 years old, regular donor, translator, E4)

The mass dissemination of this message has long had an undeniable effect: people have clearly internalized this message, citing it spontaneously when asked why they donate blood. Whether given as a reflex or because it is a socially desirable answer (Piliavin et Callero 1991), the fact remains that this motivation, strongly inspired and encouraged by blood collection organizations, underscores the practical aspect of blood, which is indeed used to save lives. Even among non-donors, this message is clearly understood.

Blood donation? It's very important. You have to donate, that's for sure.… It's absolutely necessary, I'm aware of that. I think there are also a lot of ads that raise awareness, and there are blood drives fairly regularly near where we live.

(Man, 21 years old, no donation, homosexual, student, E2)

According to Beauchamp and Childress, "To say that someone has a funda-mental need is to say that the person will be harmed or detrimentally affected in a fundamental way if that need is not fulfilled" (2001, 228). If donors consider that they are saving a life by donating blood, are they not meeting a most funda-mental need? Since donors and recipients cannot be in direct contact, it seems as if donors, aware that they have an irreplaceable substance that can meet funda-mental needs, see themselves as an intrinsic part of a structure that redistributes services to the public. In a sense, they liken their role to that of the state, repres-ented in this case by blood collection organizations.

If we combine all references to motivations emphasizing the usefulness of blood donation, 62 percent (114 respondents) appear to be motivated to donate blood due to its practical value.

The role of individual and social motivations

The role of individual motivations is the main theme studied by researchers who draw on behavioural social psychology to study what motivates individuals to develop the intention to donate blood and to engage in the practice. However, these researchers have rarely attempted to describe the role blood collection organizations play in reinforcing personal motivations, despite frequently con-cluding their analyses with recommendations to improve institutional strategies for donor recruitment and retention, and thereby indirectly admitting that these organizations have an important role to play in reinforcing donor motivations.

As Smith pointed out in the previous chapter, Healy (2006) maintains that blood collection organizations participate in establishing a set of potential moti-vations from which donors can pick and choose. For example, by stressing the fact that few people donate blood, they transform those few into special individuals, even heroes who save lives. Our analyses reveal that these organizations also reinforce donors' motivations by fueling people's pride in donating blood. This pride is often what encourages donors to continue their practice. Their donor identity is reinforced by elements that make them feel valued and that distinguish them from others who do not donate blood, making them exceptional individuals.

Sixty-three of the respondents (34%) talked about their pride in donating blood. Pride was mentioned mainly by younger respondents,[7] which points to the importance of the factor of pride both in the identity-construction process at the start of adulthood and in the development of a blood donor career. The latter is also borne out by the fact that more regular blood donors (39%) than former donors (20%) discussed their sense of pride in the practice. Such pride is reinforced by the fact that donating blood is rare in today's society, though the greatest source of pride is often individual blood characteristics. Donors are proud to be "universal donors" or to have blood belonging to a rarer and more sought-after blood type, and that their blood can be used to help babies.

> It's a kind of pride. I'm O negative. I think that's important. Anyone can be given my blood. That's a good thing. Of course if I were A or B I'd probably donate as much, but let's just say it's not as impressive [bursts out laughing].
> (Woman, 27 years old, regular donor, research professional, E2)

> They told me during my interview.... They said: "Oh, you're AB negative, your blood type is very rare. Pediatrics – after testing, your blood is almost certain to go straight to pediatrics.
> (Man, 36 years old, regular donor, teacher/firefighter, E4)

Donors' sense of pride is further reinforced when Héma-Québec staff call them to tell them they are needed.

> So I know it's one of the types they need the most. They often tell me that when they call, so yeah, of course. It's not a chore. I'm happy to do it.
> (Woman, 45 years old, regular donor, head cosmetician, E4)

> Héma-Québec seems to have my number on a special list.... Every 14 days, they make a point of calling me. Sometimes they call me because they have a specific patient, so they change donor priority to give me a spot. Most of the time it's because I'm Rh+ and that's a versatile platelet that can be given to many people.
> (Man, 51 years old, platelet and plasma donor, department head in the health sector, E3)

> I'm O negative, and that's a universal donor, which seemed like a good thing [laughs]. It was a blood type that was needed, and that made me feel

valued. A few years later, the Red Cross called me and told me that I had the kind of blood babies needed, "Sir, we need your blood. It's used for babies." That made me feels even more important.

(Man, 56 years old, regular donor, civil servant, E3)

In short, it is clear that the information provided by Héma-Québec through its direct appeals and repeated encouragement fosters blood donor pride and their sense of belonging to a select group, a sort of elite whose achievements are fully deserving of recognition.

Blood collection organizations also help reinforce individual blood donor identity by establishing potential targets associated with marks of recognition. Some donors mentioned that they were highly motivated to continue donating blood because of the challenge of reaching such objectives (e.g., 100 or 200 donations) and emphasized Héma-Québec's role in this regard.

I have my 40th [pin] with me, it's on my coat. Wow, I show it off and everything. It's like unusual for someone to get to "40." … When I reach 100, I'll wear it on my forehead.

(Man, 25 years old, platelet and plasma donor, restaurant employee, E2)

Platelets are demanding, the donation takes almost two hours. But when we went to our first Héma-Québec recognition evening for 100, 125 and 175 donations, they gave us a certificate. The 200th donation is a sort of Plex-iglas trophy and my spouse said, "Oh, that's beautiful. That would be nice." OK, but you can't just buy one at the store. You need to bleed yourself dry to get it. One hundred donations, that was my goal, and once I reached it I wanted to keep going, but less intensively. My spouse, whom I love, and I said to ourselves, "We're going to get that nice drop-shaped trophy." So that's how we kept on shooting for the drop. I'm going to get it soon. I've been invited this week to the whole recognition thing. I hope it's for the 200th and not the 175th.

(Man, 56 years old, platelet donor, foster care centre evaluator, E3)

A number of authors (Healy 2006; Piliavin et Callero 1991; Simpson 2011; Smith, Chapter 5, this volume) state that if individuals cite altruistic motivations for donating blood, it is because blood collection organizations have produced this vocabulary, based on the ideal vision of the voluntary, altruistic, and anonymous donor promoted by international agencies (e.g., the WHO and the Federation of Red Cross and Red Crescent Societies). The more donors frequent blood drives and agency staff, the more their altruistic identity may be reinforced.

Indeed, 63 of the respondents (34%) justified their blood donation in terms illustrative of "generalized altruism" (directed toward an unknown Other). They expressed themselves using relatively abstract language: I donate blood to do something good, to do a good deed, out of generosity, to give to my fellow man, to make a difference, to pass on good values, to compensate for those who don't donate. Our study does not, however, confirm that the rhetorical discourse used by blood supply structures is the main source of inspiration for donors in this regard. In fact, altruistic motivations seem to be the result of many influences. Some donors' comments reveal the presence of religious values, while others reflect a sense of community or civic belonging. Such motivations can be fostered by social as well as institutional influences. Generally speaking, donors' motivations are a combination of altruistic justifications, religious obligations, civic duty, and community solidarity.

> It's a combination of a generous act and an obligation, for you and the community. People need blood and nothing else is going to provide it. We are only going to get it from other people.
> (Man, 56 years old, regular donor, employed in the financial sector, E1)

> Giving blood means giving your life for others. I prefer to see it as an act of solidarity and generosity.
> (Man of Honduran origin, donor in Central America, no donations in Canada – temporary exclusions, priest, E1)

> My mother often told me I was O–. I wasn't pressured, but I felt I had a civic duty to do it.
> (Man, 19 years old, regular donor, student, E2)

Analysis of the social motivations for blood donation highlights the strong influence of family, close acquaintances, and the community. How can the influence of blood collection organizations be expressed in this context? In the previous chapter, Smith revealed the important role played by blood donation "ambassadors" from these organizations. These individuals work to create local cultures conducive to blood donation in local businesses and organizations. In this way blood collection organizations encourage the organization of blood drives in workplaces, counting on friendly pressure between colleagues to convince even the most reluctant individuals to donate blood. Our survey results show that 29 respondents donated or had donated blood in drives organized in their workplace (16%).

> I always [donate blood] at work. I don't make a special trip.... My motivation? First, I see people donating, my co-workers. If no one else is donating, I won't either.
> (Man of Vietnamese origin, regular donor, police department employee, E4)

> I take advantage of their presence and of the fact that my company encourages us to give blood.... I only donate when Héma-Québec comes to where I work.
> (Man, 32 years old, regular donor, engineer, E4)

By facilitating the organization of blood drives in primary and secondary schools (Charbonneau *et al.* 2014), blood collection organizations also seek to mobilize children's family and social circles, encouraging them to donate blood. Initiatives that involve partnering with various local associations to organize blood drives are also clearly aimed at leveraging the influence these associations have over their members to convince the latter to become blood donors.

In short, some organizations, such as Héma-Québec, choose to rely more on mobile blood drives than on fixed blood collection sites, travelling to meet individuals in their day-to-day environments, businesses, schools, associations, or home neighbourhoods. A number of donors expressed satisfaction at being able to count on such blood drives being held near where they carry out their main activities.

> Of course, if I had to go all the way across town ... I don't tend to go to the [permanent] blood collection centre because it's not necessarily accessible.... You're not going to drive there. It's like it has to be in your neighbourhood.
>
> (Woman, 37 years old, former donor, doctor, E4)

Difficulty accessing blood drives is, in fact, often cited as one of the main obstacles to blood donation (Bednall and Bove 2011). Twenty-one donors (11%) mentioned practical issues regarding access to blood drives. Middle-aged individuals (31–50 years old) appeared to be most affected by this problem, which is not surprising, since this is the segment of the population that struggles most frequently to reconcile their blood donation practice with other everyday responsibilities.

> I donate every time they come here.... I have three children, so outside work, it's harder to free up time that I would lose with my family.
>
> (Man, 39 years old, regular donor, computer specialist, E4)

Blood collection organizations therefore play a decisive role in adapting blood donation conditions to the everyday lives of blood donors by providing the best possible access to blood drives, both in terms of proximity to donors' everyday activities and in terms of scheduling. As Smith argued in the previous chapter, the aim of the employees of such organizations is to produce "satisfied customers." This was especially important to the 31- to 40-year-old age group.[8] Fifty-nine respondents (32%) directly mentioned convenient access to a blood drive when justifying their blood donation practice.

In addition, donating blood at mobile blood drives may itself serve as a pretext for socializing, meeting new people, or reconnecting with acquaintances. Thirteen respondents directly mentioned this aspect.

> I could have donated in [the town of] Saint-Hyacinthe, I could have gone anywhere else to donate, but I liked going to the town of Sainte-Madeleine better, as I knew the whole gang there and could chat with everyone at once.
>
> (Woman, 46 years old, former donor, E4)

Out in the country, things are close knit. We go there, we have coffee and we donate blood at the same time. It's like a little social club.

(Woman, 44 years old, former donor, day care teacher, E4)

I go alone most of the time. But there's always someone over there to talk to.... People chat, I find it fun.

(Woman, 27 years old, regular donor, research professional, E2)

In short, it is precisely by taking into account the possibilities and constraints related to individuals' everyday lives in their social contexts, and by encouraging the organization of mobile blood drives which offer opportunities for developing and maintaining social relationships, that organizations manage to foster and reinforce individuals' social motivations to donate blood. As we will see in the final part of this analysis, the practice of blood donation is strongly conditioned by its surrounding institutional conditions.

The institutional conditions that promote blood donation

All the elements we have mentioned thus far underline the importance of the role of organizations in motivating individuals to donate blood and in encouraging them to take part in blood drives. Our analyses also revealed the presence of other important inducements, such as when organizations invite target populations to donate blood to meet specific needs for rare blood, as is the case for black communities and sickle-cell anemia (Tran *et al.* 2013). They also follow up with donors to remind them when it is time to make their next blood donation. Telephone recruitment services phone donors at the end of the 56-day waiting period or when rare blood from a specific donor is needed. Other methods are also used: donor cards, ads in the media, and small posters in the vicinity of blood drives. Forty-eight respondents (26%) mentioned the importance of such methods in motivating them to donate blood.

I don't know if Héma-Québec has a record of all donors, with all their information. When they see that someone hasn't donated often, they call you. So if it's time for me to donate, they'll call to remind me. But it's not that they harass you either. It's just a way to remind you [about it].

(Man of Chilean origin, 46 years old, regular donor, carpenter, E1)

It's mainly because of the posters they put up everywhere at the college. They're everywhere, and when you walk by sometimes, you can see that there are a lot of people.

(Man, 23 years old, no donations – 2 donation attempts, E2)

I keep my little card in my wallet, showing when I can donate next. If there's a blood drive in the area, for sure I'll go donate.

(Woman, 27 years old, regular donor, research professional, E2)

Sometimes they call me.... Often they suggest a nearby blood drive, I think that's nice. Of course, for me, getting the call helps motivate me.... Basically I think they should really keep on calling people.

(Man, 27 years old, regular donor, student, E2)

As we have seen in the previous chapter, blood drive employees and volunteers are in large part responsible for donor satisfaction, other than regarding physical repercussions that may affect donor health (faintness, fainting, etc.).

Really nice. They gave me a "new donor" sticker and everyone was so nice to me. They explained everything and reassured me about all sorts of things. They're doing tests. "Don't worry, this won't take long. Here's what to do." It was really great. There were nice ladies telling us stories and reading us the paper and our horoscopes.

(Woman, 21 years old, one donation, student, E3)

Employees are also responsible for properly managing cases of temporary deferrals as, when things do not go well, individuals will not show up again to donate blood.

To help reconcile the practice of blood donation with the multiple demands of everyday life, organizations also offer donors the possibility of making an appointment to donate blood. Some donors expressed a great deal of satisfaction with this arrangement, as it was the only way for them to incorporate blood donation into their personal schedules.

Now, they often call me for blood drive.... With an appointment, it's really – it's fantastic. When it works out with my schedule, well, I go.

(Woman, 45 years old, regular donor, head cosmetician, E4)

In short, blood collection organizations listen attentively to donor preferences so that they can offer donors the best possible donation experience and encourage them to come back to donate again.

Conclusion

Blood donors have many different motivations. Factors from varied and complementary sources foster the development of the intention to donate blood and help convince individuals to start donating and to continue to do so over time. Of course, individuals first need to be made aware of the cause of blood donation. As our analyses have shown, this awareness does not only come through social circles. Above all, individuals must understand the blood supply and collection system, and the blood collection organization itself needs to have instilled enough trust in individuals for them to choose to become involved in such a cause.

As research in behavioural psychology has shown, a positive initial experience with blood donation fosters the sense that donating blood is something the individual is capable of doing. The resultant satisfaction must be stronger than anticipated fears or any discomfort experienced. Our analyses' results suggest, however, that to commit to a career as a regular donor, donors have a strong need to be supported and encouraged by blood collection organizations, which play a role in shaping their personal convictions, and also need to be convinced of the practical value of blood donation.

Our analyses reveal that certain factors may be key in fostering commitment to long-term donation: (1) a social environment which promotes socialization during donation and which offers ongoing incentives in various forms; (2) an institutional rhetoric which reinforces the sense that blood donation has an essential and useful function, that it meets concrete needs, and that, as a result, those who give blood have every reason to be proud of donating; (3) practical arrangements, such as nearby blood drives in particular, which help individuals overcome the growing obstacles of everyday life that come with founding a family. The presence of blood drives in the workplace can effectively provide an effective substitute for blood drives in educational institutions when young people leave school and their day-to-day lives become more complex.

With time, a deeper commitment to the cause of blood donation can lead some donors to switch to apheresis donation, which is more demanding in terms of donation length and frequency. This type of experience can foster the development of more personal ties with blood drive employees and volunteers. However, in order for donors to engage in this practice, organizations must disseminate information on it, since this type of donation is not well known to the general public. In sum, our analyses reveal that institutional conditions are essential at every step of the blood donor's career. All donors interviewed clearly emphasized the essential and ongoing role of blood collection organizations.

Acknowledgments

This study was made possible by a grant from Héma-Québec, the Héma-Québec Foundation, and the Social Sciences and Humanities Research Council.

Notes

1 In Chapter 4, Chauveau shows that these associations played a much more active role in France up until the 1980s, but the 1992 reforms limited them to the function of promoting blood donation.
2 Owing to the specificity of each of the surveys' objectives, which resulted in the selection of "non-donors" with targeted profiles, these respondents cannot be considered representative of non-donors in general. One might in fact ask what a non-donor profile might be, given that the vast majority of the population has never donated blood.
3 Some youth activists or volunteers were also blood donors.
4 Six "non-donors" in the parent–child dyads had previously donated blood, but had been deferred. They were considered to be former donors for the purposes of analysis.
5 The data analysis procedures for each of the surveys is presented in Charbonneau *et al.* (2015).

6 When medical reasons were cited, they were mostly temporary restrictions (iron levels, allergies, elevated pulse rates, etc.).
7 Fifty-six percent of 19- to 30-year-olds, compared to 22 percent in other age groups.
8 Forty-nine percent among 31- to 40-year-olds, versus 22 percent among 19- to 30-year-olds.

References

Alessandrini, M. 2006. "Social Capital and Blood Donation." *The International Journal of Interdisciplinary Social Sciences* 1(1): 103–115.

Armitage, C.J. and Conner, M. 2001. "Social Cognitive Determinants of Blood Donation." *Journal of Applied Social Psychology* 31(7): 1431.

Bachmann, R. 2001. "Trust, Power and Control in Trans-organizational Relations." *Organization Studies* 22(2): 337–365.

Barman, E. 2007. "An Institutional Approach to Donor Control: From Dyadic Ties to a Field-level Analysis." *AJS* 112(5): 1416–1457.

Beauchamp, T.L. and Childress, J.F. 2001. *Principles of Biomedical Ethics. Fifth Edition.* Oxford: Oxford University Press.

Bednall, T.C. and Bove, L.L. 2011. "Donating Blood: A Meta-analytic Review of Self-reported Motivators and Deterrents." *Transfusion Medicine Reviews* 25(4): 317–334.

Berger, P.L. and Luckmann, T. 1966. *The Social Construction of Reality; A Treatise in the Sociology of Knowledge.* Garden City: Doubleday.

Boudon, R. and Filleule, R. 2012. *Les méthodes en sociologie.* Paris: PUF.

Caillé, A. 2000. *Anthropologie du don. Le tiers paradigme.* Paris: Desclée de Brouwer.

Charbonneau, J. and Fainstein, B., in collaboration with Daigneault, S. 2014. *Suivi de la trousse pédagogique "Rouge Sang". Rapport final de recherche remis à Héma-Québec.* Montréal: Université INRS.

Charbonneau, J. and Tran, N. 2015. "The Paradoxical Situation of Blood Donation in the Haitian-Quebec Community." *Canadian Ethnic Studies* 47(2): 71–96.

Charbonneau, J, Cloutier, M.S., Quéniart, A., and Tran, N. 2015. *Le don de sang: un geste social et culturel.* Québec: Presses de l'Université Laval.

DiMaggio, P.J. and Powell, W.W. 1983. "The Iron Cage Revisited: Institutional Isomorphism and Collective Rationality in Organizational Fields." *American Sociological Review* 48(2): 147–160.

Ferguson, E. 1996. "Predictors of Future Behaviour: A Review of the Psychological Literature on Blood Donation." *British Journal of Health Psychology* 1: 287–308.

Ferguson, E., Taylor, M., Keatley, D., Flynn, N., and Lawrence, C. 2012. "Blood Donors' Helping Behavior is Driven by Warm Glow: More Evidence for the Blood Donor Benevolence Hypothesis." *Transfusion* 52(10): 2189–2200.

France, J.L., France, C.R., and Himawan, L.K. 2007. "A Path Analysis of Intention to Redonate among Experienced Blood Donors: An Extension of the Theory of Planned Behavior." *Transfusion* 47(6): 1006–1013.

Giddens, A. 1984. *The Constitution of Society Outline of the Theory of Structuration.* Berkeley, CA: University of California Press.

Giles, M. and Cairns, E. 1995. "Blood Donation and Ajzen's Theory of Planned Behaviour: An Examination of Perceived Behavioural Control." *The British Journal of Social Psychology* 34: 173–188.

Godin, G., Conner, M., Sheeran, P., Bélanger-Gravel, A., and Germain, M. 2007. "Determinants of Repeated Blood Donation among New and Experienced Blood Donors." *Transfusion* 47(9): 1607–1615.

Hall, P.A. and Taylor, R.C.R. 1996. "Political Science and the Three New Institutionalisms." *Political Studies* 53: 936–957.

Healy, K. 2006. *Last Best Gifts. Altruism and the Market for Human Blood and Organs.* Chicago, IL: The University of Chicago Press.

Henrion, A. 2003. *L'énigme du don de sang. Approche ethnographique d'un don entre inconnus.* Liège, Université de Liège, faculté de philosophie et lettres, mémoire.

Laurent, A. 1994. *L'individualisme méthodologique.* Paris: PUF, coll. Que sais-je?, No. 2906.

Lemmens, K.P.H., Ruiter, R.A.C., Schaalma, H.P., Abraham, C., Veldhuizen, I.J.T., Dehing, C.J.G., and Bos, A.E.R. 2009. "Modelling Antecedents of Blood Donation Motivation among Non-donors of Varying Age and Education." *British Journal of Psychology* 100(1): 71–90.

Masser, B.M., Bednall, T.C., White, K.M., and Terry, D. 2012. "Predicting the Retention of First-time Donors Using an Extended Theory of Planned Behavior." *Transfusion* 52(6): 1303–1310.

Meyer, J.W. and Rowan, B. 1977. "Institutionalized Organizations: Formal Structure as Myth and Ceremony." *AJS* 83(2): 340–363.

Misje, A.H., Bosnes, V., Gasdal, O., and Heier, H.E. 2005. "Motivation, Recruitment and Retention of Voluntary Non-remunerated Blood Donors: A Survey-Based Questionnaire Study." *Vox Sanguinis* 89(4): 236–244.

Piliavin, J.A. and Callero, P.L. 1991. *Giving Blood: The Development of an Altruistic Identity.* Baltimore, MD: Johns Hopkins University Press.

Simpson, R. 2011. "Blood Rhetorics: Donor Campaigns and their Publics in Contemporary Sri Lanka." *Ethnos* 76(2): 254–275.

Scott,W.R. and Meyer, J. 1983. "The Organization of Societal Sectors," in Meyer, J. and Scott, W.R. (eds), *Organizational Environments: Ritual and Rationality.* Beverly Hills, CA: Sage.

Smith, A., Matthews, R., and Fiddler, J. 2011. "Blood Donation and Community: Exploring the Influence of Social Capital." *International Journal of Social Inquiry* 4(1): 45–63.

Sojka, B.N. and Sojka, P. 2008. "The Blood Donation Experience: Self-reported Motives and Obstacles for Donating Blood." *Vox Sanguinis* 94(1): 56–63.

SOM Recherches et sondages. 2013. *Suivi de l'image d'Héma-Québec. Sondage Omnibus (Le SOM-R).* Présenté à Héma-Québec. Montréal.

Tran, N.Y.L., Charbonneau, J., and Valderrama-Benitez, V. 2013. "Blood Donation Practices, Motivations and Beliefs in Montreal's Black Communities: The Modern Gift under a New Light." *Ethnicity and Health* 18(6): 508–529.

Veldhuizen, I., Ferguson, E., De Kort, W., Donders, R., and Atsma, F. 2011. "Exploring the Dynamics of the Theory of Planned Behavior in the Context of Blood Donation: Does Donation Experience Make a Difference?" *Transfusion* 51(11): 2425–2437.

Weber, M. 1913. *Essai sur la théorie de la science. 3e essai. Essai sur quelques catégories de la sociologie compréhensive.* http://classiques.uqac.ca/classiques/Weber/essais_theorie_science/essais_theorie_science.html (last accessed December 16, 2014).

Wuthnow, R. 1991. *Acts of Compassion: Caring for Others and Helping Ourselves.* Princeton, NJ: Princeton University Press.

7 Religion, risk, and excess in the Indian blood donation encounter

Jacob Copeman

Introduction

This chapter provides an overview of certain devotional connotations of blood donation as it is practiced and experienced in North India. After giving a sense of the diversity of locations in the region in which people are mobilized to donate their blood, the chapter considers how gurus have become increasingly important within the movement to obtain voluntarily donated blood. Indeed, one of the most remarkable aspects of the blood donation situation in India is the success of blood bank medics in "appropriating" gurus' devotees as a kind of shortcut method of filling large gaps in supply. Blood donation has thus become a devotional act and a key component of devotees' religious lives. However, though in many ways a success, the collaboration raises some difficult questions to do with risk and wastage, which will be detailed in the second part of the chapter.

As noted above, over recent years, religious movements, in particular those led by gurus, have become critically important providers of voluntarily donated blood throughout India. The devotees of guru movements vie to donate the most blood in a kind of national league of virtuous beneficence. The successive setting and surpassing of world records has turned the collection of blood by religious movements in India into something akin to a system of "alternating disequilibrium," as described by Andrew Strathern (1971, 222), one group achieving the record and being dominant until another group breaks it, and so on.

But their exploits extend far beyond mere national boundaries. These devotional orders seek international recognition by way of achieving entries in *The Guinness Book of World Records* for most blood donations made in a single day. For instance, if you were to open the 2005 edition of *The Guinness Book of World Records* at the Medical Marvels section, which includes such entries as most fetuses in a human body, most surviving children from a single birth, most operations endured, and most hand amputations on the same arm, you would learn of the achievement of a North Indian devotional order in collecting the most units of blood in a single day: the 12,002 450 millilitre units collected by the Dera Sacha Sauda devotional order, the entry reads, "is the equivalent of 67 bathtubs of blood!"

Doctors express both delight and distaste at these great spectacles of blood giving. Many of them are highly critical of the excessive donation of blood at mass donation events; one doctor, for instance, described them to me as "blood massacres" because of the high level of wastage that results (either because such an extraordinary quantum is simply not required, with many units consequently expiring, or because of a relaxing of medical standards that results in a preponderance of "quality not sufficient" units). At the same time, however, doctors remain dependent on these movements for their blood supply and so felicitate them at awards ceremonies, where they lavish the gurus with thanks and praise, thus revealing the conflicting nature of their professional selves.

What makes the fervor of devotional blood-giving events all the more striking is the extreme aversion to blood donation of the population at large. This helps explain why albeit infuriated doctors are simultaneously in awe of these great spectacles of blood giving. They have spent their professional lives trying unsuccessfully to persuade people to donate their blood, and now, there is this extraordinary surfeit of it. Such devotion-inspired avidness raises critical questions to do with asceticism, religious merit, and public policy (particularly in respect of risk), which I address below.

Context of donation

The backdrop to my ethnographic research on Indian blood donation practices (Delhi 2003–2005) was recent legislation initiated by the Indian medical establishment seeking to stop blood banks accepting blood on the basis of payment to individual donors and also demanding an end to the prevailing ad hoc family-based system of provision. The public policy orthodoxy informing the legislation asserts that the safety of donated blood is far greater when derived from voluntary, non-remunerated donors in an anonymous system of procurement. The banning of paid donation and the phasing out of replacement donation has required innovative strategies on the part of blood banks to radically increase voluntary blood donation.

The project to foster voluntary blood donation is thus necessarily expansive; new constituencies of donor must be sought and enrolled. The Red Cross, with which I was associated during my stay in Delhi, takes its donor beds to donors, each day driving its "blood mobile" to college, corporate, and religious settings in order to collect blood as they do in other countries.[1] Political parties also donate blood at their rallies in order to demonstrate their largesse and willingness to engage in "service" (*seva*) of their constituents (actual or potential). Donation events take place in a diverse array of environments and can range from the relatively quiet, methodical, and mundane in corporate office locations to open-air, carnival-style events at which Rajasthan steel bands preside and political party activists join hands around the prostrate figure of a donating politician while chanting, "long live Sonia Gandhi," or whoever. Blood donation is indeed a key site of political expressivity in modern India.

Figure 7.1 depicts a donation event staged by the Congress political party on the death anniversary of former Indian Prime Minister Rajiv Gandhi. His garlanded portrait is visible above the donating party members. A Tamil Tiger

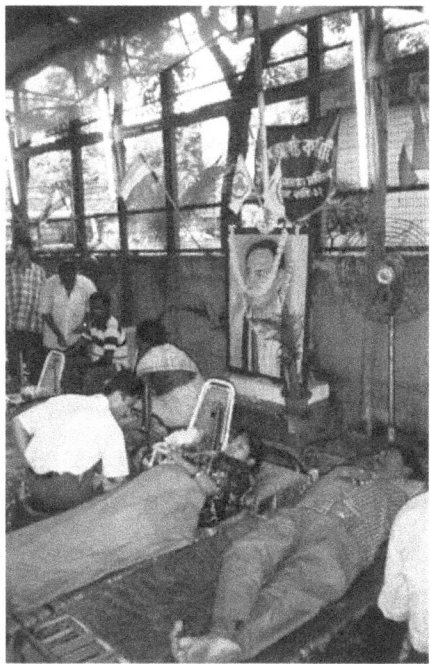

Figure 7.1 Donation event staged by Congress political party in 1991.

suicide bomber assassinated Rajiv Gandhi in 1991. It should be noted that the commemoration of bloodshed through acts of blood donation is a marked feature of blood donation events in India. For example, for donor recruiter Dr. Ajay Bagga from Hoshiarpur, Punjab State, it is "the memory of the bullet-ridden, blood-soaked body of his father [a political leader in the Punjab Pradesh Janata Party, who was assassinated by militants in 1984] which propelled him towards the blood donation movement."[2] Further, Indian soldiers who died in the 1999 India–Pakistan Kargil conflict are now remembered annually through blood donation camps staged in their honour. As I argue in my book on these matters (Copeman 2009), blood donation events staged in honor of soldiers considered to have shed their blood for the nation share with those held in memory of assassinated politicians such as Indira Gandhi and her son Rajiv Gandhi and follow a fairly familiar sacrificial template: commemorative blood donation retrospectively bestows the original death with capacities of regeneration, the victim bringing forth new life via the blood donations enacted in his or her memory.

Figure 7.2 shows Jawaharlal Nehru, the first post-independence prime minister of India and Rajiv Gandhi's grandfather, donating blood in 1942. At the time, there was an outcry: *Time* magazine reported that "Jawaharlal Nehru, 56, drew a rebuke from followers for donating to a blood bank." His health, they protested, is "national wealth, which should be preserved." He should really

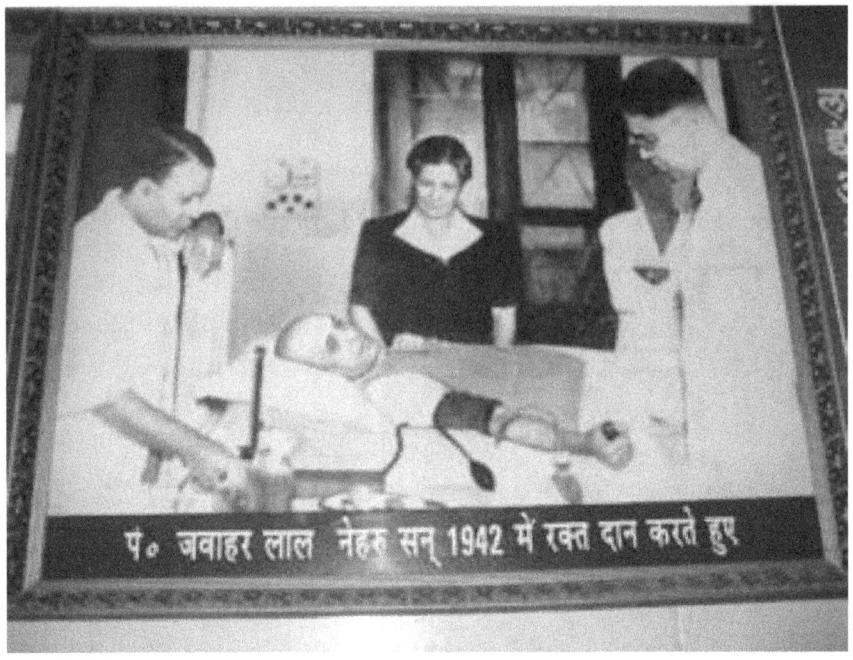

Figure 7.2 Nehru, Prime Minister of India, donating blood in 1942.

"abstain from such destructive sacrifices."[3] Nehru probably believed that he was sacrificing for the nation, but his "followers" viewed his donation as unpatriotic in presuming its harmful effects on his health. Nehru's donation, so his followers believed, because of his political indispensability, was a sacrifice *of* rather than *for* the nation. As I have mentioned, however, donating blood has now become a key mode of articulating ethical and patriotic citizenship, with gurus and politicians vying to organize donation events and, in the case of politicians, disclosing on their CVs the number of times they have personally donated.

I have sought thus far to give an indication of the diversity of locations in which blood donation events are staged and to show how the Red Cross and other medical organizations seek actively to encourage new blood donor constituencies. As one might imagine, this is resulting in the rapid proliferation of new relationships between medical institutions and other societal segments; and the sheer multiplicity and diversity of the actors involved has led to a striking plurality of understandings arising around blood donation (see Copeman 2009).

However, despite the assortment of government and NGO campaigns to boost voluntary, non-remunerated blood donation in the country, family-based replacement donation (where relatives donate for one another) still accounts for more than 50 percent of all donated blood in India, as is the case in many developing countries.[4] In Delhi, where I worked, the figure is far worse, with less than 19 percent of the total collection comprising voluntary donation.[5] The reasons for this are diverse, ranging from an abject lack of coordination between different blood banks to a widespread perception that blood donation is a dramatically unhealthy, even life-threatening activity. The "prick" of donation is particularly terrifying. As one donor told me: "When I got vaccinated and my skin was pierced I felt it was bursting my body and everything inside would spill out. It will never stop."[6] Many blood donors find the vision of their blood leaving their bodies and flowing into bags highly disturbing. Doctors in several blood banks cover blood bags with a cloth while they fill in order to avoid donors pulling away from the needle when they see the bag fill with their blood.

Fears of impotence and infertility are also often cited as reasons why people prefer not to donate their blood. More than once I was told by those reluctant to donate that the reason they could not donate was because they were getting married the following month, the implication being clear. There is a litany of other grounds for declining to donate which range from fear of resulting blindness to unamenable weather conditions; indeed, some hold that the summer heat dries up their blood. The most important reason, however, is the widespread understanding of blood loss as leading to permanent volumetric deficit. This was frequently expressed to me in the following way: "If I donate blood I will need a transfusion, so why should I give?" In an effort to counter this perception, doctors compare blood donation to having one's hair or nails cut: blood, they say, like these other detachable substances, re-forms and returns.

Devotion and donation

Although the set of campaigns to foster voluntary donation has faltered, there is, on the face if it, one important success story: devotional movements – particularly those in what is known as the *Sant* tradition – have in recent years become enthusiastic providers of donated blood. The *Sant* Nirankari Mission *alone* provides as much as 20 percent of the capital's voluntarily donated blood. The *Sant* tradition is not exclusively Hindu or Sikh but venerates the teachings of *Sant*s who have been important and influential in each religion. In the devotional contexts I have been exploring, distinctions between Hindus and non-Hindus, and indeed, distinctions of caste and other internal differentiations of "community," are downplayed in favour of shared devotional attachment to a spiritual master. The fourteenth and fifteenth centuries saw an efflorescence of *Sant* poets such as Kabir, Nanak, Ravi Das, and Nam Dev. Most espoused versions of *bhakti* (often glossed as devotion). This religious attitude implies a "participation" in the deity and a love relationship between the individual soul and the Supreme Lord, *Bhagavan* (Vaudeville 1974, 97). While initiates are derived from a very wide stratum of caste and class groups, the majority of *Sant* devotees are fairly economically disadvantaged.

I have referred to the widespread perception in the subcontinent that blood donation results in a permanent volumetric deficit. According to such a view, giving blood is not so different from donating a kidney – it is lost forever. That so many *Sant* devotees donate their blood would appear to suggest that they have been persuaded by doctors' argument that blood donation is a safe procedure. But this is not the case – and yet they continue to donate their blood. This is because they feel protected from the ill effects of extraction by the blessings of the guru, believing that true devotion results in a replenishment of a substance that would not otherwise occur. What transpires, in other words, is divinized replenishment. As one devotee, having donated, declared to me: "I feel fresher and well. *Shakti* [strength] has come from Baba Ji's [the guru's] blessings. We pray for more blood so we can give again." Another devotee expressed her view that "after seven days Baba [the guru], through his blessings, replaces the blood."

Thus it is not that these devotees differ from the majority of Indians in viewing blood donation as a safe activity but rather that they see themselves as being exempt from the ill effects that would ordinarily ensue. So in my work, I have taken up Lawrence Cohen's (2004) idea of "*as if* modernity." In donating their blood, devotees appear to evince confidence in the claims of medical science about the harmlessness of blood donation to the donor. Many devotees, however, are extremely dismissive of such claims and yet continue to donate precisely *as if* they had undergone a transformation of reason.

Devotees are particularly eager to donate their blood either in the guru's presence or in front of photographs of the guru, since it is from the guru's divine image that his protective blessings are typically thought to emanate: this is called gaining the guru's *darshan*. Blessings derived from vision of the guru are integral to the divinized replenishment I mentioned above.

Devotees say that blessings stream from the guru's eyes and hands. The eyes, in popular Hindu religion, are energy centres and energy transmitters; hence, the meeting of eyes between master and devotee is a moment of dramatic spiritual interaction (Juergensmeyer 1991, 84). Since it is precisely energy that many Indians think blood donation drains from them, it is not surprising that devotees, many of whom remain unconvinced by doctors' claims about the safety of donation, seek a direct connection to the guru's replenishing vision as they donate. Energy, as it were, simultaneously exits and enters through veins and eyes respectively. Devotees "drink" energy through their eyes even as it drains from the prick in their arms.

The ingenuity of blood bank doctors has been in recognizing the power and intensity of the relationship that exists between gurus and their devotees and enlisting it for their own collection ends. Doctors realize that if they are able to persuade particular gurus to endorse blood donation and hold donation events in their devotional centres, they can cut down on the difficult and laborious task of issuing generalized appeals for blood donors from the population at large: once the guru is motivated, recruiters assume that devotees will automatically comply. Doctors treat gurus' devotees as a shortcut method of acquiring blood, the recruitment of the guru constituting the *en masse* recruitment of his many followers.

What I have sought to emphasize in my work, however, is that this is not merely a story of doctors' one-sided appropriation of the guru–devotee relationship in order to fulfill their own requirements. The story, rather, is of the mutually beneficial interdependence, or "interoperability," that exists between *Sant* movements, which employ voluntary donation as a means to enrich and transform the experiential basis of their followers' religious lives, and the project of fostering voluntary (non-remunerated) blood donation, which tactically mobilizes the devotional relationship as a critical source of its blood.

Nirankari devotees treat blood donation as a form of spiritual perfectionism. Central to this is their view that blood giving is an operation with *moral* as well as physical consequences for recipients. Devotees frequently told me that they see their donated blood as a vessel for the conveyance of their moral and affective qualities of love and *gyan* (spiritual knowledge), which they see as forming the basis for patients of transformative transfusions of spirit. The emphasis, as it were, is as much on changing recipients as saving them. Devotees say their love is in their blood; affect is tangible. And this liquid love is adhesive, viscous love which will cause recipients to become attracted to the Nirankaris, despite not knowing from whom the blood they receive is derived. This adhesiveness gives blood donation expansive potential as a subtly transformative means of contributing to the growth of the Nirankari devotional order.

The role of substance in instantiating involuntary conversion – conversion that, so to speak, takes places "beneath the skin" – is well known to Indianist scholars. The final spark that precipitated the 1857 Indian Mutiny is widely believed to have been soldiers' belief that the cartridges provided by the British had been greased with fat from cows and pigs. The soldiers had been told that the object of their foreign masters was to make them all Christians. The first step in the course to Christianity was to deprive them of their caste through the defilement produced by biting greased cartridges. Having become out-caste, they must, in despair, accept the religion of their masters. There are many more recent, similar examples of this highly charged politics of substance. Nirankari devotees say things like: "The recipient will get the gene of a Nirankari and join our group. We can join to his body so he can join this mission." One devotee told me: "We feel love always. We feel love inside and the genes in our blood become loving genes. This loving blood will go to others and affect them so they will also follow truth and love." And an elderly female devotee informed me:

> If there is some sugar in a box, from that box you won't take out chillies, and from a box with chillies in you won't take out sugar. If you have good knowledge (*accha gyan*) then your blood is also good. If you do daily *worship* you are full of god's knowledge, your blood and your heart is pure, and that's why the doctors take it from us.

This assertion that doctors select Nirankari blood for the moral qualities contained therein portrays biomedicine as a project of moral perfectionism.

These are a particularly interesting set of perceptions since they represent a positive revaluation of the politics of substance on the part of devotees. It is well known that in many Hindu villages throughout India, caste boundaries are maintained through restrictions on who eats and drinks with whom (see, e.g., Lambert 2000). It follows from this that the disruption of these restrictions may produce disruptions in status. What the Nirankaris do is to put a very similar logic of substance and transformation to work, but in order to create an opposite, universalizing effect, they want to be related to *everybody*, to draw *anybody* toward themselves through donating their blood. Voluntary blood donation is anonymous: donors do not know to whom their blood travels, and recipients have no idea as to the origins of their transfusions. In donating their blood, Nirankari devotees disseminate their viscous love and spirit into unknowable locales, thereby generating a sense of continual spiritual expansion. The very means of preserving particularity and distinctiveness – restrictions on flows of substance – is subverted by the Nirankaris and made to open up onto the universal.

Transmissibility

But there is a problematic flipside to these ideas about the transformative properties of substance. Anthropologists have presented data from diverse parts of India which show that the receiving of unreciprocated gifts is frequently regarded as an extremely morally ambiguous activity. While acts of giving may demonstrate largesse and kingly qualities, recent Indianist scholarship has drawn attention to the physically and spiritually dangerous consequences for recipients of receiving gifts. Giving is a way of expiating sin, but not in the Christian sense of its being a spiritually uplifting act of charity. Rather, the sins and impurities of donors are objectified in the gift and transferred to recipients. Anthropologists have described how in North Indian villages, inauspicious gifts are given by high- to low-caste groups with the effect of endlessly reinforcing the dominance of the high-caste groupings. One anthropologist has put this particularly graphically: ultimately, the accepting by Brahmin priests in Banaras of pilgrims' gifts will lead to "sin emerg[ing] as excrement vomited at death; it causes the body to rot with leprosy, seeps into the hair, and on death [this sin] makes the corpse particularly incombustible" (Parry 1989, 68–69).

Now, given their potential to threaten life through passing on infection, blood donations seem on one level to literalize such understandings about the dangerous contagiousness of the Indian gift. After all, as the above quotation from Parry indicates, terrible disease is understood by Banaras priests to be the ultimate effect of accepting pilgrims' gifts. However, I do not merely draw an analogy here between the transmission of infection from pilgrims to priests (leprosy, primarily) and that which is all too often transmitted from blood donors to transfusion recipients (AIDS, hepatitis, malaria, and so on). I found evidence that in certain circumstances, the expelling of sin has become an aim of blood donation. The Maharashtrian guru Narendra Maharaj, for instance, encourages his followers to give blood at mass donation events organized precisely in order for his devotees to have an opportunity of removing their sins and "cleansing" themselves. A Delhi-based blood bank doctor provided me with a more detailed example. She told the story of a Sikh man whose wife was suffering from mental illness. He was told by his guru to give three gifts from his body as a means of restoring her sanity. As a Sikh, he did not consider giving his hair. He subsequently attempted to give blood at a Delhi blood bank on three consecutive days. Three months, however, is the officially sanctioned length of time meant to elapse between donations. The man was recognized by blood bank personnel attempting to give for a second time on the second day and barred from making further donations. There is the strong suggestion here that he was attempting to give three gifts of medically usable blood as a means of removing the inauspiciousness afflicting his family. The possibility of removing sin via blood donation would seem to make it attractive to precisely those it most needs to repel (i.e., those who have "sinned" in the conventional senses of engaging in sexual promiscuity or drug use). "*Karmic*" sin potentially collides here with actually transmissible infection. If both the non-material accumulated sins of past actions *and* medically detectable infection are transmissible through blood donation, then the attempt at removing the former obviously heightens the risk of the transmission of the latter – with clearly destructive consequences for transfusion recipients.

There is a further, connected, way in which the devotional approach to blood donation constitutes a problematic kind of "solution" to the shortage of voluntary blood donors. In his classic comparative work on different systems of procuring blood, *The Gift Relationship* (1970), policy analyst Richard Titmuss argued that systems of paid blood donation foster the creation of the "avid donor" – so keen to give that he conceals personal information that, if revealed, would disqualify him from giving. What the Indian situation demonstrates is that such avidness may be fostered not only by material reward but by the desire to build up a store of spiritual merit; in other words, spiritual as well as monetary returns are liable to create the avid donor which Titmuss sees as being so detrimental to the quality of donated blood.

Nirankari devotees' donation fervor was abundantly apparent at each donation event I attended. At one event in north Delhi, a female devotee, on being told of her disqualification on the grounds of low haemoglobin, wept, exclaiming, "Take my blood! Take my blood or I can't go home. Baba Ji says give blood, I must give blood!" At another Nirankari event, a 75-year-old man attempted to give blood. When told that donors must be under 60, he said: "My blood must be taken! Others must live at my expense. What am I? What am I? Take my blood; take my blood, why don't you take my blood?" In an attempt to calm him down, a blood bank technician eventually pricked his finger to produce a drop of blood. (Pricking the fingers of rejected devotee-donors to produce small quantities of blood is a pacification technique practiced by many doctors. It allows disqualified devotees to say that they too have bled for their guru on what they call his day of donation.) Similarly, at an event in New Delhi, a couple in their fifties were both declared ineligible to donate. The man had recently undergone bypass surgery and the woman had recently suffered from jaundice. To the Red Cross doctor who disqualified them, they said: "You are rejecting us

but we will donate today at another blood bank. Today is my guru's day of donation." The exasperated doctor turned to me and said, "They think I have come
here only to reject them. But we do it because it is bad for them as well as the
one who receives the blood. They will suffer too."

Harmonizing denial

What the above examples demonstrate is the obvious point that the blood donor
screening process is designed to eliminate not only donations that would harm
recipients but also donations that would harm donors. Donating blood in the pos-
session of such knowledge carries a suggestion of self-denial. In fact, it would
appear that some donors actually welcome the thought that their physical frail-
ness may make blood donation physically taxing or dangerous for them. They
are thus inclined to treat blood donation as an austerity similar to those practiced
in the form of fasts and other meritorious acts of self-denial. Attempts made by
physically frail devotees to donate are, of course, viewed extremely negatively
by medics. However, if one's priority is to achieve spiritual benefits through
meritorious acts of bodily austerity, such a situation may appear as a welcome
opportunity.[7]

Such self-denial is frowned upon by medics for the obvious reason that it provides an incentive for the medically unfit to donate their blood, and they, wel-
coming it precisely *because* they are unfit to donate, may thereby endanger the
ultimate recipients of their largesse. The irony, however, is that self-denial is a
profoundly important aspect of blood donation "ideology": self-denial is necessary but, in the cases discussed, misplaced. International arbiters of health
policy, such as the World Health Organization (WHO) and the Red Cross, make
specific demands on donors which I see as translating blood donation into a
mode of ascetic practice. The blood donation ideology they espouse requires that
the blood donor enacts self-care as the simultaneous care of the Other (the transfusion recipient). This brand of asceticism is encapsulated in the common exhor-
tatory slogan, "Safe Blood Starts with Me," originally formulated by the WHO,
which has been adopted by various medical authorities and institutions worldwide, including those in India. What it suggests is that donors' conduct and
desires must be subjected to habits of control and self-surveillance. Voluntary
donors, so the slogan implies, must abstain from actions such as drug use or
sexual promiscuity that may lead to the transmission of infection to recipients.
Moreover, the two primary functions of the first World Blood Donor Day, held
on June 14, 2004, were to thank donors and *to promote healthy lifestyles* among
them.

Now consider the tenet, contained in a French Voluntary Blood Donors Code
of Honour, which states: "I declare on my honour to remain worthy of being a
Voluntary Blood Donor, respecting the rules of morality, good behaviour, and
solidarity with fellow human beings" (cited in chapter 4, 84). This French Code
is reminiscent of the formal vows undertaken by initiate renouncers, and the
ideology of voluntary blood donation does indeed make ascetic demands on

donors, with asceticism defined here as "a regime of self-imposed but at the same time authoritatively prescribed and ordered bodily disciplines" (Laidlaw 1995, 151). A key symbol of the Indian renouncer's (or *sannyasi's*) world renunciation is his mastery of sensual desire. Blood donor ascetics must similarly control their desires and pledge – implicitly or explicitly – to enact "responsible" corporeal trusteeship. The following example again recalls the renouncer's vow: when the son of a friend of mine in Delhi turned 18 he made a pledge to donate blood three times a year until the age of 70, recognizing that it is was his responsibility to live healthily and take precautions to avert the causes of hypertension, diabetes, or any other disqualifying condition that could make him an agent of the transmission of infection. To be a blood donor, then, is to enter a subtle complex of duty and obligation – one is asked to safeguard that part of oneself which may become part of another.

The mode of religious asceticism described above in reference to the *Sant* Nirankaris differs from "blood donation asceticism" in that it is undertaken for the purpose of self-perfection and subsequent freedom from rebirth. Blood donation asceticism, conversely, possesses an outward-directed quality: donors engage in bodily discipline for the protection of future possible recipients of their donated blood. And yet there need not be a conflict between these modes of asceticism. The following citation, from an article on attempts to encourage blood donation among Buddhist monks and novices studying at a temple school in Chiang Mai, Thailand, suggests that if the acquisition of spiritual merit courtesy of ascetic procedures is correlated with the *effect* rather than with the *act* of donation, then it may actually help safeguard rather than endanger the safety of donated blood:

> Before a statue of the Buddha, they vow to respect their blood as "community blood" and look after it on behalf of the community or anyone who may need it in the future. As monks and novices, they already practice celibacy so there is little or no risk of infection.... In this way, they are not only assuring a supply of untainted blood, but are also applying traditional values and culture, and indirectly encouraging youth and community members to abstain from any behaviour that could put the "community blood" at risk of infection. And, in accordance with their tradition, they are accumulating merit that could help them in this or future lives.[8]

In this example, what I have called blood donation asceticism (i.e., the requirement of constant moral and physical commitment from donors in order to protect their as yet un-donated blood, which is held in trust for future recipients) is brought into line with the ascetic restraint demanded of Buddhist practitioners. The taking of a solemn vow not to endanger their blood, made before a statue of the Buddha, bears comparison with the Voluntary Blood Donors Code of Honour cited above, which exhorts signatories to remain worthy of being a voluntary blood donor, "respecting the rules of morality, good behaviour and solidarity with human beings." The Buddhist example suggests that merit would ensue less from the specific act of donating blood than from ensuring the safety of transfusion recipients, implying that merit would result from refraining from attempting to donate if, for example, the donor had recently suffered from malaria or hepatitis. Such a configuration of the relationship between merit, act, and effect in a way that foregrounds the enactment of responsibility for transfusion recipients as the very condition of obtaining merit demonstrates how the safety requirements of blood donation and devotees' concern with merit might be fruitfully reconciled. It could in consequence serve as a kind of ascetic template for helping to reorient the engagement of Indian devotional orders like the Nirankaris with blood donation procedures.

Conclusion

In concluding this chapter, I will focus on the role of blood donation at *the end*. What I mean by "blood donation at the end" is a kind of millennial or end-time blood donation. My aim in introducing, at "the end," the idea of end-time blood donation is to leave the reader with a sense of the sheer diversity of religious significance that is being read into practices of blood donation in India. As was seen above, the *Sant* Nirankaris treat blood donation as a form of spiritual perfectionism – as a means of guru-worship and the enactment of sacrificial devotion; what I was witness to, in other words, was the formation of an emergent theology of blood donation. But the *Sant* Nirankari Mission is by no means the only emergent guru-inspired theology which foregrounds blood donation.

Aniruddha Bapu lives in a seven-storey building called Happy Home in an affluent area of Mumbai. His devotees consider him, in their own words, the "highest percentage" incarnation of the god Vishnu since Krishna. Vishnu is the preserver and sustainer of the world. Bapu prophesizes that between 2007 and 2025 there will be untold natural and manmade disasters, brought on by man's wretched moral decline. The world will be seriously threatened but will not end – in 2025 the calamities will cease and "*ramrajya,*" Bapu's heavenly kingdom on earth, will appear. In his weekly spiritual discourses (*pravachan*), he warns his predominantly middle-class devotees that the frequency of disasters is increasing, ready for the deluge of 2007 to 2025, and that only devotion to him will protect them from their ravages.[9] Devotees report his warning: "Whoever follows me will survive – those who do not, I don't know." For Bapu and his devotees, disasters the world over are studied and seen as evidence that the events foretold by Bapu are gathering apace. Mumbai is particularly prone to terrorist attacks, communal riots, and flooding, and it can be no accident that it is here that this theology of disasters has been developed. But disasters further afield are also scrutinized, with the September 11 attacks on New York having attained particular importance both as a sign of what is to come and as a demonstrative example of the need to offer *bhakti* (devotion) to Bapu and obtain his protection: one United States-based devotee is said to have had a job interview planned in the World Trade Center for the morning of September 11, 2001. In a telephone call to Bapu prior to the interview to ask for his advice and blessing, he is reported to have instructed her to cancel the interview, claiming that she would die if she did not. She cancelled it and was "saved."

Bapu's devotees are first in the queue to donate their blood after bomb blasts in Mumbai, but they also donate *in preparation for forthcoming disasters.*[10] As one devotee told me: "We need gallons and gallons of blood for the disasters which are going to come." At a donation event I attended in Mumbai, another donor informed me that "soon there will be rivers of blood flowing so we are donating to get ready for that. This [blood donation] is for 2007: 2007 is the crack point maximum. So many people are going to die, and we can't help that. But those who survive can take our blood." Another devotee told me: "Bapu says, if you donate blood for me once, you will never need to take blood, and neither will your next seven generations." With the prospect of an imminent period of bloodshed and disaster, it is easy to see the appeal of this!

There is a sense in which this focus on forward planning and medical rationality seems to place Bapu and his organization in perfect accord with so-called "scientific modernity." And yet, to say the least, Bapu fosters utility and planning very much on his own terms. If, in broad brush strokes, classical utility may be understood to be largely concerned with production and conservation, conservation is at the heart of Bapu's concerns; *just as with any incarnation of Vishnu – preserver and sustainer of the world – it must be.* In donating their blood – a consummate action of medical conservation – devotees partake of the guru's sustaining role and therefore his divinity. Mumbai's particular proneness to disaster makes it easy to see why its citizens might urgently seek some form of protection – and in this case, it is a spiritual guru who has stepped forward to offer it in "theologized" form. There is more than one orientation to protection presented here: in embracing Bapu, devotees insure themselves against the coming ravages; in donating blood as an act of preparedness, they insure others against them too. In addition, these acts for the protection of others "feed back" spiritually to devotees in a manner which bears a poetic similarity to the action which initially brought it about, with their actions for the protection of others further fortifying them against impending catastrophe.

In this chapter I have tried to give an indication of the ways in which blood donation has developed into a site of religious creativity and dynamism in India. The devotees whom I have discussed harbour a multiplicity of motivations concerning their gifts of blood. I certainly do not claim that they do not ever give with beneficent intentions, that all they are concerned about is expelling sin in the direction of unwitting transfusion recipients. Rather, I have been trying to give a sense of some of the subtle motivations and ideas at play in these contexts, which are certainly not reducible in some simplistic way to *either* giving for personal gain *or* for altruistic reasons. Doctors have been successful in "appropriating" gurus' devotees as a kind of shortcut method of filling large gaps in supply. But this is not the whole story. I have sought to understand the ways in which devotees and their gurus employ a biomedical procedure as a rich corpus of conceptual substance from which to shape their religious lives while also highlighting some problems at the heart of this otherwise productive collaboration, centring on potentially heightened risk (to bother donors and recipients) and wastage.

Notes

1 See previous chapters.
2 *Tribune*, September 25, 2006.
3 www.time.com/time/asia50/c_people.html (last accessed April 14, 2011).
4 See Chapters 3, 10, and 11.
5 The *National Guidebook on Blood Donor Motivation* (Ray 2003), an Indian government publication, estimates India's blood need as eight million units per annum. The constant stream of new, blood-requiring treatment techniques causes this figure to increase year on year. The total annual collection figure, says the *Guidebook*, is four million units, with approximately two million of these units being voluntary donations and two million replacement (Ray 2003, 203). The gap between demand and supply is extremely serious and results in many preventable deaths; however, these are not as many as the figures may suggest – there are several established alternatives to transfusion, and doctors are reported to over-prescribe blood (Bray and Prabhakar 2002, 477).
6 Arnold (1993) records the acute anxieties harboured by many nineteenth-century Indians about the extractive aspects of Western medicine as practiced by their colonial masters.
7 The problem for Nirankari donors is that medical disqualification reveals the body's inability to fulfill the guru's wishes and therefore a lack of spiritual progress. Their gifts of blood are expressions of devotion. Traditionally, in Indian ascetic contexts, the more of a gift that a recipient accepts, the better the regard the recipient is showing for the giver. Acceptance of a gift is therefore a kind of judgment on a donor's general moral probity. It follows that many Nirankari devotees experience physical disqualification as *moral* disqualification. Many scholars have similarly draw attention to a strong correlation between physical and moral states in India (e.g., Osella and Osella 1996: 41). This recalls the interpretation that has been made by homosexuals between physical disqualification and social citizenship exclusion (see Chapter 9).
8 This citation is drawn from a posting by Laurie Maund made on November 11, 2005, to an e-group called SEA-AIDS, hosted by www.healthdev.org/eforums. Its title is "Living Blood Bank: How Thai Buddhist Monks are Helping their Communities Prevent HIV."
9 Other than attending *pravachan*, devotees enact worship through performing a *puja* called *paduka*, involving Bapu's footwear.
10 Most devotees were not aware of blood's perishability: refrigerated red cells expire after 30 days, platelets after six days. Only frozen plasma can last indefinitely.

References

Arnold, D. 1993. *Colonizing the Body: State Medicine and Epidemic Disease in Nineteenth-Century India*. Berkeley: University of California Press.

Bray, T. and Prabhakar, K. 2002. "Blood Policy and Transfusion Practice – India." *Tropical Medicine and International Health* 7(6): 477.

Cohen, L. 2004. "Operability: Surgery at the Margin of the State." In *Anthropology in the Margins of the State*, ed. V. Das and D. Poole, 165–190. Santa Fe: School of American Research Press.

Copeman, J. 2009. *Veins of Devotion: Blood Donation and Religious Experience in North India*. New Brunswick, NJ: Rutgers University Press.

Juergensmeyer, M. 1991. *Radhasoami Reality: The Logic of a Modern Faith.* Princeton, NJ: Princeton University Press.

Laidlaw, J. 1995. *Riches and Renunciation: Religion, Economy, and Society among the Jains.* Oxford: Clarendon Press.

Lambert, H. 2000. "Sentiment and Substance in North Indian Forms of Relatedness." In *Cultures of Relatedness,* ed. J. Carsten, 73–89. Cambridge: Cambridge University Press.

Osella, F. and Osella, C. 1996. "Articulation of Physical and Social Bodies in Kerala." *Contributions to Indian Sociology* 30(1): 37–68.

Parry, J. 1989. "On the Moral Perils of Exchange." In *Money and the Morality of Exchange,* ed. J. Parry and M. Bloch. Cambridge: Cambridge University Press.

Ray, D. 1990. *National Guide Book on Blood Donor Motivation.* Delhi: Directorate General of Health Services, Ministry of Health and Family Welfare, Government of India.

Ray, D. 2003. *National Guidebook on Blood Donor Motivation.* Delhi: National AIDS Control Organisation.

Strathern, A. 1971. *The Rope of Moka: Big-Men and Ceremonial Exchange in Mount Hagen, New Guinea.* Cambridge: Cambridge University Press.

Titmuss, R.M. 1970. *The Gift Relationship: From Human Blood to Social Policy.* London: LSE Books.

Vaudeville, C. 1974. *Kabir,* Vol. 1. Oxford: Clarendon Press.

Part III

The governance of blood donation

The authority of state control

8 Linking medicine, industry, science, and politics

The history of French blood donor deferral criteria[1]

Renaud Crespin and Bruno Danic

Introduction

Selection criteria for blood donors have existed since the beginnings of blood transfusion, but their form, shape, content, and objectives have been largely redefined since the 1950s. In France, this dynamic has been closely linked to a series of health crises, as has been presented in Chapter 4. Since the 1990s, those crises led to profound reforms in the organization and administration of public health (Benamouzig and Besançon 2005). Like other areas of public health, blood transfusion has not escaped this process, since – given the principle of "health safety" – modes of action and activities have been reoriented in line with a logic of preventing risks likely to harm the health of populations (Setbon 2004; Tabuteau 2002).

According to Robert Crawford (2004), this culture of prediction and prevention offers a way of characterizing the "healthicization" of certain areas of activity, especially where such a dynamic is accompanied by individuals being positioned within a frame of collective risk that aims to make them aware of their responsibility in order to anticipate the health hazards associated with various social practices (Barthe and Gilbert 2005; Peretti-Watel and Moatti 2009). This is the case for blood donors. While this type of analysis emphasizes the values and norms conveyed by healthicization, notably in order to underline the insecurity inherent to the desire for a safer world, it neglects the instruments and techniques by which this healthicization is concretely operationalized. To propose a history of blood donor selection instruments is therefore to attempt to understand how this healthicization has colonized blood donation, in particular by using epidemiology to redefine the hazards associated with this practice (Berlivet 2001). It is also an attempt to describe certain effects that healthicization has had on the process of defining exclusions, while acknowledging that this translation cannot be ascribed solely to public health professionals (Williams 2004).

In this text, we will approach the history of the deferral criteria of potential blood donors as that of a dynamic of instrumentation (Lascoumes and Le Galès 2007), which means that we will concentrate on the problems raised by the choice and use of the tools, standards, and techniques that allow donor selection to be effected. This approach will lead us to distinguish between the successive regimes' having developed the standards that are used as frameworks for the selection of donation candidates and to award (or withhold) them donor status. This approach extends an invitation to focus on those spaces, players, knowledge, and techniques that mobilize (or are mobilized) in this production process (Hacking 2001). The notion of regime will allow us to analyze how various clinical, biological, epidemiological, and political trends have gradually been "superimposed" within this framework, resulting in its current form. Grasping this dynamic of instrumentation is therefore inseparable from analyzing the movements of actors, knowledge, disciplines, and standards that have marked the standardization process for this instrument of public action (Crespin 2009).

For the past 50 years, the medical device for selecting blood donors, constructed as a list of situations that serve to exclude people from blood donation, has been constantly reinforced. Today, it is complementary to the biological selection of collected blood as well as to the various physical and chemical techniques capable of inactivating transmissible agents potentially present in blood products.[2] In France, the donor selection process is supported by the affirmation of the free and voluntary nature of blood donation, written into law on January 4, 1993.

Although this text seeks mainly to discuss the medical selection of blood donation candidates, our analysis cannot be undertaken without reference to those developments that have marked biological selection. Today, in France, the process of medically selecting blood donors comprises a series of three steps: the first involves pre-donation information; the second entails completion of a questionnaire preparing the potential donor for a medical interview geared toward preventing transfusion-related incidents and accidents, as well as adverse reactions resulting from the collection of blood; the third and final step is the provision of post-donation information, asking the donor to contact the *Établissement Français du Sang* (EFS)[3] in case of any event following the donation (infection or other medical event, whether or not it is linked to the donation) or of any uncertainty about answers given during the medical interview (Danic and Beauplet 2003). In the course of these three steps, the donor is asked several sets of questions aimed at reducing uncertainty surrounding the situation of the donation for the transfusion system (Chalas *et al.* 2009). The medical selection may thus be seen as an apparatus in a sense close to that given by Michel Foucault (Rabinow and Rose 2003): namely a social, material, and technical assemblage aiming (in our case) to identify the risks surrounding the donor and future donation. This identification is achieved through a brief clinical examination and questions regarding the donor's lifestyle, state of health, and health history. The content of the exams and questions is defined on the basis of a framework of exclusion criteria whose form (involving what standards?) and content (involving what knowledge?) will be examined in this text.

To account for the construction of deferral criteria is also to reflect on the process by which a health agency operator, such as the EFS, administratively produces policy using medical and biological categories that must be deciphered (Fassin 1998; Rose and Novas 2005).

From early practice to "mass" blood donation: toward standardization of deferral criteria

Since initial practices involved acts of urgent surgery, the question of supply has been central ever since the very beginnings of transfusion: the intent was to avoid the death of a parturient, or an injured soldier as a result of losing blood, around the end of the nineteenth century, then during World War I (Picard and Schneider 1996). Transfusion practices (very marginal during this war, and used only in a few dozen cases) involved a medical-technical method referred to as "arm-to-arm," in which the donor – often a fellow soldier or health professional – was directly and physically connected to the recipient. Transfusion was also limited by blood clotting in the device. The risk of transmitting infectious diseases (e.g., syphilis and malaria) was soon identified, but the priority was to save the patient's life in a desperate situation.[4] The first transfusions used a technique of direct transfusion requiring anastomosis between the radial artery of the donor and the vein of the recipient. The risk taken by the donor fully justified the "sacrificial" description of these first altruistic acts.

In the 1920s, emergency transfusion continued to dominate the first civil practices, developed in Paris. The donor's "physical and moral" appearance was the chief criterion for selection, in order to reassure the patient directly receiving blood from a stranger. In addition to asking donors to provide a sworn declaration regarding their state of health, the hospital implemented a medical examination every three months to ensure continued donor ability. In the 1950s, arm-to-arm transfusion was officially abandoned, thus establishing distance between the recipient and the point of blood collection. Early techniques exposed donors to significant vascular and infectious risk, and as a result of this – and also because of the fear of scarcity of blood induced by rapidly increasing demand – more attention was gradually paid to donors. This donor centrality also arose out of legal proceedings in the wake of syphilis contaminations. Indeed, following these disputes, donors would be required to "loyally provide untainted blood" – making any contamination an offense establishing the right to compensation (Hermitte 1996).[5] Thus challenged, blood transfusion was forced to structure donor selection. This was to be accomplished in May 1956, when, for the first time, a decree set out the rules and modalities governing donor selection.

At that time, regulations focused selection toward "screening illnesses that exclude from the giving of blood." This consisted of a clinical examination, biological tests, and the consideration of certain social practices.[6] In the 1960s, exclusion regulations were again updated by various notices issued by the *Commission consultative de la transfusion sanguine*, integrating developments arising out of advances in new blood collection techniques. This prescriptive framework did not, however, impose country-wide standardized procedures.

Indeed, the autonomy granted to various blood transfusion centres (*Centres de Transfusion Sanguine* (CTS)) led them to use this prescriptive framework to define their own selection criteria according to their experiences and demand for blood products. It is worth noting that the chief safety concern at the time was still to have the blood available in order to provide transfusions to patients.

Since the 1950s, there has been a massive rise in blood collection, fuelled by increasing demand for blood products. From 137,000 donations in 1950, the figure rose to nearly 3.5 million in 1971 and some four million in 1974. In the mid-1970s, these new needs led the health system to engage in a veritable industrialization of its production, even as it adapted to improved quality and safety standards that raised questions about its organization, as well as to the definition of country-wide norms and standards.[7]

As the 1970s drew to a close, a reflection began on how to harmonize collection practices and redefine selection guidelines for blood donation. This work was initiated on the sidelines of the official blood transfusion organizations within the *Amicale du Groupement des Responsables des Prélèvements* (AGERP). This association brought together a number of doctors in charge of collection services who, while belonging to various CTS, shared both professional experience and similar questions as to their professional practice. Within this association, a study group – the *Groupe d'Études et de Recherches sur le Prélèvement* (GERP) – was established at the initiative of two collection coordinators: Charles Aubert of the Créteil CTS and Alain Beauplet of the Rennes CTS, who were introduced by Bernard Genetet, then director of the Rennes CTS. The original kernel, composed of a dozen individuals, soon expanded to include other collection coordinators and held regular meetings. The objective was to promote collection in order to confer new legitimacy on those involved in it. To do so, the GERP channelled energy into a rationalization process aimed at harmonizing attitudes to be adopted toward donors and at standardizing collection procedures through the use of documented protocols. One of the first goals of the GERP meetings was the development of a model questionnaire that could be addressed to all donors presenting at a CTS. The questionnaire emerged from a simple question that arose during group discussions: Why did some CTSs turn away certain donors, whereas others accepted them, and how could this discrepancy be resolved?

It was not long before this work attracted the interest of the *Société Nationale de Transfusion Sanguine* (SNTS). Indeed, it was back in the early 1980s that the SNTS had put together a small group of executive members and collection coordinators; this group was also in charge of creating a "one size fits all" questionnaire. Originally piloted by B. Habibi and M. Chassaigne (Tours), the group also included A. Beauplet. Between 1982 and 1984, M. Beauplet's membership of both groups fostered exchanges. GERP brought to the table its experience and know-how, especially with regard to the complex problem of formulating questions and limiting their number in order to arrive at a questionnaire that was truly effective. The SNTS, for its part, was interested in taking advantage of the expertise of the GERP practitioners in order to be able to harmonize practices at national level. In 1983, this dialogue led to the creation of the *Donneur Santé Publique* (GDSP) group within the *Société Française de Transfusion Sanguine* (SFTS), chaired by A. Beauplet and composed of several members of the GERP.

Beginning in the early 1980s, the process of developing the guidelines and questionnaire picked up speed, spurred on by a circular (June 20, 1983) advocating the self-exclusion of potential blood donors at risk of developing AIDS. This work continued until 1989, which saw the publication of what is known as the "first monograph" that was to serve as a common framework for donor selection guidelines. In concrete terms, how were these criteria developed? First, the process took account of problems encountered in the field by those performing pre-donation interviews. At the time, these interviews were conducted by medical students, based on the medical consultation model. The donor was approached for a diagnosis. The pre-donation interview was constructed as a medical observation, which was the only reference available to students, who transferred to blood collection what they had learned in hospitals. Once the donor diagnosis was complete, the student was able to reflect on the potential blood-borne transmissibility of any observed pathologies. For example, could the presence of cancer cells, allergies, auto-immune diseases, or medical treatments constitute deferral criteria from donation? Could the collection of blood from an individual presenting a given pathology lead to medical risks that could disrupt the collection site? The GERP members addressed these questions and reasoned from a clinical standpoint, constructing their arguments based on donor pathology rather than known transfusion risks. For each of the pathological situations identified by the study group, a letter was addressed to one or more academic physicians specializing in this pathology, asking them about possible risk for donor and/or recipient. The answers thus obtained were used to develop deferral criteria. The GERP carried out most of this work, although there were regular exchanges with SFTS "donor" and "retrovirus" groups. It was in this context of exchanges between several SNTS groups that "a global conception of transfusion safety" was developed, with an emphasis on biological knowledge.[8]

The method used had multiple consequences for both the form and content of deferral criteria. First, it led to an increase in their number since, in the event of an absence of information or any uncertainty as to what effects a pathology diagnosed in the donor might have in either recipient or donor, the donor was turned away and the pathology became inconsistent with blood donation. A single case could lead to a criterion of deferral.[9] This clinical reasoning was therefore only indirectly consistent with the orientation of preventing risks among recipients, since it was the donor-centred clinic that served as the foundation for developing deferral criteria.

This primacy given to the clinic was tempered by the 1983 circular, which introduced the notion of epidemiological criteria. The circular stemmed from a report on the state of available knowledge on AIDS and blood transfusion, requested from the SNTS by the *Commission Consultative de la Transfusion Sanguine* (CCTS). Presented on June 9, 1983, the findings of the report adopted a nuanced position on transfusion risks. Based on observations made in the

United States, it referred to a "possibility of interhuman transmission by blood and certain blood products." According to the authors, in the absence of documented cases, "the risk of AIDS transmission in France by transfusion [was] not based on any tangible data," except with regard to hemophiliacs (Habibi *et al.* 1983). Nevertheless, given the gravity of AIDS and the absence of a specific test, an attitude of caution was adopted. The authors underscored the need to identify at-risk donors by using a clinical exam aimed at identifying homosexual, drug addicted, and African- or Haitian-origin populations, as well as those who had made trips to Africa or Haiti.

Following the report, discussions at the CCTS revealed that the questionnaire had become an awkward issue for those in charge of transfusion. Points of view clashed regarding whether an information note should be provided or whether donors should be questioned directly. This last option raised concerns, since it ran the risk of undermining blood drives, not only because of the sexual dimension of the questionnaire, with which medical students and doctors were unfamiliar, but also because of potential accusations of racism. A work group was formed to prepare the circular. Signed by Director General of Health Jacques Roux and published on June 20, 1983, the circular referred to the "suspected, but not established" transmission of an infectious agent likely to be responsible for AIDS. It also stated that in the absence of a test, the CTS had to take donor selection measures and ask potential donors to declare whether they belonged to at-risk groups: persons with clinical signs indicative of AIDS; homosexual or bisexual individuals with multiple partners; intravenous drug addicts; and persons originating from Haiti or equatorial Africa, as well as the sexual partners of individuals belonging to any of these groups.

For various reasons, these epidemiological criteria were poorly applied or not applied at all.[10] Moreover, subsequent regulatory texts – and especially the 1986 decree – did not reintroduce epidemiological criteria, remaining limited to the definition of a medical exam, clinical approach, and medical contraindications to donating blood; this last term in fact inspired the title of the monograph published in 1989.

1991 to 1996: the advent of health security and the primacy of the recipient

A pivotal period began in 1991 with the profound reorganisation of the transfusion system as a result of a series of health crises relating to epidemics in human immunodeficiency virus (HIV) and hepatitis C virus (HCV).[11] The beginning of the contaminated blood affair was marked by the publication of the Casteret article in *L'évènement du jeudi* magazine, as well as the 1992 report of the *Inspection Générale des Affaires Sociales* (IGAS) on HCV and the works of Aquilino Morelle (Morelle *et al.* 1992; Morelle 1993) and Michel Setbon (Setbon 1993), which directly questioned the system used to select donors. This context of suspicion and mistrust toward transfusion resulted in a dramatic fall in demand for blood products. In December of the same year, the French blood agency (AFS), created in 1992, added new criteria concerning the prevention of Creutzfeldt-Jakob disease (CJD) transmission because of iatrogenic cases diagnosed in people who had been treated with the human growth hormone. At the same time, the AFS produced regulations called "good collection practices," in reference to the "good manufacturing practices" of the pharmaceutical industry. This process led to the 1994 publication of a second edition of the monograph published in 1989. Consistent with the need for health security characterizing the reorganization of the health system and the creation of health agencies (Benamouzig and Besançon 2005), this new monograph made safety of the transfusion chain the central axiom of selection. Even so, is it possible – in light of the reasoning adopted, knowledge used, and players who took part in redefining the deferral criteria – to refer to this as a second regime for the production of exclusions?

The first element of note in this regard is the reinforcement of logic of donor exclusion, supported by views that were critical of the clinical arguments on which the criteria had been based up until then. This criticism was not really new, since it began to emerge as soon as biological screening tests for HIV (1985) and HCV (1990) were brought into use by the transfusion system. This criticism focused, for example, on the fact that existing selection systems based on essentially clinical criteria were unable to identify contaminated individuals. Within the transfusion system, the identification of a few cases only served to reinforce the uncertain nature of selection primarily based on human observation. Thanks to the tests, some of the uncertainty was lifted, since the human aspect of selection was complemented by the scientific objectivity underpinning biological knowledge and techniques. As a result, right from their very first use, these tests and their results enabled the population of donors to be labelled "at risk" and constituted a form of quality control for clinical selection, by revealing that donors were not being selected using valid criteria. The biological tests not only revealed risks faced by recipients but also became instruments for guaranteeing the safety of recipients – and of the transfusion chain. In addition, the biological analyses performed on blood donations using the tests bore out epistemological data showing that certain donor populations exhibited more risk than others – in particular, drug users and men having sex with other men (MSM).

By scientifically validating the existence of at-risk populations, biological knowledge and instruments legitimized epidemiology, all the while contributing to discrediting the existing systems, founded on the clinical selection of donors. Giving blood thus became less of a risk for a donor who was now "at risk" than for a recipient whose health and safety were the new priority of a transfusion system that needed to ensure its own sustainability. It may be hypothesized that this discrediting of clinical knowledge and systems reinforced the social and professional discrediting of clinicians within the transfusion community.

Out of concern for health security, those who collected blood were handed the mission of compensating for the sensitivity-related flaws of the tests; that is, addressing the problem posed by the window period for seroconversion. From the beginning, this objective proved extremely difficult or impossible for the clinical system of donor selection for two reasons. First, how was it possible to establish zero risk, validated by the absence of a marker of infection in a blood donation, when exposure may have occurred unbeknownst to the donor candidate, in the context of an at-risk relationship in the past? Second, how was it possible to clinically identify subjects during a seroconversion period[12] when these subjects did not show specific clinical signs? The other difficulty was that this requirement was addressed to the clinic in the context of a reorganization of the collection system that was aimed at reinforcing medicalization, whereby donor selection was now entrusted to donation physicians. While such physicians were sometimes students who, having worked in CTS, now sought to become specialized in this area of activity, newcomers most often had professional backgrounds that were unrelated to transfusion. In many cases, the decision to enter the field of donation medicine had more to do with a shortage of alternative hospital positions than any particular sense of vocation. Most donation physicians began working in this field before being completely trained for an occupation that was subject to procedures for ensuring the safety of the transfusion chain.

In sum, in a context of successive health crises, criticism aimed at the clinical selection of donors had consequences at several levels. Biological knowledge gradually became the yardstick for transfusion safety. This standard appeared to be *the* solution since, free of the subjectivity of clinical interpretation, it was based on objective results produced by scientific screening instruments. Clinical practice endured but was accorded a place only by default. Within the context of the health safety framework, it was justified only because biology alone could not identify which donors had entered a seroconversion window period. The clinic was also subservient to the health safety imperative by becoming scientifically equipped to identify at-risk donors as "objectively" as possible. The medical selection system thus gradually adopted the tools and knowledge of epidemiology, such as the category of "at risk" groups.

A further consequence was the revision, as a matter of urgency, of the 1989 framework and the publication (June, 1994) of the second edition of the *Guide to Medical Contraindications to Blood Donation*. Article L.668–3 of the act, dated January 4, 1993, concerning health in matters of blood transfusion and medication,[13] stated that "blood establishments must be equipped with good practices whose principles are defined by a regulation set forth by the AFS, approved by decree of the Ministry of Health and published in the *Journal Officiel de la République française.*" The act was finally published on January 30, 1993, with the decree being issued on September 22, 1993, and featuring the "good practices" in an appendix. Blood establishments (or ETS) were to comply with the directive within six months. These "good practices" mandated that the SNTS' "monograph of contraindications to blood donation" must serve as the reference for donor selection. Yet this monograph had not been revised since 1989. Owing to a lack of expertise from outside the AFS, it was the *Groupe Donneurs Santé Publique* that was commissioned by public authorities to undertake this revision. The group included a large number of GERP members, including its president,

A. Beauplet. The urgency generated by the succession of health crises was therefore compounded by the need to revise deferral criteria. This urgency may be explained by two factors.

First, in keeping with the wishes of the French Ministry of Health Cabinet, the criteria had to be available prior to the date of enforcement of the decree. Moreover, they had to be fully consistent with the "health safety" framework advocated by the new political majority elected in March 1993. In addition, for GERP members, it was an important issue, since it added weight to their work of rationalizing blood collection activities while taking full advantage of the legitimacy conferred by the law. However, the revision got off to a poor start. The clinicians and specialists called upon in drawing up the first monograph no longer cared to answer the questions asked of them by the GERP. The context of the contaminated blood affair, in which medical knowledge was publicly called into question, discouraged the participation of medical scholars contacted by the GERP during the writing of the first monograph. In the absence of expertise from these scholars, GERP members used whatever means remained available in order to proceed.

This process could be analyzed as something of a "*mise en rapport*" effort as conceptualized by Florian Charvolin (1993). This concept, which may be translated into English as "putting things into relation," means that the GERP, as a group, had to assemble heterogeneous and spatially dispersed disciplinary knowledge, as well as develop a document that could be used as a reference for donor selection. GERP members used three tactics in this process. First, they drew upon databases and available scientific bibliographies published in specialized periodicals and other works. Although these bibliographies sometimes proved very old, these references granted access to American blood transfusion standards as well as to the work of epidemiologists dealing with viral and microbial risks.[14] The use of this body of scientific literature and expertise aimed to meet the health security imperative by scientifically drawing up deferral criteria in order to make them more objective. The second tactic (closely related to the first) was to give a more prominent place to experiences in other countries. Lastly, GERP members leveraged networks of clinicians with whom they were familiar, even establishing friendships.

The "second monograph," published in June 1994, was twice as long as the 1989 version. Thanks to a genuine effort to find solutions through a sort of meta-analysis of existing literature, more than 80 deferral criteria were elaborated, with a strong focus on safety and security, aimed at demonstrating that the recipient was to receive significantly closer attention. "Clinical reasoning" once again endured, while being scientifically supported and reoriented toward safety of the recipient, in line with the principle of precaution – the operational matrix for the health security imperative (Borraz 2008). Epidemiology was introduced, though only in the annexes. It remained absent from the body of the text, in which the "methodology by methodology, pathology by pathology" approach was not questioned.

The salient feature to note in this second regime is that the uncertainty linked to a crisis of confidence in blood transfusion was expressed through a decrease in the demand for blood products and the reversal of certain principles that had prevailed in the development and use of deferral criteria for blood donation. In the space of a few years, a shift was made from the primacy of the donor to that of the recipient. According to this new logic, the recipient became the party that needed to be "protected" in order to both ensure the quality of blood donations and stimulate demand, with a view to ensuring the sustainability of the transfusion system. As a result, the donor became the focus of fresh attention (not to say suspicion): the donor was to be supervised and controlled.

Multiplication of regulatory spaces and actors: new constraints in the development of selection criteria?

As of 1995, the *Groupe Donneurs Santé Publique* of the AFS ceased to hold meetings, though the reflection on and construction of donor exclusion criteria continued in other spaces and integrated other arguments. In 1997, the fact that a potential donor had previously received a transfusion was turned into a permanent deferral from blood donation. The reasoning here was specific. Following on from works undertaken by the *Comité de suivi de la sécurité transfusionnelle*, the permanent deferral of transfusion recipients marked a break from the clinical reasoning that had prevailed up until then and resembled a form of hybridization between biological and epidemiological reasoning and knowledge.[15] Although no connection was ever mentioned, this measure was taken during the emergence of the variant of Creutzfeld-Jacob disease and was implicitly based on a statistical modelling of the spread of HCV between the late 1960s and early 1990s. As fears of seeing this disease transmitted by transfusion grew, the risk assessment remained theoretical and pursued two objectives: first, to avoid worrying deferred donors; and second, to learn more about the role of transfusion in the transmission of CJD.

The exclusion of donation recipients was mainly a precautionary measure, since the reasoning behind this exclusion was to lower a risk that had yet to materialize, based on a hypothetical construction: what was needed was to turn away a population with theoretically higher than average risks of being exposed to a blood-borne agent, so as to break the potential chain of blood-borne transmission. This measure had two chief consequences for the public health management of transfusion risks. First, it implicitly legitimized the concept of modelling a risk, which assumed the feasibility of managing transfusion safety by anticipating emerging risks. Second, by legitimizing the notion of a "sentinel population," it enabled justification (by biological science rather than epidemiology alone) of the exclusion of populations said to be "at risk." This second consequence thus constitutes a major obstacle to any evolution toward the notion of "at-risk behaviours" in order to draw up, or revise, certain deferral criteria concerning homosexual men.

In the 2000s, the development of deferral criteria generated new decision-making paths. In December 2000, to address the experimental transmission of bovine spongiform encephalopathy in sheep, the State Secretariat for Health imposed the deferral from blood donation of persons having resided in the British Isles for a total of more than one year between 1980 and 1996. This decision was based on proposals from a group of experts brought together by the AFSSAPS (*Agence Française de Sécurité Sanitaire des Produits de Santé*, now renamed ANSM).

In 2002, at the initiative of EFS President Christian Charpy, a work group proceeded to revise the deferral criteria. This revision led to elaborating a new framework that was to be the first internal reference document produced by the EFS: the *Document Referencing ContraIndications* (DRCI). Development of the new framework was entrusted to the new president of the GDSP[16] Gilles Folléa, in a context marked by the growing protest against the ban preventing male homosexuals from giving blood.

In October 2000, a number of organizations fighting AIDS and defending individual freedoms contested the contents of certain internal EFS information documents for blood donors, which put homosexuality, prostitution, and drug use on the same level as grounds for permanent deferral from blood donation. Taking a stand in the fight against discrimination, these associations asked the EFS for explanations, as well as for replacement of the "at-risk population" category by that of "at-risk practice" in order to select donors. To contain this growing protest, C. Charpy responded to the associations by saying that, given that the length of the pre-donation medical interview could not exceed ten minutes, it was difficult for the doctor to assess the private behaviours of each donor. A commitment was nevertheless made to review the writing of these documents and to redefine exclusion criteria for blood donation. At the end of 2001, the contents of pre-donation information were placed under review by the *Comité Consultatif National d'Éthique*, which, in a notice issued in early 2002, recommended that the EFS avoid stigmatizing male homosexuality in its literature.[17]

In spite of all this, the DRCI – rather than revising previous elements – remained consistent with previously adopted reasoning, proving to be a vehicle for scientific consolidation of deferral patterns. Indeed, neither biology nor epidemiology clearly replaced clinical reasoning. However, knowledge and data stemming from these disciplines developed the scientific baggage used to elaborate deferral criteria. In conformity with the new expert determination which, in health agencies, was intended to guarantee greater transparency, the approach adopted by the new EFS/SFTS work group was above all to "document" guidelines by establishing the traceability of references used as grounds for scientific justification of exclusions. Once again, the mining or extraction of solutions from various available bibliographies was the primary method used to reference experiences in other countries and to underline the difficulty of transposing them in France.[18] This "putting into relation" also implied specifically writing down criteria that would, henceforth, need to conform to the standards of new administrative and scientific procedures in matters of health expertise.[19] Ultimately, the DRCI did not revise any existing criteria[20] and, according to G. Folléa, took up "95% of the work of the GDSP presided by Alain Beauplet." In 2006, the DRCI would be revised in order to integrate a European directive dating back to 2004.[21] Although compliance with the European text was the key issue in this revision, the revision process involved two phases. The first concerned a politicization of deferral policy following a public controversy as to the legitimacy of some of these criteria. The second concerned standardization through a relocation of the decision-making process into new spaces, establishing the role of agencies and the weight of health arguments in producing deferrals guidelines.

As in 2002, the revision process opened with the issue of MSM exclusion. In February 2006, the *Haute Autorité de Lutte contre les Discriminations et pour l'Egalité* stated that "it appears the decision to definitively exclude a person from giving blood must be taken based on risks arising from their behaviour" rather than sexual orientation. Seizing the opportunity of the integration of the European directive referring to "behaviour" rather than to "at-risk population," several associations publicly reaffirmed their opposition to using this epidemiologically based category to justify exclusion from blood donation (Rose and Novas 2005). This criticism was underpinned by two levels of argument. The first denounced the social prejudices of epidemiology: were homosexuals the only ones to engage in at-risk behaviors? The second drew on legal arguments: the exclusion of homosexuals was stigmatizing and discriminatory. In May 2006, developing this criticism, former minister and socialist deputy Jack Lang addressed a letter to Minister of Health Xavier Bertrand in which he requested openness to blood donation from homosexuals and a reconsideration of grounds for exclusion, so that these might be based on the criterion of "at-risk behaviours" and would no longer stigmatize a population or sexual orientation.

On May 17, 2006, the Minister of Health answered that he had not only requested the opinions of numerous experts but had also brought together, along with his Cabinet, a number of associations representing the gay community as well as members of the EFS, the AFSSAPS, and the Ministry of Health. Noting that the principle of transfusion safety remained crucial, the Minister refuted the idea of discrimination, stating that homosexuality did not "in itself constitute a criterion for deferral from blood donation," since experts fixed deferral criteria on epidemiological, rather than sociological, grounds. The available epidemiological data showed that the prevalence of HIV infection in the active male homosexual population was 12.3 percent, in contrast with 0.2 percent in the general population. He concluded that it was not homosexuality itself but rather sexual relations between men that constituted a deferral from blood donation.

Consultations continued through the spring. On July 11, 2006, just as the presidential campaign was beginning, Xavier Bertrand, in an interview for *Le Monde* newspaper, stated that permanent exclusion targeting "MSM" seemed unsatisfactory to him, since it stigmatized "de facto a population rather than behaviours. It will therefore disappear." He also added that he intended "to avoid future reference to *at-risk populations* in favour of *at-risk sexual practices*," particularly in the questionnaire. This position allowed Xavier Bertrand to adopt a posture as a defender of rights and as an opponent of discrimination. It met with disagreement from a number of agencies opposed to abolishing the principle of deferral in the absence of data on the consequences for health safety. Faced with a deadlock, public authorities delayed, deciding that the appendix to the 2004 European directive would have to be subject to a ministerial order and adopted through regulations.

After the presidential election, Roselyne Bachelot, the new Minister of Health, followed up on the regulation process. The AFSSAPS, which up until this point had seemed to wish to draw on the FDA model, resolved to limit itself to giving a mere opinion on the ministerial order, as set out in its regulatory texts. On the initiative of the Ministry, an ad hoc group of experts was formed, representing the main agencies and organizations concerned by blood transfusion (EFS, *Centre de Transfusion Sanguine des Armées* (CTSA), *Institut National de la Transfusion Sanguine* (INTS), AFSSAPS, *Institut National de Veille Sanitaire* (INVS), and the Ministry of Health).

Within this new, exclusive space of expertise, two main questions guided debates on the consequences of opening blood donation to men who, in the official terminology, "had sex with men" (MSM). The first of these focused on the risk this represented for transfusion safety: would such an opening not run the risk of increasing the number of contamination cases, creating uncertainty within and around the health security system? The second question was based on the observation that systematically deferring MSM was a misunderstood, poorly accepted, and above all circumvented criterion for selection.

Indeed, the available data showed that between 2005 and 2008, half of HIV seroconversion cases discovered on the occasion of a blood donation involved donors who acknowledged that they had engaged in homosexual practices only when told by EFS doctors that they were HIV positive. These figures were a source of concern, in particular for the EFS.[22] The second question was therefore to find out whether better compliance by MSM might be achieved by modifying the content of the pre-donation questionnaire; that is, no longer asking donors about their belonging to a group considered "of itself" to be "at risk," but rather about at-risk behaviours, which would have to be specified. This last question appeared all the more legitimate, since it seemed to comply with the approach promoted by the European directive, which called for the deferral of behaviours deemed to be "high risk."

In the ensuing discussions, available epidemiological data proved decisive in understanding – at least in part – the decision ultimately adopted. Indeed, the yearly analysis of HIV-positive discoveries performed by INVS showed that the incidence of HIV infection diagnosis was about 200 times higher in the male homosexual population, in comparison with the heterosexual population (Cazein 2009). The prevalence of HIV infection reached 18 percent in meeting places in Paris (enquête Prevagay 2009), in contrast with 0.2 percent in the general population. The model proposed by INVS concluded that there was a risk of one to four additional transfusion-related contamination cases per year, out of three million donations. Based on this epidemiological data, the Minister's office, with the approval of the Ministry of Health, came to a decision and justified the maintainance

of permanent deferral for MSM. Yet it seems worth considering that public interventions by patient associations also played a role in maintaining the status quo.
This was, for example, the case of the *Association Française des Hémophiles*,
which publicly reiterated the Minister's responsibility were new contamination
cases to arise.[23]

In 2011, during the last French presidential campaign, the debate took on new
momentum when socialist candidate François Hollande made an electoral
promise that he would allow homosexuals to give blood. Once elected, this
promise was reaffirmed on World Blood Donor Day, June 2012, by the new
Health Minister Marisol Touraine, who declared that the "sexual orientation criterion is not in itself a risk" and that she would be working toward moving this
situation forward in the coming months. In December 2012, seemingly in antici-
pation of a resolution from the Council of Europe, the Minister did a U-turn: "as
long as no-one gives me an absolute guarantee that this will not result in
increased risk for those who receive transfusions, I am unable to lift this ban."
These words have attracted fierce criticism from homosexual organizations, yet
they are close to the resolution passed by the Committee of Ministers of the
Council of Europe on March 27, 2013.

Based on the findings of experts, this resolution recognizes that although
certain behaviours do not carry any risk, it is first of all necessary to be able to
scientifically prove the absence of risk prior to establishing – as the UK did in
2011 – a principle of temporary rather than permanent exclusion of MSM. In
France, public action continues as we await new scientific data. This essentially
entails calling upon two sources of expertise. The first of these is via the parliamentary channel: in March 2013, Jean-Marc Ayrault, Prime Minister, entrusted
a young doctor and socialist representative with conducting a reflection on the
overall organization of the blood supply chain in line with the ethical (voluntary,
altruistic, free-of-charge) principles of self-sufficiency and health security. The
report submitted in mid-July 2013 suggests a sort of compromise between the
electoral promise and the European resolution: on the one hand, it recommends
an end to the focus on donor sexual orientation in favour of using the questionnaire to identify individual high-risk behaviour; and, on the other hand, it considers exclusion from donation, unless scientifically founded, to be potentially
perceived as discriminatory. The second source of expertise called upon is that
of the National Consultative Ethics Committee (CCNE), which has been asked
to provide an opinion on elements that might enable a regulatory framework for
the opening of blood donation to MSM. Caution should be exercised, especially
given that the CCNE's conclusions (regardless of what they may be) will have to
be discussed with all blood transfusion stakeholders in a configuration, which
will be specified only once the CCNE has submitted its conclusions.

Although the political decision seems to have been handed back to expert and
scientific opinion, the issue of blood donation for male homosexuals may yet
find resolution in the legal system. Indeed, in a decision of October 1, 2013, the
Administrative Tribunal of Strasbourg deferred ruling on a case in which a donor
has brought an action against the EFS after having been refused the option of

giving blood on grounds of homosexuality. Prior to making its ruling, the Strasbourg Tribunal is waiting for the Court of Justice of the European Union (CJEU) to issue its interpretation of Directive 2004/33/CE of the European Parliament and of the Council, on which the order of January 12, 2009 (specifying donor selection criteria), is based. The CJEU will then have to interpret the directive on the two categories for exclusion from blood donation it establishes: temporary and permanent. The question is whether French application of this directive – which has always considered MSM to belong in the permanent exclusion category – is just or unfounded.

What are the salient features in this last regime? First, we can observe that political authorities regained control over the deferral criteria decision-making process. The state has emerged as the ultimate guarantor of health safety in the name of a principle of precaution – a principle that did not prevent policy action. Indeed, public authorities continued to take action in a situation of uncertainty with regard to the European directive, while integrating considerations other than scientific expertise alone, since the demands of associations were taken into as well as, it would seem, structured debate between experts were taken into account in the decision-making process. And yet, this expertise was exercised in an ad hoc and confined space in which the only actors present were those responsible for the management of transfusion risks. Is it really possible to speak of an extension of expertise to outside protagonists, based on the models proposed by the designers and promoters of technical and health democracies, in order to improve understanding or educate the public about decisions in these areas (Callon *et al.* 2001; Tabuteau 2008)? It is important to note that the principle of precaution did not lead the political world to distance itself from the advice of experts but rather, on the contrary, to use it to enlist science in justifying a decision that rested not only on assessing health risks but also on anticipating the political risks taken in the event of contamination (Borraz 2008).

In sum, it appears that a democratization of health-related decisions results less from the procedure of making health decisions itself than from the effects of the publicity now accorded to debates between experts (Granjou 2007). This publicity – or public "staging" – of debates offers a way of ensuring acceptance of a decision from which various concerned ministers stand to obtain undeniable political gain. It allows them to appear responsive to the demands made by associations while presenting themselves as being at the forefront of a struggle against discrimination that may be sanctioned by law. By basing themselves on epidemiological expertise that, thanks to science, neutralizes potential ideological confrontations, it also authorizes them to show themselves to be guarantors and protectors of health – which constitutes a powerful legitimizing tool in political action (Fassin 1996; Dodier 2003).

Conclusion

This examination of regimes for developing deferral criteria from blood donation has highlighted the distribution and hierarchy of knowledge in order to grasp the evolving dynamic of the medical selection apparatus, as well as to better understand some of its relationships with its environment. We have shown that the development of deferral criteria is based on the gradual integration of knowledge and know-how stemming from different disciplines and modes of reasoning, with a view to controlling the uncertainties that weigh on transfusion activities. While the clinical approach is still the foundation for the development of deferral criteria, its place in the selection device seems to have become increasingly tenuous, even marginalized, as the framework has become "healthi-cized" through the integration of a range of knowledge, especially epidemiologi-cal and biological. Thanks to this knowledge, the action of "putting at risk" the uncertainty surrounding donors could draw, and be based, on data and figures that confer objectivity (Porter 1996).

Although health knowledge has colonized transfusion activities, the incorpo-ration of heterogeneous knowledge today raises uncertainty as to the hierarchy and role of this knowledge, as well as about relationships between the transfu-sion system and its environment. Within the context of health safety and the principle of precaution, all emerging threats are today translated into transfusion risks, as is the case for prion, the West Nile virus – but this was also the case for Severe Acute Respiratory Syndrome (SARS), dengue fever, chikungunya fever, H1N1 flu, etc. Two sources of uncertainty thus arise. The first has to do with the production sites of this putting-at-risk. For 15 years, the fragmentation of decision-making spaces and the heightened intervention of actors external to the transfusion system in producing exclusion policy have increasingly obscured the decision-making processes for deferrals criteria that transfusion professionals must apply (and defend) in the field, in order to ensure transfusion safety. Some deferral criteria are poorly understood, and their permanence even more so, since the patterns underlying their development remain unclear. This is the case for permanent exclusions concerning transfusion recipients and travellers who have resided for one year or more in the British Isles between 1980 and 1996.[24]

The second source of uncertainty stems from how the selection apparatus actually works. It was originally based on a relationship of trust which, when accorded to a donor, allowed transfusion to "save" the life of a recipient. As new risks have emerged, this relationship has changed. Today, the search for optimal safety gives rise to a relationship of systematic suspicion toward the donor, which constantly extends to new entities (viruses, prions, medications) and various populations (MSM, transfusion recipients, travellers), reinforcing the mistrust already looming over certain so-called "at-risk" populations. This is the case, for example, with MSM, who are still perceived as carriers of risks that are incompatible with the safety of the transfusion system. Because it is increasingly contested in the public sphere, this deferral policy, perceived as a social exclu-sion, even discrimination, gives rise to further uncertainty, since the transfusion system fears that debates on its legitimacy will encourage potential donors to conceal their homosexual practices. In addition, this attitude of suspicion results in areas of uncertainty being displaced and multiplied. Today, according to EFS sources, on the basis of existing deferral criteria, the rate of donation refusal is such that one regular donor out of ten and one new donor out of four is turned away. In a context of growing demand for blood products, areas of uncertainty may be found in both the prevention of risks relating to existing and emerging infectious diseases and the possibility of ensuring the supply of blood products.

Areas of uncertainty have also developed around compliance with the protocols that come with implementation of the health security framework and standards. Their multiplication has led to fine standardization of collection-related activities. The strict control used to enforce procedures and protocols has become an increasing source of ambiguity for transfusion centre staff and directors. Each incident, however minor, tends to call into question the whole selection process. Hence, once again, the question arises of how to increase collection procedure efficiency. More specifically, according to EFS internal discussions on risk management, these questions focus on whether professionals in charge of donor selection over- or under-select donors based on the same questionnaire, as substantial disparities have been observed from one region to another, within the same region, from one centre to another, and from one doctor to another within the same centre. The regulation of procedures is thus inseparable from a movement of standardizing medical competence and rationalization of staff in health bureaucracies (Di Maggio and Powell 1983; Vinck and Weisz 2007). As a result, the question now arises as to whether the ongoing evaluation of collection activities and donor selection – by still further diminishing the uncertainty inherent to human interpretation of safety standards – should logically lead to eliminating the need for donation physicians.

Notes

1 A previous version of this chapter has been published in Johanne Charbonneau and Nathalie Tran (eds). 2012. *Les Enjeux du Don de Sang dans le Monde*. Rennes: Presses de l'EHESP. However, this chapter, originally published in French, has been updated, and additional ideas have been included in the analyses and conclusions.
2 The biological screening of donations is limited by the availability of tests and by the window period following contamination, which can vary between ten and 56 days depending on the nature of the test used, and over the course of which the test is, misleadingly, negative. Physico-chemical techniques still have very relative effectiveness limited to plasma and platelet concentrates. Donor selection therefore remains important for controlling known – and especially emerging – risks.
3 The EFS's mission and responsibilities are presented in Chapter 4.
4 Blood transfusion was last-chance treatment, under the constant threat of hemolysis owing to blood incompatibility, consistent with a rule of "make or break." However, the alternative was death for a soldier or for a woman suffering from delivery hemorrhage.
5 All translations from French into English in this text are ours.
6 The following were turned away from blood donation: women who were pregnant, had given birth fewer than six months prior to the donation, or were breastfeeding; subjects carrying a progressive disease (e.g., arterial hypertension or hypotension); persons with tuberculosis, rheumatic arthritis, cancer, brucellosis (fewer than two years prior), or jaundice (fewer than five years prior); persons who had been vaccinated or revaccinated for smallpox (fewer than 15 days prior); persons who had received a diphtheria anti-toxin or anti-tetanus serum (under one month prior); and

subjects whose hemoglobin levels were under 12 g/dL for men and 11 g/dL for women. Finally, for certain strength-intensive or dangerous occupations, blood preferably had to be collected at the end of the day so that the donor would have to wait until the following day to resume work. In September 1971, a new decree added Ag Australia detection to the list of biological examinations required before each donation.

7 See Chapter 4.

8 To support this hypothesis, several documents may be cited, along with the minutes of a meeting held on Monday, July 4, 1988, in the Cabanel Chamber, attended by the *Groupe Donneurs* and the *Groupe Rétrovirus*.

9 This was the case for sarcoidosis for the recipient or neurofibromatosis for the donor.

10 See Chapter 4.

11 See Chapter 4 for more details on this topic.

12 That is, contaminated by the virus but still negative when they took the screening test.

13 *Loi n° 93–5 du 4 janvier 1993 relative à la sécurité en matière de transfusion sanguine et de médicament.*

14 This was the case, for example, for the bibliography concerning hepatitis C contamination related to a digestive endoscopy.

15 The group was composed of three members: Françoise Brun-Vézinet, virologist at Bichat Hospital; Janine Goudard, epidemiologist at INSERM; and Patrick Hervé, former Medical and Scientific Director of the AFS, pediatrician, and hematologist.

16 The group was renamed *Médecine du don* (donation medicine).

17 In compliance with these recommendations, information on transmissible diseases and at-risk behaviour for transfusion was henceforth reserved for the pre-donation interview.

18 As was the case for English statistics that were able to be developed based on ethnic criteria.

19 On this point, it should be noted that the presentation of deferral criteria in the DRCI was written using a model borrowed from the legal world, presenting the argument in the form of preambles. As D. Benamouzig and J. Besançon have pointed out, this type of presentation aims to ensure the quality and tracability of the product of expertise in order to promote transparency.

20 With the exception of a possible allergy to a medication.

21 Since 2002, three European directives have been published with a view to defining the rules for minimal safety in the countries of the European Union. The 2004 directive includes an appendix setting out minimal criteria for selecting donors in order to ensure transfusion safety. Part of this text discusses the risks of infectious diseases that could be transmissible by blood transfusion. It addresses two types of exclusions: the first concerns "persons whose sexual behavior or professional activity exposes them to risks of contracting severe and blood-borne infectious disease" and is temporary. The second concerns "people at high risk for the transmission of a blood-borne disease" and is a permanent exclusion. Each country of the European Union had to transpose these directives into their national law and to interpret these two situations according to their own epidemiological data.

22 These figures were analyzed on a yearly basis as part of the epidemiological supervision of blood donors organized by the *Institut de Veille sanitaire* (INVS) based on de-identified data communicated by the EFS.

23 Or the AIDES association, which showed that it was barely convinced of the value of a measure that would strongly risk stigmatizing the homosexual community if even a single contamination case were to result from lifting the permanent and systematic deferral of MSM.

24 Over and beyond the absence of documented cases on the possible role of transfusion in spreading new variants of Creutzfeld-Jacob disease, it is in particular the one-year

period that raises questions. A clinician in charge of a collection centre stated in an interview that,

> In the case of travellers (in the British Isles), we get the impression that we are responding to a political concern from a minister; the exclusion criteria is not based on epidemiological knowledge, but a political assessment of the lifestyles of all people. In this case, medical authority is being asked to legitimize political precaution.

References

Barthe, Y. and Gilbert, G.C. 2005. "Impuretés et compromis de l'expertise, une difficile reconnaissance. À propos des risques collectifs et des situations d'incertitude." In *Le recours aux experts. Raisons et usages politiques*, edited by Dumoulin, L., La Branche, S., Robert, C., and Warin, P., 43–62. Grenoble: Presses Universitaires de Grenoble.

Benamouzig, D. and Besançon, J. 2005. "Administrer un monde incertain: les nouvelles bureaucraties techniques. Le cas des agences sanitaires en France." *Sociologie du travail* 47: 301–322.

Berlivet, L. 2001. "Déchiffrer la maladie. Épidémiologie et cultures de santé publique." In *Les cultures de la santé publique*, edited by Dozon, J.-P. and Fassin, D., 75–102. Paris: Balland.

Borraz, O. 2008. *Les politiques du risque*. Paris: Presses de Sciences-Po.

Callon, M., Lascoumes, P., and Barthe, Y. 2001. *Agir dans un monde incertain. Essai sur la démocratie technique*. Paris: Le Seuil.

Cazein, F. 2009. "VIH-sida: les hommes homosexuels particulièrement touchés en France et en Europe." *Bulletin épidémiologique hebdomadaire web* 2: 1–15.

Chalas, Y., Claude, G., and Vinck, D. 2009. "Saisir la question de l'incertitude à partir de la pratique des acteurs." In *Comment les acteurs s'arrangent avec l'incertitude*, edited by Chalas, Y., Gilbert, C., and Vinck, D., 7–16. Paris: Études des archives contemporaines.

Charvolin, F. 1993. "'La mise en rapport' des pollutions et nuisances (1964–1967). Inscriptions, affaires publiques et changement d'échelle environnemental en France." In *Les raisons de l'action publique. Entre expertise et débat*, edited by CRESAL, 137–153. Paris: L'Harmattan.

Crawford, R. 2004. "Risk Ritual and the Management of Control." *Health* 8: 505–528.

Crespin, R. 2009. "Quand l'instrument définit les problèmes. Le cas du dépistage des drogues aux États-Unis." In *Comment se construisent les problèmes de santé publique*, edited by Gilbert, C. and Henry, E., 215–236. Paris: La Découverte.

Danic, B. and Beauplet, A. 2003. "La collecte de sang en France: organisation et difficultés." *Hématologie* 9: 231–240.

DiMaggio, P.J. and Powell, W.W. 1983. "The Iron Cage Revisited: Institutional Isomorphism and Collective Rationality in Organizational Fields." *American Sociological Review* 48(2): 147–160.

Dodier, N. 2003. *Leçons politiques de l'épidémie de sida*. Paris: Editions de l'EHESS.

Fassin, D. 1996. *L'espace politique de la santé. Essai de généalogie*. Paris: PUF.

Fassin, D. 1998. "Les politiques de la médicalisation." In *L'ère de la médicalisation*, edited by Aïach, P. and Delanoë, D., 1–14. Paris: Editions Economica.

Granjou, C. 2007. "Quand le risque devient un objet politique: expertise scientifique et démocratie sanitaire." *Chantiers politiques* 5: 102–112.

Habibi, B., Jean-Pierre, A., and Couroucé, A.-M. 1983. "Transfusion sanguine et le syndrome d'immuno-dépression acquise." *Revue française de Transfusion sanguine et Immuno-hématologie* 26: 447–465.

Hacking, I. 2001. *Entre science et réalité: La construction sociale de quoi?* Paris: La Découverte.

Hermitte, M.-A. 1996. *Le sang et le droit. Essai sur la transfusion sanguine.* Paris: Seuil.

Hood, C. 1986. *The Tools of Government.* Chatman: Chatman House.

IGASS/IGSJ. 1992. *Joint Report of the Inspection Générale des Affaires Sociales and the Inspection Générale des Services Judiciaires*, November. Rapport d'enquête sur les collectes de sang en milieu pénitenciaire. Paris: IGASS/IGSJ.

Lascoumes, P. and Le Galès P. 2007. "Introduction: Understanding Public Policy through its Instruments – From the Nature of Instruments to the Sociology of Public Policy Instrumentation." *Governance: An International Journal of Policy, Administration, and Institutions* 20: 1–21.

Morelle, A. 1993. "L'institution médicale en question. Retour sur l'affaire du sang contaminé." *Revue Esprit* 195: 5–51.

Peretti-Watel, P. and Moatti, J.-P. 2009. *Le principe de prévention.* Paris: Seuil-La République des Idées.

Picard, J.-F. and Schneider, W.H. 1996. "L'histoire de la transfusion sanguine dans sa relation à la recherche médicale." *Vingtième Siècle* 49: 3–17.

Porter, M.T. 1996. *Trust in Numbers: The Pursuit of Objectivity in Science and Public Life.* Princeton, NJ: Princeton University Press.

Prevagay. 2009. www.invs.sante.fr/presse/2009/communiques/resultas_enquete_prevagay_171109/resultats_prevagay.pdf (last accessed December 16, 2014).

Rabinow, P. and Rose, N. 2003. "Introduction. Foucault Today." In *The Essential Foucault: Selections from the Essential Works of Foucault, 1954–1984*, edited by Rabinow, P. and Rose N., 7–35. New York: New Press.

Rose, N. and Novas, C. 2005. "Biological Citizenship." In *Global Assemblages. Technology, Politics and Ethics as Anthropological Problems*, edited by Ong, A. and Collier, S.J., 439–463. Oxford: Blackwell.

Setbon, M. 1993. *Pouvoirs contre sida.* Paris: Seuil.

Setbon, M. 2004. *Risques, sécurité sanitaire et processus de décision.* Paris: Elsevier.

Tabuteau, D. 2002. *La sécurité sanitaire.* Paris: Berger-Levrault.

Tabuteau, D. 2008. "La décision en santé." *Santé Publique* 20: 297–312.

Vinck, D. and Weisz, G. 2007. "Les mutations de l'action publique sanitaire. Quelle histoire et quelle place donner aux régimes de production des connaissances?" In *La gouvernance des innovations médicales*, edited by Virginie Tournay, 5–15. Paris: PUF.

Williams, S.J. 2004. "Beyond Medicalization-healthicization? A Rejoinder to Hislop and Arbert." *Sociology of Health and Illness* 26: 453–459.

9   Blood donation in Australia

Altruism and exclusion[1]

Kylie Valentine

Introduction

Australia's blood donation system meets the criteria described by Richard Titmuss (Titmuss *et al.* 1997) as enabling altruistic, non-commoditized giving to a stranger. Donors are volunteers, unpaid, and give anonymously. They also represent a very small proportion of the pool of potential donors. Although recent specific data are not available, a much-cited figure is that donors represent 3 percent of the population – compared to the 30 percent who will require blood at some point (Stephen 2001). This is both a significant concern for transfusion medicine and the subject of most of the scholarly literature on Australian blood donation. What is it that motivates donors in Australia to donate, what are the factors that determine whether or not the intention to donate is translated into action, and what place does donation have in the broad context of social capital, social inclusion, and altruism? These questions are important and have been the focus of research, some of it funded by the Australian Red Cross Blood Service (Alessandrini 2005; Chmielewski *et al.* 2012; Fletcher *et al.* 2003; Hollingsworth and Wildman 2004). Individual and structural barriers to donating are a public policy concern, and social marketing efforts are being harnessed to address these barriers.

Yet motivation and barriers are not the only significant questions around blood donation. The lifelong exclusion or deferral of particular groups of people is also important: for the feelings of exclusion and further disenfranchisement in some of these groups; for the relationships and allegiances between advocacy and research communities; and for the meanings of intimate, embodied civil activity.

This chapter describes Australia's national systems of blood donation and their governance arrangements, the characteristics and attitudes of donors, and deferral policies. My primary focus is on the impact and political meanings of deferral policies, especially as they relate to marginalized groups. In recent years the civil and political significance of blood donation has become particularly visible in Australia, in part because of the contesting of the deferral policies relating to gay men. I argue that the social solidarity and altruism which is so important to blood donation, and so highly valued, has a concomitant devaluing effect on those who are excluded from deferring. I also argue that the technologies of screening and testing which ensure blood safety are also necessarily social, and so both reflect and produce the meanings and dimensions of citizenship and participation beyond the donating space.

The national blood system

Australia's first transfusion service was set up in 1929, and the Australian Red Cross has managed blood transfusion services since their inception. In recent years, the most significant policy developments have been the result of a review of the Australian blood banking and plasma product sector, commissioned by the Australian government and convened by former Governor General Sir Ninian Stephen. The report of that review was delivered in 2001, it recommended the development of a national blood authority, to be responsible for managing the supply of blood and blood products (Stephen 2001). In response to this review, the National Blood Authority was established under the National Blood Authority Act 2003.

The National Blood Authority manages purchasing and planning on behalf of all Australian governments (prior to its formation, state and territory governments had responsibility for the supply and delivery of blood and blood products). The Therapeutic Goods Administration (TGA), however, is also responsible for regulating the sector, including donor deferral directives. The TGA is a division of the Australian government's Department of Health and Ageing, and regulates all medicines and therapeutic goods. The Australian Red Cross Blood Service (ARCBS) is the national "face" of blood donation and is responsible for donor screening and blood testing. A highly trusted non-government organization, internationally and in Australia, the Red Cross's stewardship of Australia's blood donation system is partly responsible for the faith placed in blood donation's safety. The current review of deferral policies was commissioned by the Red Cross, and complaints that the deferral policies amount to discrimination have been levelled at the ARCBS, not the Australian government. However, as the regulating body of the ARCBS, the Australian government also has a direct role in deferral policies. The complex governance arrangements of Australia's blood supply are a product of the moves toward privatization and the contracting of government services in Australia, and the shared responsibilities for enacting regulation between the government and the ARCBS, a non-government organization.

Donors and donating

Donation in Australia occurs in ARCBS premises or mobile donor centres, which are set up in large workplaces and public places. The centres are staffed by enrolled (one-year trained) and registered (three-year trained) nurses and assistant staff, who are responsible for administering the screening questionnaire, phlebotomy and blood collection, as well as preparing the blood and samples for transfer to the processing centre. The screening questionnaire is completed by the donor and contains 56 items for new donors and 37 for returning donors. It includes items on general health, medications, recent medical and dental procedures, family histories of specific illnesses (vCJD, fatal familial insomnia, Gerstmann-Straussler-Scheinker syndrome), travel history, HIV and hepatitis C, recent tattoos and piercing, recent sexual activity, and any lifetime injecting drug use.

The National Blood Authority reports that in 2012 to 2013, almost 579,000 people donated blood – the Australian total population is around 23 million, of whom those aged 15 to 70, the approximate age range eligible to donate blood, comprise 16.5 million (ABS 2013; NBA 2013). The ARCBS website presents information on donating in the form of infographics with this text: "1 in 3 Australians will need blood or blood products in their lifetime; 1 in 30 Australians donate each year" (ARCBS 2013). A 1999 donor survey conducted by the ARCBS found that three-quarters of donors were aged 35 years or older (Stephen 2001, 62). Frequency of donation is prescribed by the TGA, based on guidelines from the Council of Europe, so strategies for increasing the pool of donors focus on recruiting new donors and retaining existing donors.

Given the importance of retention and recruitment, studies of donors in Australia have focused both on the intentions of non-donors to donate and on donors' views about non-monetary incentives and rewards. Studies have found that fears around the risk of contamination in Australia are not significant either for donors or for non-donors (although fear of needles may be a barrier) and that the voluntary nature of donation is regarded as extremely important (Reid and Wood 2008; Alessandrini 2005). Time and distance to donor centres are thought to be more important barriers, in line with Kieran Healy's (2000) analysis of the importance of blood donation regimes to donor rates, although the non-donor population is so large and diverse that it is difficult to identify the most important barriers to donating.

Donor deferral policies

Australia's regulatory approaches are similar to those in Europe. These include criteria for donation and deferral policies. Donors must be "fit, healthy and not suffering from a cold, flu or other illness" at the time of donation or in the previous seven days; be aged between 16 and 70 years; and weigh more than 45 kg. Other criteria are based on demographic and behavioural risk categories, and are estimated to exclude around 30 percent of the Australian population from donating at any one time (AFAO 2010) (Box 9.1).

As I have argued elsewhere (Valentine 2005), these groups are diverse. This diversity relates not to the exclusivity of categories – it is entirely possible that people could belong to more than one of these excluded groups – but to their political and social identity. For example, sexually active gay men have been excluded from donating since 1983, following the emergence of the HIV pandemic and the transmission through blood transfusions of HIV and hepatitis C

***Box 9.1* Criteria and period of exclusion for blood donation in Australia**

Category	Criteria	Period of exclusion
UK residency	Residency in the UK for a period of six months or more between 1980 and 1996, or recipient of blood in the UK	Permanent
Donor health	Epilepsy	Three years since most recent seizure
	Hepatitis B or C	Permanent
	Angina or heart attack	Permanent
Drug use	Intravenous drug use	Permanent
Sexual activity	Men: sex with another man*	12 months
	Women: sex with a man who has had sex with another man	
	Sex with a partner who has HIV or hepatitis C	
	Sex with a partner who has hepatitis B, unless vaccinated or immune	
	Sex with a partner who has ever injected drugs	
	Sex with a male or female sex worker	

Note
* In this chapter, "gay men" should be read as an inclusive category, incorporating men who have sex with men but do not identify as gay.

(HCV) to a number of patients. The decision to exclude gay men from donating led to contestation and protests (Sendziuk 2001), as has been the case in other countries.[2] In contrast, the decision in 2000 to exclude people who had resided in the UK, due to the risk of vCJD transmission, generated no public response at all. Residency in the UK does not have the same political salience or significance as gay sexual activity, and the political histories of HIV fear and homophobia charged the exclusion of gay men from donating in a manner that had no parallel in the histories of vCJD.

Blood donation in Australia, as elsewhere, has a foundation of volunteer donors who are motivated by altruism and unremunerated in any way. So central is voluntary donation to the donation system that it was not considered by the 2001 Stephen Review, which was instructed to take this policy position as a given (Stephen 2001, 66). The motives of donors are therefore universally understood to be related to altruism, social solidarity, and public contributions. Their motives are relevant, in other words, to civic and social participation, and the exclusion of particular groups from donation amounts to their exclusion from this participation. Whereas the exclusion of people who have lived in the UK (including UK-born residents of Australia) has little or no political meaning, especially as it is only those who lived in the UK for a proscribed length of time in a given period, the exclusion of people who are already marginalized has much greater meaning. The exclusion of injecting drug users from donating can work to reinforce public prejudices against them and confirm them as something less than full citizens. Blood donation is strongly marketed as an act of public altruism, and most people understand it in those terms. At the same time, the criteria for altruistic donation are relatively narrow, and those who donate without meeting those criteria are portrayed as very far from altruistic: as risky, unsafe, and placing others in danger (Valentine 2005).

The impact of this on excluded groups is recognized, to a certain extent, by the ARCBS, although, of the two "fact sheets" on specific deferral policies, only that for previous residents of the UK acknowledges that the policies may be "disappointing" (ARCBS n.d.a, n.d.b). There is no fact sheet for drug users, and the fact sheet for gay men makes no acknowledgment of the unintended effects of the policy. It is gay men, however, who have been most active in contesting the policies that exclude them from donating, and the activism of gay men has illuminated the links between altruism, citizenship, and inclusion in the context of blood donation.

Active citizenship, social exclusion, and risk

In 2004, a gay man named Michael Cain attended the ARCBS in Launceston, Tasmania, intending to donate blood. In accordance with ARCBS and TGA regulations, Mr. Cain was asked to complete a donor declaration, answered each of the questions honestly, and in accordance with policy, his blood was not taken for donation. Subsequently, Mr. Cain brought a complaint against the Australian ARCBS to the Tasmanian Anti-Discrimination Tribunal. The basis of his complaint, as reported in the Tribunal's decision report, was that:

> The Red Cross discriminated against him as a homosexual and in relation to his lawful sexual activity. His case is that altruistically minded homosexuals in stable, monogamous relationships posing no realistic risk of HIV infection ought to be permitted to donate blood.
>
> (ADT 2009)

In its defence, the ARCBS claimed that it was not providing a service, so Mr. Cain was not being discriminated against by being denied that service; that there is no stigma associated with not donating; and that the differential treatment experienced by Mr. Cain was reasonable, because of the duty of the ARCBS to protect the safety of the blood supply.

The decision of the Tribunal was that the ARCBS did not discriminate against Mr. Cain and that even if it had, such discrimination would be legitimate because the conduct of the ARCBS was required by law. Despite this ruling, the Tribunal acknowledged the harms done by the deferral policies:

The Tribunal considers that the deferral of Mr. Cain amounts to a dis-advantage to him that is not trivial.... Mr. Cain lost an opportunity to perform a community service valued by our society.... Mr. Cain was deprived of an opportunity to perform an altruistic act – an act that is recog-nised and valued by society. There is also a risk for homosexual donors that they may be stigmatised by society, reinforcing misconceptions that they, as individuals, are high risk carriers of HIV and other blood borne diseases and that their blood is unsafe and reinforcing negative discriminatory notions of homosexuals as posing a risk to the community.

(ADT 2009)

Counter to the defence of the ARCBS that donation is not a service to the donor and that there is no stigma attached to non-donors, the Tribunal recognized that the value of donating has a corollary in the harms done when the opportunity to donate is denied. Harm is done, as the Tribunal acknowledged, to stigmatized and marginalized groups by policies that exclude them from donating. The harm arises from denying these groups the opportunity to participate in the highly valued act of donating blood. Although campaigns to encourage donation emphasize the value of donor altruism to blood recipients, altruism is also valu-able to those who donate, a fact that is rarely acknowledged except in the context of deferral policies and their impact.

Harm also arises from the reinforcement of perceptions that gay men pose risks to others, particularly of contamination with HIV. Similarly, a qualitative study with African migrants in Victoria found that many of the study particip-ants felt excluded from donating, either because they assumed that deferral pol-icies were in place against them or because of the reaction of ARCBS staff when they did donate. The study found that "participants' experiences of discrimina-tion encompassed social marginalisation in employment, income, education and media and bodily marginalisation, resulting in a perception that their blood would not be wanted" (Polonsky *et al.* 2011, 339). There are no specific deferral policies in place for people who have spent time in Africa, but the study parti-cipants' experiences of social exclusion led them to feel not only emotionally disconnected from socially altruistic acts such as blood donation but specifically excluded from it. The authors note: "participants felt that their blood would be rejected, which compounded their sense of alienation" (2011, 341). Social exclusion and perceptions of blood donation become a feedback loop: exclusion from social participation leads to disconnection from social altruism, which reinforces feelings of social exclusion. This is the case for groups such as African migrants who experience discriminatory attitudes from healthcare workers even where policies are not discriminatory. It is also the case for groups like gay men and injecting drug users, who are specifically excluded by deferral policies.

In the case of African migrants (findings which could likely be extrapolated to other ethnic groups), the findings of the research study, partly funded by the ARCBS, include recommendations that marketing campaigns for new donors should have a greater representation of Africans and better information about African communities' specific requirements for donated blood. This latter point is related to ABO and rhesus grouping: as the donor population in Australia tends to be older and Anglo-European, their blood types are often incompatible with the blood requirements of some migrant communities. The study also recommends better communication of the fact that the donations are appreciated; better messages, that is, about the altruism and social benefits of donating (Polonsky *et al.* 2011).

In the case of gay men, the implications of the Tasmanian Anti-Discrimination Tribunal's findings are different. While finding that the harm done to Mr. Cain and other gay men is justified by the imperative to ensure the safety of the blood supply, the Tribunal also emphasized the need for ongoing vigilance in assessing deferral policies, in order to ensure that these policies have a sound scientific basis.

One of the consequences of the Tasmanian case was a national review of the deferral policies relating to sexual activity (ARCBS 2009). The review was set up by the ARCBS but conducted by an independent committee, constituted by medical experts and affected community representatives: an infectious disease physician; an immunologist; a hemophilia patient advocate; an ethicist; an epidemiologist; a donor representative; gay and lesbian group representatives; an HIV patient group representative; and a public health clinician. The review reviewed submissions from the public and epidemiological data in 2010/2011, and reported in 2012 (Review Committee *et al.* 2012). Its terms of reference were "to review the ongoing appropriateness of exclusion of donors on the basis of current and/or past sexual activity to ensure the ongoing safety of blood and blood products provided in Australia" with a particular focus on the following:

a   The appropriateness of ongoing exclusion of men who have sex with men and in particular:

 i   Whether it is possible to define sexual activities that should result in exclusion from donation.
 ii The level of protection afforded by regular condom use and whether this is sufficient in the context of transfusion transmission to avoid exclusion.
 iii Whether (in the context of routine blood donation operations) it is possible to consistently identify a set of criteria by which individuals might be identified as at greater risk of acquiring blood-borne infections than that of the wider population.
 iv The appropriate period (if any) of any exclusion.

b   Consideration of possible additional approaches to protect the donated blood supply from the risks associated with HIV acquired through heterosexual activity, with a particular emphasis on risks associated with sexual activity with people living in or from geographic areas of high prevalence.

c   The relative risk of male-to-female versus male-to-male sex.

d   The appropriateness of excluding current and former sex workers and the appropriate period of any exclusion.

e   Whether the potential for sexual transmission as a route of infection in an as yet identified (i.e., new or emerging) pathogen should impact upon the duration of current deferrals for sexual activity.

f   Advise on the development of effective communication tools to improve overall compliance with the sexual activity-based donor criteria and to explain their ongoing use.

(ARCBS 2009)

Submissions to the review included those from non-government organizations representing gay and lesbian communities, people living with HIV,[3] and Christian groups (Review Committee *et al.* 2012, 23). Unsurprisingly, Christian groups support the status quo and argue for the maintenance of deferral policies. Perhaps unsurprisingly, HIV organizations also support a deferral policy, although one that applies only to men who have anal sex, and for a much shorter period, as HIV testing technologies are far more time- and cost-efficient than when the deferral policies were devised and enable identification of the HIV virus within days, not months, of infection (AFAO 2010).

What are the reasons for the anti-discrimination cases and appeals to review policy deferrals? Given that such a small proportion of the Australian population donates blood, why has the exclusion of sexually active gay men been taken up as an instance of discrimination? In contrast with marriage, another contemporary area of activism and arguments for equality in Australia, blood donation is not a mainstream activity, nor a significant part of many lives. The answers to these questions lie in two areas. The first, described already, is the recognition that blood donation is a highly valued, highly regarded symbol of social solidarity and that exclusion from donation has effects on the meanings of citizenship, especially but not only for those who are excluded. The second is in the history of HIV in Australia and in the active role that affected communities played in formulating Australia's policy response.

The 1980s blood "scandals" of France, Japan, and Germany, where governments were slow to act on urgent information about HIV and HCV contamination, was quite unlike the rapid response in Australia, which was also one of the first countries in the world to adopt universal screening of all blood products (Sendziuk 2001). Changes in donor policy were the responsibility of managers and governments. Australia's overall response to HIV, however, was driven by affected communities themselves, particularly gay men and drug users. As in other parts of the world, governments sought out members of affected communities to participate in policy-making, including representation on parliamentary and ministerial committees. Australia, however, was a world leader in not only ensuring that affected communities had input into policy development but also that those affected communities' practices of negotiating risk and safety were taken up by policy (Kippax and Race 2003). The development of policies and processes was a reflexive process, whereby affected communities were recognized not only as "expert stakeholders" but as engaging in apparently unsafe practices and strategies that were in fact safe for particular people in particular circumstances (Kippax and Kinder 2002). Internationally, gay men's activism was targeted at not only traditional social and political instruments (discrimination and civil rights, access to healthcare) but also the conduct of basic and clinical research. As Steven Epstein (1997, 692) writes in his account of clinical trials of AIDS drugs in the 1990s, these trials:

> are distinctive not only because of the militancy of many of the patients, but because their representatives have mobilised to develop effective social movement organisations that evaluate knowledge claims, disseminate information, and insert laypeople within the process of knowledge construction.

The history of gay men, blood donation, and HIV in Australia is, in other words, not simply a history in which affected communities were consulted as part of policy development. Instead, the risk management practices developed by communities were incorporated into medical and policy knowledge, while community organizations developed and disseminated medical and policy knowledge. This activist, medically engaged, relational history, a form of biological citizenship (Rose and Novas 2005), is at odds with the blanket deferral policy for sexually active gay men – a top-down, bureaucratic, un-negotiated rule. The review should be seen as part of this history, although its concluding remarks mis-state the nature of this history: "Blood donation is not considered a human right and the deferral of groups on the basis of infectious risk does not represent any direct threat to an individual's privacy or freedom of sexual choice" (Review Committee *et al.* 2012, 47). This statement originates in the framing of exclusion from donation as discrimination, and, perhaps, in the rhetorical power of appeals to human rights. The political histories of blood donation in Australia, however, are best understood not in the legal or universalist language of rights but in specific and negotiated practices and knowledge.

New research on the attitudes of Australian donors indicates that this mode of engaged partnership is also relevant to those who are not excluded from donation. Rather than being viewed as passive customers, donors are active members of the blood donation and delivery system: "they act more as strategic supply chain partners in maximizing net benefit for the blood service, rather than as self-interested parties in a traditional market exchange" (Chmielewski *et al.* 2012, 9). While the findings of this research have ready application to the recruitment and rewarding of donors, they also suggest that our understandings of donation and social solidarity need to include these perceptions of active partnership.

Conclusion

Blood donation in Australia is tied, as it is in other countries, to World War I. The Australian Red Cross Society was formed in 1914; the first donors were

Australian soldiers at military casualty stations. A consideration of blood donation is therefore a consideration of the national medical and security apparatus, and of the mobilization of biological citizenship by the state. This history is embedded in the governance of the national blood supply, which also reflects, as noted earlier, contemporary forms of relationships between government and non-government organizations in the funding and delivery of services.

However, it is social citizenship, rather than patriotism, that dominates most representations of donation. In contrast with Singapore, where the national blood service was explicitly connected with the modernization of the state (Reubi 2010), Australian efforts to recruit donors and Australian research (and, as noted earlier, research is often in support of those efforts) focus on altruism and reciprocity. The oldest form of transplant, blood also remains distinct in its capacity for donation. Newer forms of live donation have been enabled by technological improvements, including oocytes, bone marrow, kidney, and liver. All of these involve considerable expense, or pain, or obvious limitations (a kidney can only be donated once), or all of these. The straightforwardness of blood donation, and the widespread public approval of voluntary donation, underpins the attempts to bridge the gap between people who *could* donate and the people who actually *do*: most public appeals emphasize blood as an extraordinary resource: both indispensable in medicine and – because donation is safe, painless, fast, and repeatable – potentially limitless.

Despite this, challenges relating to the safety and supply of the national blood system remain. Australia's blood supply has been sufficient and safe since the 1980s, but securing both is seen to require ongoing vigilance: for example, the NBA devised a National Blood Supply Contingency Plan in 2008 for use in the event of critical blood shortages. Australia's changing demographics and aging population are likely to both increase the proportion of people ineligible to donate because of age restrictions and augment the need for blood to treat people who are living longer with chronic conditions. For both of these reasons, as we have seen in other chapters in this book, the question of supply is likely to become more pressing.[4] The tension between supply and safety has had specific enactments in the recent histories of deferral policies and their relationship to discrimination law.

The ARCBS website (www.donateblood.com.au/) exemplifies this tension. On the one hand, it is one arm of the deferral policy, and is designed to screen ineligible applicants prior to their attendance at a clinic or mobile centre. The website is also, however, a key site for the recruitment and encouragement of potential donors, and abounds with recruitment messages that are placed in conjunction with the detailed pre-donation screening questions: "Australia Doesn't Have Enough Blood: Roll Up Your Sleeves and Give Today"; "When you give blood, you give life"; "People who give blood are united by their generosity and the desire to give something back to the community."

When aspirant donors do attend a centre with the intention to donate, the screening questionnaire contains questions that for most people will be anodyne ("What was your country of birth?"), intimate ("Within the last 12 months have you had sex with a man who you think may have had oral or anal sex with another man?"), and potentially confusing or confronting ("Within the last 12 months have you worked in an abattoir?", "Do you know of anyone in your family who had or has Fatal Familial Insomnia?"). It is administered as a self-completion questionnaire on paper but is then checked and verified by one of the ARCBS staff. Whatever the basis of deferral policies, their implementation is enacted at the level of a personal interaction: it is possible for potential donors to exclude themselves based on the website pre-screening information, but anyone who does turn up to donate will have to speak with a healthcare worker about where they have been, what they have taken, and with whom they have had sex. Even those who are regular donors report being nervous about the screening process and worried that they will be turned away because of something "wrong" with their blood (cited in Valentine 2005).[5] Those who are told, by policy or through the discriminatory attitudes of staff, that there is something wrong with their blood feel the sting of rejection keenly. Race, sexuality, health, and other perennial markers of social standing and status are never eliminated from donation; the act of donation is necessarily about real-life encounters between individuals, not the impersonal implementation of policy. Whatever clinical rationales are in place for deferral policies, they also exemplify the ineluctably social, political dimensions of donation.

Notes

1 A previous version of this chapter has been published in Johanne Charbonneau and Nathalie Tran (eds). 2012. *Les Enjeux du Don de Sang dans le Monde*. Rennes: Presses de l'EHESP. However, this chapter, originally published in French, has been updated, and additional ideas have been included in the analyses and conclusions.
2 See previous chapter.
3 On April 15, 2010, gay activist Rodney Croome made a pointed distinction between organizations representing gay men and AIDS Councils, because the latter group have until recently supported existing deferral policies. www.rodneycroome.id.au/weblog?id=C0_97_1 (last accessed December 16, 2014).
4 The ARCBS website points out in a number of places that around one-third of blood recipients are cancer patients, in an explicit attempt to emphasize the breadth of need and to counter perceptions that its primary use is for accidents and other trauma.
5 See also Chapter 6 for similar results in Canada.

References

Alessandrini, M. 2005. "Understanding Australian social capital and blood donation." *Third Sector Review* 11(2): 35–58.
Australian Bureau of Statistics (ABS). 2013. *4102.0 – Australian Social Trends, July 2013*. www.abs.gov.au/AUSSTATS/abs@.nsf/Lookup/4102.0Main+Features30July+2013 (last accessed December 8, 2013).
Anti-Discrimination Tribunal (ADT). 2009. Anti-Discrimination Decisions [2009] TASADT 03: Cain, Michael v. The Australian Red Cross Society. Hobart: Magistrates Court of Tasmania.
Australian Federation of AIDS Organisations (AFAO). 2010. Submission to the Review of Australian Blood Donor Deferrals Related to Sexual Activity.

Australian Red Cross Blood Service (ARCBS). 2009. Review of Australian Blood Donor Deferrals Relating to Sexual Activity. www.bloodrulesreview.com.au/ (last accessed December 16, 2014).

Australian Red Cross Blood Service (ARCBS). 2013. Info for students. www.donate-blood.com.au/files/J097%20- %20website%20diagrams%20FINAL%20Nov%202013. pdf (last accessed December 16. 2014).

Australian Red Cross Blood Service (ARCBS). n.d.a. *Male to Male Sex Fact Sheet.* www. donateblood.com.au/files/images/Male%20to%20male%20sex%20Fact%20Sheet_June% 202010.pdf (last accessed December 16, 2014).

Australian Red Cross Blood Service (ARCBS). n.d.b. *Residency in UK 1980–1996 Fact Sheet.* www.donateblood.com.au/files/pdfs/Residency%20in%20UK%201980-1996%20 Fact%20Sheet.pdf (last accessed December 16, 2014).

Chmielewski, D., Bove, L.L., Lei, J., Neville, B., and Nagpal, A. 2012. "A new perspective on the incentive–blood donation relationship: Partnership, congruency, and affirmation of competence." *Transfusion* 52(9): 1889–1900.

Epstein, S. 1997. "Activism, drug regulation, and the politics of therapeutic evaluation in the AIDS era: A case study of ddC and the 'surrogate markers' debate." *Social Studies Of Science* 27(5): 691–726.

Fletcher, A., Guthrie, J., and Steane, P. 2003. "Mapping stakeholder perceptions for a third sector organization." *Journal of Intellectual Capita* 4(4): 505–527.

Healy, K. 2000. "Embedded altruism: Blood collection regimes and the European union's donor population." *The American Journal of Sociology* 105(6): 1633–1657.

Hollingsworth, B. and Wildman J. 2004. "What population factors influence the decision to donate blood?" *Transfusion Medicine* 14(1): 9–12.

Kippax, S. and Kinder, P. 2002. "Reflexive practice: The relationship between social research and health promotion in HIV prevention." *Sex Education* 2(2): 91–104. doi: 10.1080/14681810220144855.

Kippax, S. and Race, K. 2003. "Sustaining safe practice: Twenty years on." *Social Science and Medicine* 57(1): 1–12.

National Blood Authority (NBA). 2013. *National Blood Authority Annual Report 2012–13.* Canberra: National Blood Authority.

Polonsky, M.J., Brijnath, B., and Renzaho, A.M. 2011. ""They don't want our blood": Social inclusion and blood donation among African migrants in Australia." *Social Science and Medicine* 73(2): 336–342.

Reid, M. and Wood, A. 2008. "An investigation into blood donation intentions among non-donors." *International Journal of Nonprofit and Voluntary Sector Marketing* 13(1): 31–43.

Reubi, D. 2010. "Blood donors, development and modernisation: Configurations of biological sociality and citizenship in post-colonial Singapore." *Citizenship Studies* 14(5): 473–493. doi: 10.1080/13621025.2010.506697.

Review Committee, Pitt, V., and Wilson, D. 2012. "Review of Australian blood donor deferrals relating to sexual activity." An independent review commissioned by the Australian Red Cross Blood Service.

Rose, N. and Novas, C. 2005. "Biological citizenship [electronic version]." In *Global Assemblages: Technology, Politics and Ethics as Anthropological Problems*, edited by Ong, A. and Collier, S. Malden, MA: Blackwell.

Sendziuk, P. 2001. "Bad blood: The contamination of Australia's blood supply and the emergence of gay activism in the age of AIDS." *Journal of Australian Studies* 25(67): 75–85.

Stephen, N. 2001. "Review of the Australian blood banking and plasma product sector." A report to the Commonwealth Minister for Health and Aged Care by a committee chaired by the Rt. Hon. Sir Ninian Stephen. Canberra: AGPS.

Titmuss, R., Oakley, A., and Ashton, J. 1997. *The Gift Relationship: From Human Blood to Social Policy*. Original edn, with new chapters. New York: New Press.

Valentine, K. 2005. "Citizenship, identity, blood donation." *Body and Society* 11(2): 113–128.

10 A Latin American perspective on blood donation and transfusion systems

Maria Cristina Martínez Valenzuela and Carlos Alberto Sanchez

Introduction

With an ever-increasing demand for blood products in Latin America, there is an immense need to ensure a safe and sufficient supply. Latin American countries constitute a heterogeneous group of low- and middle-income countries with different cultures, geographic characteristics, and levels of economic and social development. In some countries, the gross national product (GNP) per capita is less than US$2,000 per year. In contrast, in others, the annual GNP per capita is greater than US$10,000 (World Bank, World Development Indicators 2012). Recruiting and retaining blood donors poses major challenges for blood services. To address these problems, it is necessary to identify the social, demographic, organizational, cultural, and economic factors that have contributed to defining the different blood collection systems in Latin American countries and that influence the public's willingness to donate blood. It is vital to focus not only on individuals but also on the management of blood donation. As Kieran Healy (2006) and Piliavin and Callero (1991) have suggested, blood supply not only depends on the altruistic act of giving blood but also on the nature and effectiveness of the blood collection system established and used in a country.

An institutional analysis of Latin American collection systems

In Latin America, as on other continents consisting primarily of developing countries, blood product supply systems have not yet attained the level of stability found in most Western countries. In many countries, it would appear that the necessary conditions are still not in place. In this chapter, we will attempt to identify the main factors behind the challenges to the stabilization of this emerging field by treating the blood donation and transfusion system as an organizational field (DiMaggio and Powell 1983).

A field's stability is dependent on the dominant social actors' power and their social skill in using the resources at their disposal to maintain their position (Fligstein and McAdam 2012; Mahoney and Thelen 2009). These actors need to be able to impose their logic and their cultural frame of action (Barman 2007). They may use various forms of resources (Giddens 1984) to achieve their goals, such as technology, professional expertise, and government or legislative support. It is therefore essential that such resources be available. The field must also be able to develop a global structure based either on a hierarchical order or on a relatively stable coalition of social actors (Mahoney and Thelen 2009). The social actors involved must share a common understanding of the main issues at stake (Scott 2001). The presence of internal governance units whose actions are based on norms and rules imposed by the dominant actors is also essential for the field to work (Fligstein and McAdam 2012). These norms must benefit from a degree of legitimacy and recognition both inside the field and in public opinion. Finally, in stable systems, the state plays an essential role as arbiter (DiMaggio and Powell 1983; Hall and Taylor 1996; Scott and Meyer 1983). As previous chapters have shown, in most countries, the state has in fact been a key actor in structuring the field of blood donation and transfusion, as well as in defining its normative framework. Thus, the inability to stabilize a field may be the result of several factors. Before examining the factors behind the instability of blood collection systems in Latin American countries, we will briefly sketch a portrait of the situation on the continent.

Dissimilar social health conditions in Latin American countries

At the beginning of the twenty-first century, health conditions in the countries of Latin America continue to improve, as reflected in both national average life expectancy at birth and mortality rates (Pan American Health Organization (PAHO) 2012, 3). The global sanitary field's history is associated with social, economic, environmental, and technological advances, as well as with the increased availability of healthcare services and the effectiveness of public health programs. However, these health gains have not been uniform across all countries or for different social groups within individual countries.

An important demographic transformation occurred in Latin America with the declines in both the infant mortality rate (which dropped by 66 percent between 1990 and 2009: PAHO 2012, 3) and fertility rates (Organización PanAmericana de la Salud – OPS/Organización Mundial de la Salud. Datos básicos en salud 2011). These changes coincided with the aging of the general population and a concomitant increase in chronic and degenerative diseases. Two mortality patterns coexist: one typical of poor societal living conditions (involving viral and parasitic causes), and the other of more developed societies (involving chronic and degenerative causes). For example, malaria remains endemic in 21 countries, especially among populations living near the Amazon Basin (World Health Organization 2011). The group of so-called neglected diseases is a reflection of the inequalities affecting different population groups. There are two elements involved: a set of poverty-related pathologies (such as Chagas disease, onchocerciasis, trachoma, and geo-helminth infection) and neglected populations living in highly marginalized situations (Hotez *et al.* 2008; OPS 2009, 2012). In 2008, Paraguay reported an outbreak of yellow fever comprising 28 cases and 11 deaths (PAHO 2008). In 2007, 3.9 million people died from chronic, non-communicable diseases (CNCDs) in Latin America, with cardiovascular diseases being the leading cause of death (OPS

2012). All this is combined with high mortality from accidents and violence. Between 2000 and 2007, the death rate among men rose from 229.1 per 100,000 inhabitants to 237.8 (OPS 2011).

Migration from rural to urban areas has resulted in three-quarters of the total population being concentrated in cities (PAHO 2012, 4). In 2010, 79.4 percent of Latin American and Caribbean people resided in urban areas. The growth of urbanization has important health implications due to the increased risk of exposure to social problems such as violence, drug abuse, and motor vehicle accidents. This change also becomes a means for the increased transmission of infectious agents generally found in rural areas.

Urban–rural inequalities persist, reflecting the greater vulnerability of indigenous populations. For example, in Bolivia, infant mortality was 36 per 1, 000 live births in urban areas, and 67 per 1,000 in rural areas in 2008. In the same year, mortality in children under the age of five fell to 63 per 1,000 live births from 75 per 1,000 live births in 2003, but inequalities between urban (43 per 1,000 live births) and rural areas (87 per 1,000 live births) continued (PAHO 2012, 73).

The differences in health status between individuals with high incomes and those with low incomes persist, despite observable overall improvements (Martinez and Vinelli 2006, 182). Increases in life expectancy at birth and decreases in infant and maternal mortality have been greater in those countries with higher total health expenditure per capita, higher expenditure on health as a percentage of gross domestic product (GDP), and more equitable income distribution.

For example, Uruguay is an upper-middle-income country. By 2010, its gross domestic product (GDP) had grown by 36 percent as compared to 2004; its Gini coefficient of inequality was 0.453, and the poverty rate was18.6 percent. Total expenditure on health as a percentage of gross domestic product was 8.1 percent. The country has one of the lowest maternal mortality rates in Latin America, at 8.5 per 100,000 live births, and a life expectancy at birth of 76.1 years (PAHO 2012, 213). On the other hand, Bolivia is a lower-middle-income country. A significant proportion of the population lives below the poverty line. In 2010, its Gini coefficient of inequality was 0.563, and total expenditure on health as a percentage of gross domestic product was 5.5 percent. The country has a life expectancy at birth of 66.3 years and a maternal mortality rate of 310 per 100,000 live births (PAHO 2012, 73).

The differences in the health conditions observed within and between Latin American countries suggest that their blood supply systems will also present a contrasting picture.

Unmet needs for blood products

A key problem facing the healthcare systems in Latin American countries is the lack of adequate supplies of safe blood for hospitals. A country´s need for blood depends on how highly developed its healthcare structure is. It has generally been assumed that in developed healthcare systems, blood requirements will be met if the number of units donated annually corresponds to donations by 3 to 5 percent of the population. However, wherever the healthcare system is not well developed, determination of the need for blood components should be based not on the size of the population but on other factors that reflect the quality and extent of health services development. Population density and the number of hospital beds must be taken into account, bearing in mind that active hematology, trauma, oncology, open-heart surgery, and transplantation surgery programs may increase the demand (Szilassy 1990).

Several documents in the Pan American Health Organization's reports on transfusion medicine in Caribbean and Latin American countries indicate that countries in Latin America gradually increased the number of blood units collected from 2001 to 2009 (OPS 2005–2009; PAHO 2011) (see Table 10.1).

Additional information on the number of donations may be obtained by assessing the ratio of donations to overall population in each country (OPS 2005–2010). The donation rate has gradually increased from 127 donations per 10,000 inhabitants in 2001 to 162 donations per 10,000 inhabitants in 2009. However, this increase is still not sufficient to meet patient need. Table 10.2 contains the information provided by the PAHO (PAHO 2012, 163) on donation rates in Latin American countries for 2005 and 2009. In 2005, the average rate was 148 donations per 10,000 inhabitants, while in 2009 the rate was approximately 162.

One of the indicators of progress used for the Regional Plan of Action 2001 to 2010 was that all Latin American countries would have implemented regional blood collection and processing systems to cover the needs of patients of geographically distinct areas. The mean number of blood units processed by centres is shown to be directly correlated with availability of blood and the proportion of voluntary blood donors on a national level. In 2005, the average number of units collected in Latin American blood banks was 3,163 units, increasing to 3,974 units in 2009. The range, however, is very wide, with the Dominican Republic collecting on average 1,309 units per blood bank, whereas the corresponding figure for Brazil was 9,270 units. Nicaragua has, without question, the most efficient system, with an average of 23,274 units collected per blood bank or blood centre. In 2009, the mean number of blood units processed per Nicaraguan centre per year was 3,974, the equivalent of 12 to 15 units per centre per day. In general, other than in Nicaragua, where three centres processed 69,932 blood units, the efficiency of blood services is deficient in all Latin American countries (PAHO 2011, 155–161) (see Table 10.3).

Table 10.1 Total blood units collected, blood units donated per 10,000 inhabitants, and voluntary blood donations, Latin American countries, 2001 to 2009

	2001	*2005*	*2009*
Units collected (n)	6,256,568	7,976,737	9,077,212
Donations per 10,000 inhabitants	127	148	162
Number of voluntary blood donations	952,658	2,950,018	3,570,185
Voluntary blood donations (%)	15.2	36.6	39.3

Table 10.2 Number of blood units collected and donation rate (per 10,000 inhabitants), 2005 and 2009

Country	Blood donations per year 2005	Blood donations per year 2009	Donation rate 2005	Donation rate 2009
Argentina	365,313	926,941	94.3	230.0
Bolivia	46,764	69,073	50.9	70.0
Brazil	3,738,580	3,661,647	200.9	189.0
Chile	178,079	206,676	109.3	121.8
Colombia	527,711	692,487	122.6	151.7
Costa Rica	54,170	59,336	125.2	129.6
Cuba	495,343	403,060	442.5	359.7
Ecuador	124,724	174,960	95.5	128.4
El Salvador	80,142	82,757	132.3	134.3
Guatemala	77,290	91,554	60.8	65.3
Honduras	52,317	58,3170	75.9	78.1
Mexico	1,351,204	1,602,071	128.3	146.2
Nicaragua	54,117	69,932	99.2	121.2
Panama	42,771	51,539	132.3	149.2
Paraguay	47,060	66,873	79.7	105.3
Peru	179,721	221,266	64.6	75.9
Dominican Republic	62,120	85,169	65.2	84.4
Uruguay	95,686	92,073	287.8	273.9
Venezuela	403,625	461,481	151.0	161.4

Table 10.3 Total blood-processing centers and blood units processed per year, 2005 to 2009

Country	Number of centres, 2005	Number of centres, 2009	Number of units processed per centre, 2005	Number of units processed per centre, 2009
Argentina	480	400	761	2,254
Bolivia	22	20	2,126	3,449
Brazil	562	395	6,652	9,270
Chile	78	38	2,283	5,348
Colombia	110	91	4,797	7,604
Costa Rica	17	27	3,186	7,604
Cuba	48	46	10,320	8,762
Ecuador	22	33	5,669	5,302
El Salvador	32	29	2,504	2,853
Guatemala	47	60	1,664	1,525
Honduras	22	24	2,378	2,429
Mexico	550	560	2,457	2,570
Nicaragua	24	3	2,255	23,274
Panama	26	26	1,645	1,975
Paraguay	16	11	4,706	6,075
Peru	92	90	1,953	2,453
Dominican Republic	58	65	1,071	1,309
Uruguay	76	57	1,259	1,615
Venezuela	240	302	1,495	1,528
All countries	2,522	2,277	3,163	3,974

Table 10.4 Availability of blood components and blood donation rate, 2001, 2005, and 2009

Country	Blood donation rate per 10,000 inhabitants			Blood units separated into components (%)		
	2001	*2005*	*2009*	*2001*	*2005*	*2009*
Guatemala	41	61	65	67	84	87
Bolivia	50	51	70	53	67	89
Peru	97	65	76	75	72	79
Honduras	53	76	78	25	32	39
Dominican Republic	30	65	84	58	78	39
Paraguay	79	180	105	59	55	74
Nicaragua	90	99	121	69	78	90
Chile	154	109	121	76	95	100
Ecuador	90	96	128	74	77	NR
Costa Rica	149	125	129	84	89	94
El Salvador	111	132	134	79	93	96
Mexico	97	128	146	1	88	94
Panama	153	132	149	87	33	91
Colombia	104	123	151	NR	39	90
Venezuela	112	151	161	94	81	80
Brazil	161	200	189	NR	38	95
Argentina	90	94	230	81	87	90
Uruguay	350	287	273	NR	87	NR
Cuba	538	442	360	45	43	95

The median proportion of blood units separated into components was 69 percent in 2005 versus 84 percent in 2009. In 2009, Chile, Brazil, Cuba, and El Salvador prepared red blood cells from at least 95 percent of units collected, while Argentina, Colombia, Costa Rica, Mexico, Nicaragua, and Panama reported preparing red blood cells from 90 percent to 94 percent of whole blood units. Meanwhile, the Dominican Republic and Honduras prepared components from less than 50 percent of the blood units collected (PAHO 2011, 156). In fact, all six of the countries with availability rates below 110 units per 10,000 inhabitants in 2009 – Bolivia, Guatemala, Peru, Paraguay, Honduras, and the Dominican Republic – prepared components from fewer than 90 percent of their units, further limiting the national availability of blood components for transfusion (PAHO 2011, 156–165) (see Table 10.4).

The impact of insufficient blood collection has been made very clear by J. Cruz, who reports, "There is an inverse relationship between national blood availability rates and maternal mortality ratios in the Latin American and Caribbean countries that have information on maternal deaths" (Cruz 2007). In 1999, eight of the nine countries with maternal mortality ratios above 83 per 100,000 live births had blood availability rates below 100 per 10,000 inhabitants (OPS 2012, 47).

Persistent risks of contamination

The safety of blood and blood components also remains a continuing concern. The risk of transmission of the human immunodeficiency virus (HIV), hepatitis B virus (HBV), hepatitis C virus (HCV), malaria, or Chagas disease is still real for some transfusion recipients.

In the 1980s, the medical community recognized that contaminated blood was responsible for the transmission of HIV and that screening blood before transfusion was an effective means of prevention. During the following years, all efforts were directed toward the acquisition of blood screening equipment and testing reagents. Some of the countries' achievements in this area include more than 99 percent of blood units collected screened for HIV, hepatitis B and C, and syphilis, and 96.6 percent screened for T. cruzi, the parasite that causes Chagas disease (OPS 2012, 37).

Every year, thousands of individuals are permanently excluded from blood donation due to various infections. Because the majority of blood donors are one-time donors, it is assumed that there is no real difference in the rates of infectious disease markers between donors and donations (Schmunis and Cruz 2005).[1] A significant number of individuals are permanently lost each year from the donation process, some of them unnecessarily (OPS 2012, 36).

In 2009, the percentage of units testing positive (reactive) for markers of transfusion-transmissible infections (TTI) varied, from 1.05 percent in Chile to 16.57 percent in Paraguay (median 3.1 percent). TTI markers were detected in 292,248 (3.22%) units collected in 19 Latin American countries. The number of units discarded varied, between 1,079 in Nicaragua and 66,889 in Argentina (OPS 2006–2009).

In 2011, 36,327 donors tested positive for HIV, 31,823 for hepatitis B, and 50,628 for hepatitis C (PAHO 2011, 157). The median prevalence of HIV antibodies among donors in countries with more than 80 percent voluntary donations was 0.05 percent, while in countries with less than 80 percent voluntary donation it was 0.26 percent. For the other markers, the corresponding figures were 0.41 percent and 0.41 percent for hepatitis C, 0.28 percent and 0.31 percent for HBsAg, and 0.68 percent and 1.40 percent for syphilis (PAHO 2011, 63–64) (see Table 10.5; PAHO 2011, 56–63).

It is estimated that the 319,996 units discarded in 2009 because they tested positive for infectious markers represented a cost of US$17,919,776 (PAHO 2012, 45). Factors that contribute to the high prevalence of markers among blood donors include poor recruitment and selection processes, and inadequate laboratory testing quality (PAHO 2011, 156).

The high prevalence of infectious disease markers among blood donors contributes to the risk of transmission by blood. Large numbers of first-time donors also increase the risk of TTI.

According to PAHO/WHO data (PAHO 2011, 157), blood-borne pathogens such as HIV, HCV, and HBV are much more common in the blood of paid and replacement donors than in voluntary, altruistic donors. This is because both

Table 10.5 Voluntary blood donations and TTI markers in Latin America, 2011

Countries	Voluntary blood donations (%)		Infectious disease markers per 100 blood donations: HIV, HBV, HCV, and syphilis				
	2009	2011	HIV	HBsAg	HCV	Syphilis	
Cuba	100	100	0.02	0.32	0.63	0.59	
Nicaragua	87	100	0.06	0.24	0.20	0.77	
Colombia	76	82	0.25	0.16	0.55	1.45	
Costa Rica	65	61	0.15	0.10	0.62	0.59	
Brazil	57	60	0.33	0.17	0.32	0.81	
Ecuador	35	50	0.33	0.26	0.35	0.63	
Bolivia	33	35	0.20	0.25	0.33	0.71	
Argentina	19	34	0.26	0.26	0.52	0.74	
Uruguay	24	NA	0.13	0.15	0.37	0.49	
Chile	17	21	0.03	0.02	0.03	1.22	
Dominican Republic	24	18	0.22	0.98	0.29	0.55	
Honduras	12	17	0.20	0.20	0.52	0.79	
El Salvador	12	12	0.06	0.16	0.13	1.10	
Venezuela	4	6	0.23	0.53	0.32	1.81	
Panama	5	6	0.59	0.67	0.58	1.30	
Paraguay	14	6	0.74	0.37	0.40	8.03	
Guatemala	4	5	0.26	0.36	0.65	2.10	
Peru	5	4	0.22	0.41	0.44	1.11	
Mexico	3	3	0.22	0.16	0.56	0.51	

paid and replacement donors are more likely to hide risky behaviours from blood bank personnel than are people whose only motivation is to give the gift of blood. Testing alone could not prevent the transmission of infectious agents through blood transfusion. Through the advocacy of the World Health Organization (WHO) and PAHO, countries began decades ago to look at developing national transfusion services responsible for both the recruitment of altruistic donors, as well as for the collection, processing, and distribution of blood components. However, aside from this initial recognition of the importance of a national transfusion service, the safety and availability of blood and blood components has remained a low priority in healthcare systems. The main social actors in the health field do not, from the outset, share an understanding of the crucial importance of this issue.

The many factors underlying these problems

In short, the establishment of a safe, well-run, efficient, and cost-effective blood donation system remains a challenge for most Latin American countries. Blood transfusion faces numerous problems: highly fragmented systems, hospital-based blood banks, lack of national blood policies or coordinated blood programs, reliance on replacement donors, limited material resources, inappropriate facilities and equipment, inadequate distribution of human resources, lack of appropriate computer systems, limited knowledge of quality management, inadequate quality standards, and insufficient guidelines for donor selection, blood collection, production, and appropriate use of blood components (Martinez and Vinelli 2006, 181).

A decentralized and little-regulated system

Blood donation and transfusion were originally established in the context of hospital settings or coordinated by the national Red Cross. Thus, for many years, activities were shaped by hospitals' internal regulations or by international standards, with no perceived need for specific national legislation. Legislation was first enacted to limit the commercial exploitation of blood and blood components, which had become commonplace. The HIV epidemic forced health authorities to look at blood donation in a different light and fostered the development of explicit and obligatory donor testing requirements (Bolis 2005).

The PAHO has urged countries in Latin America to establish local legislation to prevent commercial exploitation and ensure the availability of and access to safe blood in sufficient quantities (PAHO 2006–2010). The development of blood transfusion legislation and regulations in Latin America has occurred gradually, over a long period of time. Laws and decrees first appeared in the 1950s in Uruguay (Law No. 12.072, No. 12.072, November 1953, Establishment of the National Blood Service); then, in the 1960s, in Brazil (Decree No. 53988, June 1965, National Donor Day), Argentina (Law No. 17132, January 1967, Blood transfusion and laboratory testing), and Chile (Decree No. 16720, November 1967, National Blood Bank) (Bolis 2005).

According to the PAHO, 18 countries in Latin America have national laws regulating blood banks and transfusion services. However, challenges remain with regard to the steering capacity of health authorities, even though many countries have specific units within their Ministries of Health to oversee the national blood system.

Blood transfusion norms and regulations began to appear in the 1960s in Argentina, Brazil, Chile, and Costa Rica; in the 1970s in Bolivia, Colombia, Ecuador, Paraguay, Uruguay, and Venezuela; in the 1980s in Honduras, Mexico, and Nicaragua; and in the 1990s in Guatemala, Panama, and Peru. The first norms and regulations were designed to address concerns regarding the transmission of infectious diseases, such as syphilis and Chagas disease, which were followed by worries about hepatitis in the 1970s and HIV in the 1980s. The norms and regulations have evolved over time, from initially focusing on disease screening to concentrating on voluntary donations and quality assurance.

The current legal frameworks in Latin American countries are deficient with regard to the establishment of national systems with suitable organizations, functions, and financial support. Countries in Latin America have a regulatory framework which mandates the safe use of blood and blood products through the adequate selection of donors, screening for infectious diseases, and the implementation of good clinical practices. Among the factors that may act as barriers to the establishment of a comprehensive legal framework are: lack of political commitment, lack of human and material resources needed to oversee the organization, functioning, and performance of all blood banks; weak or nonexistent regulatory bodies; and the absence or ineffectiveness of blood transfusion policy and strategy (PAHO 2011, 155).

Changes in the officials at national Ministries of Health force changes not only management but also in technical issues and priorities. In many instances, this may cause delays in the completion of programs and projects started by previous administrations (Martinez and Vinelli 2006, 183).

Human and financial resources allocated for blood transfusion at the national level are insufficient (Martinez and Vinelli 2006, 155; PAHO 2011, 183). With few exceptions, Latin American Ministries of Health lack the human and material resources needed to oversee the organization, functioning, and performance of existing blood banks, independent of how they are administered. In certain instances, Ministries of Health rely on national or international nongovernmental organizations to run the national blood program. The multiplicity of actors, coupled with limited oversight by health authorities, may represent an obstacle to the appropriate use of national resources.

Although the Ministries of Health are nominally responsible for the oversight of blood banks, the administrative and financial independence of centres not run by the Ministries makes implementation and enforcement of their norms, requirements, guidelines, and recommendations difficult. Blood services are part of a variety of institutions that may or may not be involved in patient care and are organized according to a range of models. They may be run by the Ministry of Health, the Ministry of Social Security, the Armed Forces, the National

Police, the private sector, or national or international non-governmental organizations such as the Red Cross. (Schmunis and Cruz 2005; PAHO 2011; OPS 1997). However, the prevalent model in Latin America is independent, hospital-based blood banks. Hospital-based blood banks, although part of the blood services of the national system, are structured to respond to the needs of the specific hospital, and their resources are allocated and managed accordingly.

Furthermore, blood donor recruitment in hospital settings faces unique challenges; healthy donors may be apprehensive of hospital premises and may not be willing to donate as a result. The situation is further complicated by decentralization, especially in federal countries such as Argentina, Brazil, and Mexico, where states or provinces have their own local health authorities.

The variety of institutions and the decentralized models of administration result in an excessive number of blood collection and processing sites (Schmunis and Cruz 2005), while the existence of an inordinate number of hospital-based blood banks has negative consequences for blood availability and voluntary blood donation. Many blood banks operate in total isolation, and standards vary from bank to bank. The multiplicity of blood banks hinders the implementation of quality programs on a national level. Implementing quality programs in services that collect 12 to 15 units per centre per day is expensive and inefficient. Training of personnel, maintenance of equipment, audits, and external performance evaluations demand a gigantic effort and enormous investment of already limited resources (Franco 2003).

In this fragmented system, few blood banks are able to collect and review information on capital and revenue costs. Most blood banks are therefore unable to develop adequate budgets and ways of enhancing their productivity and getting adequate numbers of voluntary blood donors. It is difficult to finance and implement suitable computer systems for managing data in both individual blood banks and national networks. Several systems have been developed locally, but in most cases, these are deficient and do not contribute to public safety (Martinez and Vinelli 2006).

Because good computer systems are expensive, blood banks rely on suppliers to fill this need. Unfortunately, some of the systems that are offered by commercial companies have not been adequately validated and cannot be used to build a national network providing a national blood system based on repeated, voluntary blood donation (Martinez and Vinelli 2006).

Given that small blood banks can be unsafe, wasteful, and costly, some Latin American governments have supported centralization. There has therefore been a reduction in the number of blood banks, from 2,522 blood-processing centres in 2005 to 2,277 in 2009 in the 19 Latin American countries (see Table 10.7). Centralization projects include the National Blood Programs in Argentina, Brazil, Chile, Nicaragua, Uruguay, Paraguay, and Colombia.

In 2009, the number of blood-processing centres in Argentina, Brazil, Chile, Colombia, Nicaragua, Paraguay, and Uruguay diminished by 351. Argentina (80 centres), Brazil (167 centres), and Chile (40 centres) accounted for 80 percent of the reduction. In Nicaragua, the Ministry of Health closed all 21 hospital-based blood banks and set up a national network with three centres managed by the Red Cross. On the other hand, Costa Rica, the Dominican Republic, Ecuador, Guatemala, Honduras, Mexico, and Venezuela reported 113 more processing facilities in 2009 than in 2005.

Obstacles to voluntary blood donation

In Latin America, blood donations are obtained from replacement donors, in a system in which patients' relatives and friends give blood in order to replace blood components already transfused to the patient or deposit blood in advance of a surgical procedure. This system places a significant burden on patients and their families, and may be dangerous, as it opens the door to hidden, paid donors.

Voluntary blood donors are a minority in Latin America, in spite of evidence that they are healthier than paid or replacement donors. The widespread requirements by hospitals for patients to provide blood replacement continue to be an obstacle to voluntary blood donation (PAHO 2011, 158). Most of the countries have failed to establish 100 percent voluntary blood donation systems.

In 2009, the largest proportions of voluntary donations were found in Cuba (100%), Nicaragua (87%), Colombia (65%), Costa Rica (76%), Brazil (57%), and Ecuador (35%), followed by Bolivia (30%). In five countries, less than 10 percent of donations were voluntary: Guatemala (4%), Mexico (3%), Panama (5%), Peru (5%), and Venezuela (6%) (see Table 10.6).

Table 10.6 Blood collection and voluntary donations: Latin American countries, 2009

Country	Number of blood units collected	Number of voluntary donations
Argentina	926,941	171,059
Bolivia	69,073	23,104
Brazil	3,661,647	2,102,834
Chile	206,676	36,030
Colombia	692,487	523,830
Costa Rica	59,336	38,593
Cuba	403,060	403,060
Ecuador	174,960	61,230
El Salvador	82,757	9,652
Guatemala	91,554	3,918
Honduras	58,317	7,108
Mexico	1,602,071	43,943
Nicaragua	69,932	60,650
Panama	51,539	2,519
Paraguay	66,873	9,095
Peru	221,266	10,597
Dominican Republic	85,169	20,770
Uruguay	92,073	22,026
Venezuela	461,481	20,167
Total	9,077,212	3,570,185

In 2011, only 3.76 million (41%) of a total 9.14 million units of blood collected in Latin America were altruistic donations. Only two countries had achieved 100 percent voluntary altruistic blood donations: Cuba and Nicaragua (PAHO 2011, 56) (see Table 10.7).

As demonstrated in Nicaragua, where replacement donation was terminated, a well-planned transition strategy that includes the active recruitment of blood donors and the participation of qualified personnel to service them can result in important changes in the blood donation system.

In 2005, the proportion of paid donations in Latin American countries was 0.2 percent. In 2009, 7,124 paid donations accounted for 0.1 percent of all donations (OPS 2006–2010, 45); remunerated donations were reported by the Dominican Republic (3300), Honduras (294), Panama (7641), and Peru (88). By 2011, the proportion of paid donors was 0.08 percent (PAHO 2011, 53) (see Table 10.8).

The stagnation in the proportion of voluntary blood donors at the regional level, the overall high rates of donor deferral, and the prevalence of infectious disease markers at the national level clearly indicate that the processes involved in blood donor recruitment and selection need improvement. This is also one of the main conclusions of socio-anthropological studies carried out in 17 countries in the Region of the Americas (Peredo *et al.* 2001; Bork *et al.* 1999; Ramirez *et al.* 2001; Bustamante *et al.* 2002; Alfonso Valdez *et al.* 2002; Villa de Pina *et al.* 2000; Cruz Roja Ecuatoriana 2000; Fuentes de Sanchez *et al.* 2000; Saenz de

Table 10.7 Voluntary blood donations: Latin American countries, 2009 to 2011

Countries	Voluntary blood donations (%)	
	2009	*2011*
Cuba	100	100
Nicaragua	87	100
Colombia	76	82
Costa Rica	65	61
Brazil	57	60
Ecuador	35	50
Bolivia	33	35
Argentina	19	34
Uruguay	24	NR
Chile	17	21
Dominican Republic	24	18
Honduras	12	17
El Salvador	12	12
Venezuela	4	6
Panama	5	6
Paraguay	14	6
Guatemala	4	5
Peru	5	4
Mexico	3	3

Table 10.8 Blood donations in Caribbean and Latin American countries, 2011

Variable	Caribbean countries	Latin American countries
Blood units collected	134,757	9,141,157
Number of voluntary donations	75,771	3,767,731
Voluntary donations (%)	56.23	41.22
Number of remunerated donations		7,124
Remunerated donations (%)		0.08

Tejada *et al.* 2000; Adjudah *et al.* 2001; Cruz Roja Nicaragüense 2000; Castillo 2002; Chaparro de Ruiz Diaz *et al.* 2000; Fuentes Rivera Salcedo and Roca 2001; Algarra *et al.* 2002; Garcia Gutierrez *et al.* 2003). These surveys shared very similar findings, which may be summarized as follows (PAHO 2009): the population has a positive attitude toward blood donation, considers that giving blood is useful, donates blood when it is necessary, is willing to help to achieve blood sufficiency, is interested in learning more about blood donation, prefers being given opportunities to donate over being offered material incentives, and requires that national blood systems be transparent. Prospective donors demand information on the requirements for becoming a blood donor, the reasons for deferral, the risks and physical consequences of donating blood, the community's need for blood, and the places, frequency, and procedures for blood donation.

Why, then, does the voluntary, non-remunerated, and anonymous system struggle so much to become established within the population? The model promoted by the WHO and the Red Cross is known to be the most prevalent in Western countries. As noted in previous chapters, in India and Africa this model must compete with local cultural models that are better recognized and seen as more legitimate by the population. The same is true of Latin American countries, where replacement donation remains the most widespread practice. To explore this subject in further detail, we used a small-scale study conducted by an undergraduate student in psychology (Martinez and Sanchez, not published) in 2013, in Concepción, Chile, to investigate young people's motivations for giving blood, the obstacles to their doing so, and the strategies used to recruit donors from this group. A self-administered questionnaire was prepared and distributed at random to donor and non-donor students at San Sebastian University. In the interests of a long-term blood supply, it may be beneficial to focus on recruiting young people. It would appear that in order to reach young people and ensure they remain committed blood donors, it could be useful to recruit young volunteers to ensure an active presence in schools and universities as young ambassadors for blood donation.

With regard to the types of event that may have triggered the decision to give blood, most young people indicated an emergency involving someone they cared about or the testimony of a person who had been saved by a transfusion. This would seem to indicate, on the one hand, a recognition of the need for blood donation and, therefore, of the reality of the situation, and, on the other hand, an awareness that potential donors need to be involved personally and emotionally in order to make the decision to donate. It is also interesting to note that the motivation for giving blood was not associated with concrete benefits.

The main reasons young people gave for not donating blood included inadequate information, fear, indifference, and laziness. Questioned about fears that might act as deterrents to giving blood, students reported being afraid of needles, or of feeling unwell or fainting after donating blood.[2] Inadequate information was recognized as one of the main obstacles to giving blood. The use of means such as social networks and SMS to encourage young people to give blood was found to be less important than might have first been thought. More than 50 percent of students preferred talking with their friends in their usual meeting places, favouring direct interaction over the use of new technologies. Our study suggests that it may be more efficient for blood collection centres to focus recruitment efforts on exploiting peer groups or using experienced spokespersons in university or school settings.

This study of modest proportions reveals that young people's chief motivation for donating blood is the desire to meet the needs of the people they care about. This is also the motivation at the heart of the replacement donation model (see Chapter 11). These young people need to be personally and emotionally involved in order to engage in the cause. Even their answers to questions about the best means by which to send them cause-related information point to the importance of interpersonal connections. In short, multiple challenges remain for the many Latin American countries striving to develop a voluntary and anonymous donation system.

Conclusion

This overview of the situation of blood donation and transfusion in Latin American countries has afforded an opportunity to identify the main factors behind challenges in stabilizing this field. It appears that in many countries, few dominant actors have been able to distinguish themselves and impose their views over the decades. A great many social actors within these decentralized systems do not share a common understanding of the issues involved and are unable to establish stable coalitions. There is also a notable lack of any hierarchical structure that may be conducive to stabilizing the field. The state itself struggles to assert its role as arbiter. In most of the countries, the absence of a national blood collection and transfusion policy, together with the limited influence of internal governance units – when they do in fact exist – are also deterrents to the emergence of dominant logics of action within the field.

The analysis demonstrates the importance of available resources when it comes to developing a stable field. In many countries, these resources are absent or highly dispersed. Local actors appropriate them for their own purposes, without coordinating with other social actors in the field. In such a context, it would appear difficult to develop a blood collection system such as voluntary, non-remunerated, and anonymous donation that does not, from the outset, benefit from strong legitimacy in the population.

The goal of blood donor recruitment and retention is to provide sufficient amounts of blood products to all patients in a country. In short, it is not possible to retain blood donors unless the national blood legislation is up-to-date and the necessary funding exists for recruiting and retaining activities. For different reasons (deferral criteria, IT solutions, exchange of blood components, purchasing, etc.), Latin American countries could benefit from the development of a unified national blood system that is also responsible for the national coordination of blood donor promotion activities, and the national and local coordination of blood collection centres.

Blood donors will not come to blood banks unless the latter are modern and efficient, and voluntary blood donors must be treated with respect. Donors expect to be serviced by trained medical professionals, who take the medical check-up seriously. Altruism is good, but respect for the donor is even better. Being efficient is the best way to show respect. Efficient service includes donor-friendly business hours that are respected, parking spaces reserved for donors, immediate service, and pleasant surroundings. Donors take the decisive step of becoming donors when another person (relative, friend) recommends it. Basically, most donors simply want to help their fellow human beings and to ensure a safe supply of blood should they, or their relatives, need blood one day. The reputation of the blood system is very important.

The experience of Nicaragua, one of the Latin American countries with the least financial resources, demonstrates that the political will of the government is vital to implementation on a national level. National blood component self-sufficiency can be achieved when a national approach is developed by the consensus of all interested parties and implemented with the leadership and support of the Ministry of Health, with the efficient processing of blood by a specialized institution with pertinent technical leadership and adequately trained personnel.

Notes

1 The comparison of prevalence estimates among countries is not straightforward, because reagents and laboratory procedures used in different countries may vary in sensitivity and specificity.
2 In this respect, the answers of the young people participating in the study are very much in line with those reported in surveys conducted in other countries (Bednall and Bove 2011; Schreiber *et al.* 2006; Sojka and Sojka 2008).

References

Adjudah, S., Logan, S., Nelson, M., and Gordon, D. 2001. *Anthropological Study of Voluntary Blood Donation in Kingston, Jamaica*. Jamaica.
Alfonso Valdez, M.E., Lam Diaz, R.M., and Ballester Santovenia, J.M. 2002. *Investigación de aspectos soci-culturales relacionados con ladonación voluntaria de sangre en Cuba*. Cuba.
Algarra,Y., Arias, M., Calderon, R., and Duran, M. 2002. *Aspectos socio-culturales relacionados con la donación de sangre en Venezuela*. Ministerio de Salud y Desarrollo Social, Dirección General de Salud Poblacional, Caracas, Venezuela.

Barman, E. 2007. "An institutional approach to donor control: From dyadic ties to a field-level analysis." *AJS* 112(5): 1416–1457.

Bednall, T.C. and Bove, L.L. 2011. "Donating blood: a meta-analytic review of self-reported motivators and deterrents." *Transfusion Medicine Reviews* 25(4): 317–334.

Bolis, M. 2005. *Comparativo de legislaciones sobre sangre segura.* Washington, DC: OPS (THS/EV2005/009).

Bork, A., Zaninovic, P., Lyng, C., Ceron, C.L., Meneses, P., and Salinas, D. 1999. *Factores asociados a la donación de sangre en la Va region.* Hospital Carlos van Buren, Universidad Católica de Valparaiso, Chile.

Bustamante Castillo, X., Fernandez Delgado, X., Garcia Solano, Z., Salazar Solis, J.L., Sanabria Zamora, V., and Solis Ramirez, M.I. 2002. *Investigación de aspectos socio-culturales relacionados con la donación de sangre en Costa Rica.* Ministerio de Salud de Costa Rica, Caja Costarricense de Seguro Social, Organización PanAmericana de la Salud, Organizacion Mundial de la Salud, Costa Rica.

Castillo, Z., Bayard, V., Cedeno de Lopez, A., de Crespo, M., Polanco, D., and Armien, B. 2002. *Investigación de aspectos socio-culturales relacionados con donación voluntaria de sangre efectuada en tres bancos de sangre en Panamá durante el período del 2 de abril al 2 de mayo del año 2001.* Panamá.

Chaparro de Ruiz Diaz, C., Romero de Centeno, A., Hermosilla, M., and Barrios de Rolon, P. 2000. *Aspectos socio-culturales relacionados con la donación voluntaria de sangre. Ministerio de Salud Pública y Bienestar Social.* Centro Nacional de Transfusión Sanguinea, Instituto Nacional de Salud, Asunción, Paraguay.

Cruz, J. 2007. "Reduction of maternal mortality: The need for voluntary blood donors." *International Journal of Gynecological Obstetrics* 98(3): 291–293.

Cruz Roja Ecuatoriana. 2000. *Investigación sobre aspectos socio-culturales relacionados con donación voluntaria de sangre en las tres ciudades principales del Ecuador.* Secretaría Nacional de Sangre, Ecuador.

Cruz Roja Nicaragüense. 2000. *Informe Preliminar. Aspectos socio-culturales relacionados con la donación voluntaria de sangre.* Nicaragua.

DiMaggio, P.J. and Powell, W.W. 1983. "The iron cage revisited: Institutional isomorphism and collective rationality in organizational fields." *American Sociological Review* 48(2): 147–160.

Fligstein, N. and McAdam, D. 2012. *A Theory of Fields.* New York: Oxford University Press.

Franco, E. 2003. "Quality control of immunological testing of blood in the Region of the Americas." *Rev Pan Am Salud Pública* 13: 176–182.

Fuentes de Sanchez, L.P., Guevara de Bolanos, A., Gutierrez Villacorta, M.D., Torres de Valencia, C.E. 2000. *Investigación de aspectos socio-culturales relacionados con donación voluntaria de sangre.* El Salvador.

Fuentes Rivera Salcedo, J. and Roca Valencia, O. 2001. *Perfil antropológico del donante de sangre en Perú. Programa Nacional de Hemoterapia y Bancos de Sangre.* Ministerio de Salud, Lima, Perú.

Garcia Gutierrez, M., Saenz de Tejada, E., and Cruz, J.R. 2003. "Estudio de factores socio-culturales relacionados con la donación voluntaria de sangre en las Américas." *Rev Panam Salud Pública* 13: 85–90.

Hall, P.A. and Taylor, R.C.R. 1996. "Political science and the three new institutionalisms." *Political Studies* 53: 936–957.

Healy, K. 2006. *Last Best Gifts. Altruism and the Market for Human Blood and Organs.* Chicago, IL: The University of Chicago Press.

Hotez, P.J., Bottazzi, M.E., Franco-Paredes, C., and Ault, S.K. 2008. *The neglected tropical diseases of Latin America and the Caribbean: A review of diseases burden and distribution and road map for control and elimination.* www.plosntds.org/article/info%3Adoi% 2F10.1371%2Fjournal.pntd.0000300\ (last accessed December 16, 2014).

Mahoney, J. and Thelen, K. 2009. "A theory of gradual change." In *Explaining Institutional Change: Ambiguity, Agency, and Power*, edited by Mahoney, J. and Thelen, K., 1–37. New York: Cambridge University Press.

Martinez, C. and Sanchez, C. Not published. *Motivations and Obstacles to Giving Blood among Young people in Concepción.*

Martinez, C. and Vinelli, E. 2006. "Setting transfusion standards in developing countries: A Latin American perspective." In *Global Perspectives in Transfusion Medicine*, edited by Lozano, M., Contreras, M., and Blajchman, M., 181–207. Bethesda, MD: AABB Press.

Organizacion PanAmericana de la Salud. 1997. "Situación de los bancos de sangre en la Región de las Américas, 1994–1995." *Bol. Epidemiol.* 18: 11–12.

Organizacion PanAmericana de la Salud. 2010a. *Suministro de Sangre para Transfusiones en los Países del Caribe y Latinoamérica en 2005. Datos Basales para el Plan Regional de Acción de Seguridad Transfusional 2006–2010.* Documentos Técnicos. Acceso a Productos de Calidad. THS\EV-2007\01 E. Washington, DC: OPS.

Organizacion PanAmericana de la Salud. 2010b. *Suministro de Sangre para Transfusiones en los Países del Caribe y Latinoamérica 2006, 2007, 2008 y 2009. Avances desde 2005 del Plan Regional de Seguridad Transfusional.* Washington, DC: OPS.

Organizacion PanAmericana de la Salud. 2011. *51er Consejo Directivo. Iniciativa Regional y Plan de Acción para la Seguridad Transfusional 2006–2010: Evaluación Final.* Documento CD51/INF/5, pp. 32–49. Washington, DC: OPS.

Organizacion PanAmericana de la Salud. 2012. *Estándares de Trabajo para Servicios de Sangre* (tercera edición). Washington, DC: OPS.

Organización PanAmericana de la Salud/Organización Mundial de la Salud. 2009. *Eliminación de las enfermedades desatendidas y otras infecciones relacionadas con la pobreza.* http://new.paho.org/hq/dmdocuments/2009/CD49.R19/20(Esp).

Organización PanAmericana de la Salud/Organización Mundial de la Salud. 2011a. *Datos básicos en salud 2011. Fecundidad.* www.paho.org/Spanish/SHA/coredata/tabulator/ newTabulator.htm (last accessed December 16, 2014).

Organización PanAmericana de la Salud/Organización Mundial de la Salud. 2011b. *Muertes por causas externas. Sistema de Información de Mortalidad.* www.paho.org/ spanish/ad/dpc/haunit-page.htm.

Organización PanAmericana de la Salud/Organización Mundial de la Salud. 2012a. *Enfermedad de Chagas. Transmisión por el principal vector.* http://new.paho.org/hq/ images/stories/AD/HSD/CD/Chagas/int_trans_vector_chagas_800.jpg (last accessed December 16, 2014).

Organización PanAmericana de la Salud/Organización Mundial de la Salud. 2012b. *Datosbásicos en salud. Mortalidad por enfermedades crónicas.* http://new.paho.org/ hq/index.php?option=comcontent&task=blogcategory&id=2391&Itemid=2392.

Pan American Health Organization (PAHO). 2005a. *46th Directing Council. Progress Report on the Regional Initiative for Blood Safety and Plan of Action for 2006–2010.* Presented at the 46th Directing Council 57th Session of the Regional Committee Pan American Health Organization, Washington, DC, September 26–30.

Pan American Health Organization (PAHO). 2005b. *Transfusion Medicine in the Caribbean and Latin American Countries 2000–2003.* Technical Documents. Access to Quality Products. THS\EV-2005\005 I. Washington, DC: PAHO.

Pan American Health Organization (PAHO). 2008. *Emerging and Reemerging Infectious Diseases 2008, Region of the Americas.* www.paho.org/hq/index.php?option=com_docman&task=doc_details&gid=7155&tmpl=component&Itemid=1994&lang=es (last accessed December 16, 2014).

Pan American Health Organization (PAHO). 2009. *Eligibility for Blood Donation: Recommendations for Education and Selection of Prospective Blood Donors.* Washington, DC: PAHO.

Pan American Health Organization (PAHO). 2011. www.paho.org/spanish/ad/dpc/haunitpage.htm (last accessed August 15, 2011).

Pan American Health Organization (PAHO). 2012. *Health in the Americas 2012 Edition. Regional Outlook and Country Profiles.* www1.paho.org/saludenlasamericas/docs/hia-2012-summary.pdf (last accessed December 16, 2014).

Pan American Health Organization (PAHO). 2013. *Supply of Blood for Transfusion in Latin American and Caribbean Countries 2010 and 2011.* Washington, DC: PAHO.

Peredo Vasquez, M., Cruz Arano, J., Cuellar Cuellar, O., Rocha Castro, R., Alvarez Aguilera, R.M., and Sanchez Teran, C. 2001. *Informe final de la investigación sobre aspectos socio-culturales relacionados con la donación voluntaria de sangre en los bancos de sangre de La Paz, Santa Cruz y Cochabamba.* La Paz, Bolivia.

Piliavin, J.A. and Callero, P.L. 1991. *Giving Blood: The Development of an Altruistic Identity.* Baltimore, MA: Johns Hopkins University Press.

Ramirez, H., Sepulveda, E., Junca, O.L., and Erazo, M.E. 2001. *Informe final. Estudio antropológico sobre donación de sangre.* Colombia.

Saenz de Tejada, E. 2000. *Investigación de aspectos socio-culturales relacionados con donación voluntaria de sangre en Guatemala.*

Schmunis, G. and Cruz, J. 2005. "Safety of the blood supply." *Clinical Microbial Review* 18: 12–29.

Schreiber, G.B., Schlumpf, K.S., and Glynn, S.A. 2006. "Convenience, the bane of our existence, and other barriers to donating." *Transfusion* 46(4): 545–553.

Scott, W.R. 2001. *Institutions and Organizations.* Thousand Oaks, CA: Sage.

Scott, W.R. and Meyer, J. 1983. "The organization of societal sectors." In *Organizational Environments: Ritual and Rationality,* edited by Meyer, J. and Scott, W.R., 108–140. Beverly Hills, CA: Sage.

Sojka, B.N. and Sojka, P. 2008. "The blood donation experience: Self-reported motives and obstacles for donating blood." *Vox Sanguinis* 94(1): 56–63.

Szilassy, C. 1990. "Calculations of present and projected blood needs." In *Management of Blood Transfusion Services,* edited by Hollán, S., Wagstaff, W., Leikola, J., and Lothe, F. Geneva, Switzerland: World Health Organization.

Villa de Pina, M., Ruiz Camacho, H.J., Erikson Santos, A., Sosa, S., Saenz de Tejada, E., Centeno, R., and Castellanos, P.L. 2000. *Aspectos socio-culturales relacionados con la donación voluntaria de sangre. Secretaría de Estado de Salud Pública y Asistencia Social, Departamento Nacional de Laboratorios y Bancos de Sangre.* Santo Domingo – República Dominicana.

World Bank. World Development Indicators. 2012. *GNI Per Capita, Atlas Method (Current US$).* World Bank Publications. http://data.worldbank.org/indicator/NY.GNP.PCAP.CD/countries (last accessed December 16, 2014).

World Health Organization. 2011. *World Malaria Report 2011.* www.who.int/malaria/world_malaria_report_2011/WMR2011_noprofiles_lowres.pdf?ua=1 (last accessed December 16, 2014).

11 "She is my blood"

Donation and reciprocity in Trinidad[1]

Vishala Parmasad

Introduction

On my first clinical rotation as a medical student in a public hospital in Trinidad, a senior doctor asked a young anemic patient, Mary,[2] whether she had any "blood chits" so she could be "topped up" (i.e., transfused) before the surgery. Having only a textbook knowledge of the mechanics of blood transfusion, I was as puzzled as Mary by this question, prompting the doctor to begin what was clearly a routine explanation. Given that her "blood count" was so low, Dr. Williams explained, Mary needed a pre-operative blood transfusion. To obtain blood for this transfusion, however, Mary would have to ask her family and friends to donate blood to a blood bank, in return for which they would receive "blood chits" in Mary's name. These chits were vital: the hospital blood bank would release blood to Mary's doctors for her transfusion only upon receiving them. This form of "replacement donation" constitutes the main means of blood procurement in Trinidad and Tobago, and this explanation soon became my own uncomfortable if routine clinical duty as a medical student and junior doctor. My discomfort arose from the inconsistency of this routine practice with the standard recommendations of international biomedicine, which advocate solely non-remunerated voluntary donation. It also arose from a more general awareness of the discourse around voluntary donation – of blood donation as a purely altruistic act, a means of saving a life, a form of patriotism, a civic responsibility. I was not alone in feeling this discomfort, either as a clinician or as a citizen. Yet, in 2011, a government-mandated attempt to transition to solely non-remunerated voluntary donation on a national scale failed miserably. Operating theaters were forced to cancel their operative lists; entire wards were temporarily closed down. The attempt lasted for only four months. By April 29, it had been abandoned for a return to the "chit system" of replacement donation.

In this chapter, I draw upon qualitative and ethnographic research conducted over the period 2008 to 2013 to explore blood donation in Trinidad in the context of a national anemia: a chronic blood insufficiency that only replacement donation has thus far been able to meet. My research consisted of participant observation as a donor, as well as multiple interviews conducted with over 50 informants. They included patients at hospitals, donors, and potential donors at the three major blood donation centres, and stakeholders involved in blood procurement, processing, and transfusion. Further research was conducted at newspaper archives, the Medical Sciences Library of the Eric Williams Medical Sciences Complex, the West Indiana Collection, and the Alma Jordan Library, University of the West Indies, Trinidad. To supplement the scarce literature regarding the historical aspects of blood donation in Trinidad, interviews were conducted with persons instrumental in the field of blood transfusion locally.

The research showed that blood donation and procurement in Trinidad are subject to structural inadequacies in the health sector that consistently militate both against the provision of an adequate supply of blood to the nation and against the implementation of World Health Organization (WHO) recommendations for solely non-remunerated blood donation. Simultaneously, at a deeper level, blood donation is embedded in complex networks of social meaning, exchange, and trust that are described by the rhetoric of "altruism" advocated by the internationalized discourse of transfusion medicine. Blood procurement and donation in Trinidad also reflects the changing social tropes that have swept its landscape: traces of both colonial and migrant histories and pasts.

The first section of the chapter contextualizes blood transfusion in Trinidad, and outlines the history of the National Blood Transfusion Service, the second section explores anthropological approaches to blood donation, and the third section summarizes perspectives elicited from interviews with blood donors over 2008 and 2009. This is followed by an overview of the failed attempt to transition to solely voluntary, non-remunerated blood donation in 2011.

Blood banking in Trinidad

Trinidad and Tobago is a multi-ethnic, multi-religious twin-island Republic in the southern Caribbean.[3] Although historically a Spanish and then a British sugar-producing colony, the main economic activity of Trinidad for the past century has been the production of oil and gas, with recent significant inputs from petrochemical and light industries. This resulted in Trinidad and Tobago being removed from the listing of "developing countries" by the Organization for Economic Cooperation and Development (OECD) in October 2011. The Government of Trinidad and Tobago provides its 1.3 million citizens with free public healthcare through local health centres and large central hospitals. Replacement donation and voluntary donation have been officially sanctioned by a National Blood Transfusion Service (NBTS) since the 1980s, with replacement donation accounting for approximately 87 percent of the total collected blood (Sampath *et al.* 2007).

Origins of blood transfusion in Trinidad

Medical records show that the first transfusions in Trinidad were performed on expatriate workers in the petroleum industry in the 1950s. Trinidad and Tobago was still a British colony at the time, and all doctors and nurses were trained in the United Kingdom, with most doctors also being expatriates (McCollin 2009).

In the 1960s and 1970s, transfusions were not yet a commonplace element in the local medical therapeutic repertoire, but they began to increase after Independence in 1962. Transfusions were performed on an as-needed basis by surgeons and physicians at the two local public hospitals: Port of Spain General Hospital (POSGH), which served the north of the country, and San Fernando General Hospital (SFGH), which served the south. Blood procurement therefore also took place on an as-needed basis at these hospitals. Blood donation was integrated into the general activities of the hospital: donors reclined in hospital beds on the wards, and testing for pathogens and processing of the blood was performed amidst the other routine activities of the hospital hematology and pathology laboratories. As blood transfusion became a more common therapeutic management and demand increased, the blood banks were developed as in-hospital departments, specifically to meet their institutional needs.

This historical process differed greatly from the UK and Europe, where blood banks had already been established as independent entities in the 1940s and 1950s in response to World War II, and their activities were nationally coordinated (Rudmann 2005). In many of these countries, directed blood procurement was phased out at the same time that blood banks were developed. The move away from replacement donation resulted from the increasing demands for blood that such donation could not meet, as the therapeutic applications of blood and blood components expanded with the rapid growth of medical science and technology. More invasive and more risky procedures required more blood, which compelled a simultaneous transformation in the procurement and storage of adequate supplies. This development had not taken place in Trinidad and Tobago over the period of British colonization, due in part to the flow of expatriate doctors through Trinidad and other colonies and then back to Britain, after they had gained experience. Thus there were few pre-existing structures around population health in place until Trinidad gained its independence in 1962.

In the 1960s, however, the newly independent government of Trinidad and Tobago was eager to mark its capacity for self-governance by providing increased secondary-level health services, resulting in a relatively rapid expansion of the public health sector. The Ministry of Health was to be assessed on multiple occasions by both local and foreign observers, who would suggest a decentralization of its activities in order to facilitate more effective function and less entrenchment of its bureaucratic procedures. Assessments of the public health sector also noted that expansion in services was not accompanied by systematic transformation of the health infrastructure to support these services.

Blood procurement in Trinidad was thus linked to immediate and directed use in hospital. Blood donors were drawn from among persons present with the patient, most often relatives or friends, and thus drew on pre-existing forms of social cohesion to meet its need. Replacement donation as the initial mechanism of blood procurement in Trinidad was thus perceived as a natural outgrowth of the early clinical settings of acute need.

Development of the National Blood Transfusion Service

The National Blood Transfusion Service (NBTS) was formed in 1988 after years of concerted lobbying by private individuals and a fledgling non-governmental organization, the Friends of the Blood Bank Association (FBBA). The FBBA was started in 1972 by a group of private citizens, including the local surgeon Mr. McDonald Jorsling, to promote voluntary blood donation in recognition that the country's needs could not be met by the sole practice of replacement donation. Apart from lobbying for the formation of the NBTS, the FBBA was instrumental in fundraising to purchase and refit an 1895 colonial-era military hospital adjacent to the POSGH, to house the NBTS.

The formation of the NBTS was unaccompanied by the passing of any legislation or governmental policy delineating the extent of its powers or its purview over blood procurement and transfusion practices nationally. Indeed, in the early years, the only direct employee of the NBTS was its Medical Director, traditionally also the Director of the FBBA, who also had responsibilities on the wards of POSGH as a practicing hematologist. In these early years, Dr. Waverly Charles, the Medical Director of the NBTS, formulated the "chit system" of replacement donation – arguably, merely formalizing the procurement practices already in use. The NBTS functioned largely as the institutional blood bank of POSGH. Over the next 20 years, with concerted pressure from stakeholders, the Ministry of Health transitioned to employing dedicated transfusion nurses and technical staff for the NBTS on a contractual basis. The FBBA has however remained an autonomous non-governmental organization, while being integrated into the functioning of the NBTS. Interviews with various stakeholders have critiqued the relationship of the FBBA, the NBTS, and the Ministry of Health as promoting ambiguity and preventing the allocation of ultimate responsibility.

The passing of the Regional Health Authorities Act in 1994 decentralized direct responsibility for the provision of healthcare services from the Ministry of Health to multiple geographically based Regional Health Authorities (RHAs). The Ministry of Health now assumed a policy-making, public-health-focused oversight role. By this time there were three major public hospitals: POSGH, SFGH, and the Eric Williams Medical Sciences Complex (EWMSC), opened in 1990. Each hospital fell within a different RHA, and its staffing and functioning fell under their purview. This entrenched the independent, non-integrated operation of the hospital blood banks, with the NBTS headquarters functioning as the blood bank for POSGH. To quote one clinician, each hospital "jealously guarded its blood supply to meet its own institutional needs."

In the 2000s, increasing attempts began to be made to integrate, standardize, and regularize the blood donation processes at the different national hospitals. A push was also made within the NBTS to encourage the transition in hospitals from the "chit-based" replacement donation system to solely voluntary, non-remunerated donation. This was attributed to a change in the Medical Director of the NBTS to Dr. Kenneth Charles, and to the passing of the Human Tissue Transplant Act of 2001. The Act defined blood as a regenerative human tissue and made its trade and barter illegal, with Section 21(1) making it an offense to have blood taken for the purposes of trading for valuable consideration for oneself or another person. The penalty imposed by law is $50,000 and six months' imprisonment. Yet this Act was not publicized outside of the blood banks, and there are no records of increased public education campaigns advocating voluntary donation at this time.

The continued absence of a national blood transfusion policy, as in other Latin American countries[4] that granted the NBTS legal authority over blood dispensation between hospitals, however, impeded efforts at integrating the blood banking system in Trinidad and Tobago. Furthermore, no specific resources were allocated to the NBTS to facilitate this integration: at SFGH and EWMSC, blood bank personnel continued to be employed by the individual hospitals under the RHAs. Neither were there official mandates recommending standardized national protocols around transfusion practices. The staff of the NBTS made efforts to ensure international standards were met for donor screening, blood collection and processing, by conducting training programs for blood bank personnel from the hospitals. These voluntary training sessions put a strain on the already limited human resources of the NBTS. Yet one stakeholder informed me that "The hospitals were not shutting down due to a lack of blood, and the Ministry of Health has long operated on the basis that one should not fix problems that do not exist."

Persons at the Ministry of Health intimated that it has consistently allocated little to no funding and personnel to public education campaigns about blood donation, as this is considered the responsibility of the NBTS. Indeed, the Health Education Division of the Ministry of Health directs its health promotion efforts to the major causes of morbidity and mortality affecting Trinidad, which are chronic non-communicable diseases and HIV/AIDS. Since the inception of the NBTS, it has been the FBBA that has engaged the public directly through public education campaigns, annual fundraisers, and voluntary blood drives utilizing its mobile unit. Despite its integration with the functioning of the NBTS, however, the FBBA has never been heavily staffed, and much of this is accomplished by a single "recruitment officer." According to a clinician, these efforts are thus "inevitably limited in breadth of reach and scope of audience." Other stakeholders questioned how funds raised through the FBBA's fundraising activity and corporate sponsorship were being used, other than meeting their limited staffing requirements and maintenance of the mobile unit and the computerized registry of voluntary donors purchased and installed at the NBTS. Meanwhile, the Ministry's budgetary allocations to the NBTS went toward meeting all other staffing and technical costs of a blood transfusion service.

By 2007, "National Blood Transfusion Service Policy and Technical Guidelines" had been formulated by stakeholders at the NBTS and submitted for approval to the Ministry of Health. These guidelines delineated the capacities of the various blood banks across the country and outlined measures to facilitate the integration of transfusion services at a national scale. Blood banking and processing facilities had been expanded over the years, coming to consist of a central laboratory, located at the NBTS Headquarters in Port of Spain; donation and testing "blood benches" at SFGH; and a donation and processing centre at EWMSC. Smaller satellite centres for blood collection only were located at the health facilities of the Point Fortin Hospital, Sangre Grande Hospital, and the Scarborough Hospital in Tobago.

Blood bank personnel at POSGH and SFGH agreed that communications between the individual blood banks and coordination of the national blood supply improved after 2006/2007. Blood products required by an individual hospital could be sourced from the NBTS headquarters or, with their assistance, from another hospital. The 2007 NBTS policy document, however, noted the continued absence of legislation regarding the national blood supply and highlighted that this translated into poor organization at all levels, including procurement. As one stakeholder stated, this had resulted in "unprofessional, dangerous, and almost criminal failures at a national level" such that blood donation could not be looked at in isolation. Nevertheless, referring to the rapid expansion of tertiary-level healthcare available both privately and, increasingly, publicly in Trinidad, one informant said, "If they [the current administration] want to develop [healthcare] at the rate they want to develop, it all comes down to the blood."

By 2008, healthcare provision in Trinidad and Tobago had changed significantly. Increasing affluence and an expanding middle class; lack of investment in the facilities of the public health institutions; and increased numbers of medical practitioners and specialists had resulted in the rise of a parallel system of private, fee-for-service health facilities (hospitals and nursing homes) alongside the public health institutions. Some of these private hospitals offered highly invasive and transfusion-dependent tertiary-level medical procedures such as coronary artery bypass grafting. Yet no private blood banks were established; the private hospitals also depended on replacement donors, and the screening, collection, and processing of blood by the public health sector blood banks. Replacement donors were sent by the private institutions to the public blood banks to donate, and the private hospitals would then collect the blood directly from the banks for surgical or medical intervention.

In my research, biomedical personnel vigorously critiqued this system. As there is no standardized national transfusion policy that specifies the maximum number of units necessary for specific surgical interventions, it was thought that some private hospitals were requesting and receiving units in excess of their patients' actual requirements. This "blood hoarding" was believed to be occurring so that private hospitals could create "informal" blood banks on their premises, with a pool of blood available for other surgical or medical procedures. Interviewees considered this to be highly dangerous, since appropriate transfusion practices could not be confirmed, given that there is no legislation allowing for governmental or medical oversight of private hospitals. A second critique was that private hospitals are not charged for the blood they obtain from the national blood transfusion services but charge their patients a fee for transfusion. This was considered to be highly unethical, since the patient ends up paying twice for a resource that has been offered up freely by their family and friends: first, through their tax dollars, and second, out of pocket. Lastly, the lack of transparency in the process of transferring blood from the public blood banks to private institutions was critiqued. More than one individual intimated that it would be easy to unfairly dispense blood obtained from replacement donors in the public health system to private hospitals, to the detriment of patients in the public hospitals. There is no current estimate of the volume of blood procured by private hospitals from the national blood transfusion services.

Local blood procurement practices

Replacement donation, as it is practiced in Trinidad and Tobago, revolves around the "blood donor chit." This inch-square piece of paper serves as the material evidence of donation and is inscribed with the intended transfusion recipient's name, the date of donation, and an institutional stamp. Each chit guarantees the recipient one 500ml unit of packed red blood cells. Blood chits are non-transferrable and expire six months after the date of donation. When the medical team of an intended transfusion recipient receives a blood chit, the doctors attach it to a request for packed red blood cells and send it to the hospital blood bank with a sample of the patient's blood. The blood bank ascertains the patient's blood group, cross-matches the unit to be transfused with his or her blood-sample, and returns a compatible unit of packed red blood cells to the medical team for transfusion. Thus, despite the act of giving blood "for" or "to" someone, as most donors in this research described donation, the circulation of blood from replacement donor to recipient is a symbolic rather than a direct process. This form of replacement donation (also referred to as "directed replacement donation") is intended to ensure a constant balance between the units of blood donated and withdrawn from the blood banks.

Blood is collected at the six blood collection centres across Trinidad and Tobago. At the processing centres, donated blood is tested for blood-borne infections (HIV, hepatitis B and C, HTLV1, syphilis, and Chagas disease), and is then grouped, processed, separated into its therapeutic components, and stored. This process takes approximately 48 hours, with blood products having a shelf life of 28 days. Pre-donation screening in Trinidad and Tobago, however, rules out or "defers" donation 36 to 44 percent of the time (PAHO 2008; Charles *et al.* 2010). According to the literature, the most common reasons for deferral include high-risk sexual activity (27.6%), low hemoglobin count (22.2%), and hypertension (17.5%) (Charles *et al.* 2010).

Replacement donation in Trinidad and Tobago occurs in conjunction with a (modified) voluntary donation system. This voluntary system was first instituted in the 1970s under the aegis of the FBBA, in an attempt to incentivize voluntary donation in the local setting of purely replacement donation. Upon making an undirected donation, voluntary donors are given a "donor card" or "donation diary" with their blood group and other information, including the "credits to their account"; that is, a running tally of the number of donations made. If the volunteer later needs a transfusion, she or he is guaranteed the same number of units donated. These may be "withdrawn" from the blood bank using the "diary," a computerized record of which is maintained by the FBBA at the NBTS headquarters. Voluntary donations are transferrable: a volunteer donor can direct a past donation to someone else in need of blood, such as a family member, and these do not expire. A voluntary donation may be collected directly at the blood banks or on blood drives conducted by the FBBA and the NBTS at various local corporations, institutions, and religious organizations.[5] The mobile blood unit does not attend an event unless a minimum of 25 donors is estimated. Interviewees from the FBBA stated that the mobile unit attempts to repeat their blood drives every six months at a specific location and that the mobile unit can conduct over 100 blood drives per year. This schedule of voluntary blood drives attempts to make up the running deficit within local blood banks. The few individual voluntary donors most often donate at the NBTS headquarters. Despite these efforts, however, voluntary donations have been found to contribute less than 15 percent of the total yearly donations (Cruz and Perez-Rosales 2003).

In public hospitals, patients who have received life-threatening traumatic injuries and intra-operative, gynecological, or obstetric emergencies always receive blood to meet the urgent therapeutic need. The family of the transfused patient is later advised to replace the blood their relative has received by donating an equivalent number of units. Not unexpectedly, given that the patient has already been transfused, this replacement rarely occurs. In some other extenuating circumstances, units of blood may be issued by the blood banks in excess of the chits provided, or despite their absence. A common example is that of children suffering from thalassemia major, and who require transfusions of up to four units of blood on a monthly basis for life. Interviews with the families of thalassemic patients revealed that it was the norm for families to "run out of" people to ask to be directed replacement donors within the first few years after the child's diagnosis. Yet, even in the absence of donors, most pediatric thalassemic patients receive blood from sympathetic blood banks, though they often remain perpetually under-transfused. Many research participants with chronic blood requirements indicated that there is in a thriving black market in blood in Trinidad and Tobago. Indeed, remunerated replacement donations may contribute a much higher percentage of total blood collected than is officially recognized, with one senior doctor with many years' experience estimating it at 40 to 50 percent.

The WHO and its regional arm, the Pan American Health Organization (PAHO), and the International Federation of Red Cross and Red Crescent Societies recommend the collection of 50 units per 1,000 population per year for an adequate national blood supply. Thus Trinidad and Tobago would require 65,000 units annually for its population of 1.3 million. However, only 11.6 units per 1,000 population were collected in 2003 and 10.4 in 2005, and the estimated average annual collection is 20,000 units (Cruz and Perez-Rosales 2003; PAHO 2008). Yet, within just one of the three major tertiary public hospitals in Trinidad, 500 units of packed red blood cells are requested each week. Thus, it is estimated that 70 percent of the country's transfusion needs are not met in full (Sampath *et al.* 2007). Furthermore, less than 1 percent of the population is currently responsible for donating all the blood used medically in Trinidad and Tobago. In 2011, the attempted transition to solely voluntary, non-remunerated donation failed to even maintain the previous percentage of donors.

Research by the WHO has shown higher rates of infections in blood procured by replacement or remunerated means. As we have seen in previous chapters, this has resulted in an international discourse in transfusion medicine that promotes blood procurement solely from voluntary, non-remunerated donors (Cruz and Perez-Rosales 2003; Glynn *et al.* 2006). It may be argued that the emphasis on voluntary donation is based on a conceptualization of blood as a resource that should be shared for "altruistic" reasons and to develop "civic-mindedness" among populations, as Valentine has argued in Chapter 9, a perspective propounded by one of the seminal writers on blood donation, Richard Titmuss (1997). Despite the WHO recommendations, however, replacement donation continues to be common practice in many of the countries of the Global South.[6]

Anthropological approaches to blood donation

Many recent studies conducted in diverse geographic locations examine the discursive entanglements of blood donation with such factors as class, socio-economics, nationality, disease status, and so on. Some of these studies appraise the extractive forms of bodily donation as "good to think with" (Lévi-Strauss 1966; Scheper-Hughes 2001). Biotechnical and biomedical discourse, however, emphasizes the "reality" of the body to such an extent that one is tempted to speak to the absence of social theory, to compose arguments in response to the exclusion of crucially relevant theoretical schemas. The perspectives of biomedical practitioners outlined in the preceding discussion of blood donation in Trinidad generally excluded the social and cultural, locating donation within a purely instrumental space. In contrast, in this section, I place at the centre of my analysis the lived corporeality of the ethnographic accounts of donors and recipients, to emphasize what they consider to be at stake in the extractive blood procurement practices of Trinidad and Tobago. The following overview of theoretical approaches to donation highlights issues particularly relevant to the ethnographic context of Trinidad and Tobago.

Bodily commodification

The human body and its parts have a long history of being commodified – as religious relics, for perceived medical or therapeutic uses, or for symbolic purposes as tokens of war (see Lock (2002) for further discussion). Thus, the body and its parts have variously been perceived as inalienable, or as alienable and divisible, and commodified accordingly. In recent medical practice, the transplant of parts from one body to another has been an inalienable act, dependent upon what Lawrence Cohen (2001) has called "kin and skin" – genetic compatibility that is often kinship-related. Technologically mediated medical advances have, however, rendered bodily tissues divisible from their living donors, transforming even previously inalienable body parts to alienable, and thence to freely movable commodities (see Cohen (2001) for further discussion).

Developments in transfusion medicine after World War II similarly transformed blood into an alienable commodity. Civilians in the United States and Europe donated blood for soldiers on the front as part of the war effort, with directed donation promoted as the chance to give the "gift of life." Technological advances after the war however transformed transfusion medicine. As blood's utility expanded, so did its pool of potential recipients: donation was no longer directed (toward the war effort) or limited to "kin and skin." Blood thus became an alienated commodity. Remunerated donation became common among the poor in some cities in the United States, China, and other countries around the world. In countries that had fought in World War II, however, there continued to be an ethic of donation as an "altruistic act" done for the benefit of society rather than for personal gain. In the 1970s there was a resurgence of emphasis on volunteer donation founded on the notion of altruism.

Blood as an alienable commodity

The framing of blood donation as "altruistic" was advanced by Richard Titmuss (1997). Titmuss examined Marcel Mauss' notion of gift-giving as foundational to social cohesion and rearticulated it by proposing voluntary blood donation as the ultimate, unselfish "gifting": an altruistic act done solely to benefit society. Mauss (1923) found that gifts acted as inalienable representations of the givers that imposed an obligatory reciprocity upon their recipients, a "tyranny" of expected return that was contained in the very act of gift-giving. Mauss proposed that it was the inherent *inalienability* of the gift that created and maintained cohesive social relations. Rejecting the expectation of reciprocity in gift-giving as "selfish," Titmuss contended that voluntarily "gifted" blood, donated to and withdrawn from blood banks anonymously by multiple donors and recipients, was most true to the "altruistic" spirit of a gift, since there could be no expectation of return. Thus Titmuss proposed that voluntary donation could create and maintain social relations on a much larger scale through alienable gifting, facilitated by the anonymity of donation and receipt. Thus the selfish tyranny of obligation could be substituted by altruism. Debates about donor motivations gained greater urgency in the wake of the discovery of Acquired Immune Deficiency Syndrome (AIDS). Voluntary donation emerged as the gold standard procurement practice, through which donated blood was rendered alienable and yet not a commodity.

Equity in commodification of bodily parts

As has been said previously in this book, the rhetoric of altruism that predominates in transfusion medicine internationally focuses on the motivations of the donor – blood as a "gift of life" that is regenerated constantly within the body and may thus be given without harming the donor. Yet very little is said about the motivations of the blood banks or biopharmaceutical companies that receive this voluntarily donated blood and channel it into systems of commodification. Cohen (1999) and Scheper-Hughes (2000), among many others, have described an overall movement of body parts from the poor to the rich; countries of the Global South to the Global North; and women to men. Blood is less obviously implicated in the perpetuation of such inequities on a global scale, but the same principles of inequitable access still apply. Depending on the national health policies of the countries in question, voluntarily donated blood from what Scheper-Hughes has called the "social body" is continuously redistributed within it, transformed, and processed, most often in accordance with market forces.

Trinidadian perceptions of blood

Inalienable blood

> People don't want to give blood because they saying that if I give you blood, and something happen to my child or my family, who going to give them? That is why I [am] giving blood now, because it is for family, but if it is for some stranger why I would want to donate?

The above statement was made by Maggie, an African-Trinidadian woman aged 25, who was at the blood bank for the first time, donating for her maternal uncle. Her perspective was echoed and re-echoed in the interviews performed with donors at the blood banks: most participants linked blood donation to notions of kinship and family. The emergent concept was that "blood is donated for kin or friends." This concept took variable iterative form in over 85 percent of the interviews conducted with the non-biomedically trained study participants, and also extended well beyond the formal study population to be repeated in the media and in online websites. "Blood donation" was assumed to be synonymous with "replacement donation" in the speech and references of over 80 percent of the study population. Although this sample was not intended to be statistically representative of the overall population of Trinidad, these notions did not differ by ethnicity or religion.

When asked why they did not consider donating on a voluntary basis, the second most common response elicited was the need to keep their blood "in reserve" in case of prospective familial demand, since blood donor chits last for only six months and most donors can only donate once or twice a year. Given the synonymous use of donation and replacement donation this was not surprising. People admitted to having "heard" of voluntary donation but were uncertain of its utility. As expressed by one Presbyterian Minister: "There should be no problem with donation as far as I am aware in Trinidad because of the generally large size of the family structure."

In this and many similar statements, there was an implicit expectation that the request for donation, asked of family, would be met. Blood procurement, therefore, was repeatedly framed in relational terms: donation was the enactment of an interpersonal transaction. Thus, replacement donation drew upon Maussian social networks of reciprocity, being framed as an obligatory gift that in its giving reaffirmed the inalienable relations of kinship and friendship. What Titmuss defined as a crucial step in framing voluntary donation as an "altruistic" act, the transformation of blood from inalienable to alienable, was therefore continually contested in the practice of replacement blood procurement. Donation in Trinidad did not expand the potential pool of recipients to include an anonymous Other.

The interconnection between blood donation and kinship was also marked by confusion regarding the processes of donation. For example, an elderly Indian-Trinidadian woman named Rookmini was adamant that the only persons who could donate for a patient were his or her nuclear family: "Only the real blood relations – meaning mother, father, brother, sister." In this statement Rookmini expressed two common misconceptions uncovered in the research: first, that the blood of directed replacement donors is directly transfused into the patient in question and for that reason must compulsorily be from the patient's family members; and second, that kinship is somehow related to blood type. The common foundation to both of these assumptions is the inalienability of blood. However, the same phrase, "blood," was operational within two clearly distinct frames of reference: with regard to the act of donation, "blood" relatedness was limited to the nuclear family unit, while outside of that context "blood" relatedness implied a Hindu notion of kin, one which was derived from a tradition brought with Indians to Trinidad over 160 years previously. The rearticulation and delimiting of the concept of kinship among a significant portion of the population of Trinidad and Tobago therefore appears to contradict the emphasis placed on replacement donation within the existing biomedical paradigm.

Commodifying the inalienable

As was previously found in 2003 (Sampath *et al.* 2007), a large proportion of the study population professed a lack of awareness of any blood shortage in Trinidad. The most common reason given for not donating was that people "never saw a reason to donate." Given the inalienability of blood from larger systems of reciprocity that replacement donation reproduces, it is not surprising that undirected "need" was not perceived as a "reason." However, the problems produced by such low rates of donation within a health system in which blood is required for many therapeutic interventions are diverse.

In our study, people clearly indicated that they had first drawn upon their familial network before seeking outside of it. In part, their stories were laments about the lengths to which they had to go to obtain blood. The act of having to "buy" blood or "pay" for donors is inherently perceived as the act of someone with a restricted familial network that reflects little social capital.

An elderly African-Trinidadian woman on the wards required minor surgery but had to have a transfusion pre-operatively because her hemoglobin was already low. She had no immediate relatives in the country; however, she was supported by regular payments which her children, who were living in Canada and the United States, made to her account.

> Lucille [a live-in home caregiver] will be donating blood for me. She does donate for people all the time, and she tell me she will help me out. But I don't want her to give me her blood just so … I will pay her for doin' it, she don't owe me [anything].

The chronic low rates of donation therefore resulted in a situation in which blood was not inalienable but was a saleable item. The system of replacement drew upon ideas of reciprocity but also reiterated them, predisposing donors to the expectation of some kind of return. Yet the blood buying and selling engaged in was not at its root a profit-making enterprise. Instead, the expectation of reciprocity implicit in the gift of blood required satisfaction in some tangible way: money was used to stand in for what would otherwise be hidden bonds of kinship or friendship.

The price of a unit of blood was relatively constant in 2009, at $200 to $500 (US$30 to US$89). At times of more acute shortage, however, such as will be later described in 2011, this price was elevated when market forces intervened more dramatically. However, blood in Trinidad continues to be unsettlingly inalienable yet commodified by the market, resisting both voluntary donation and the limits of replacement donation.

Inequitable procurement

Some biomedical personnel and patients alike criticized the NBTS and the Government of Trinidad and Tobago for failing to put into place policies to institute voluntary donation as the sole legal and accepted mode of donation in Trinidad. Their experiences within and outside of the blood transfusion system had led them to think of the replacement donation system as "coercive" of vulnerable patients, ripe for profit, promoting inequity, and inherently immoral.

Patients and their families likewise questioned the equity of the system. There was a belief that only some persons required blood donor chits to obtain blood from the blood banks, while others were regularly given blood without them: "We don't know who [gets] blood just so [without needing replacement donors] and who don't." Despite the universal implementation of the chit system, there was a marked lack of trust in the blood banks, and in the health system in general. One interviewee reported on "persons in high positions," such as ministers of government, who received blood for their relatives on an as-needed basis without the need for chits. Another replacement donor, who had lined up in the sun for four hours before being turned away, pointed out, "rich people don't have no problem buying three [or] four chits a day, it don't have to mean they getting anybody to donate at all."

Similarly, the process of voluntary donation allows donors with a donation diary to receive blood on an as-needed basis and allows for transferrable donations. Yet only a very small proportion of the population is aware of this donation practice, and it is limited to what one blood donation nurse described as "the elites," later adding, "they are the only ones who have a sense of national responsibility." Indeed, the FBBA was itself started by mainly professionals and businesspeople from the upper socio-economic strata of Trinidad.

Despite the FBBA's ongoing efforts at public education and promotion of voluntary donation, fewer than 10 percent of the research subjects were aware of the advantages of voluntary donation and the incentive of receiving "credits." One stakeholder in the transfusion service described this as resulting in a situation in which a few members of the public – those intimately connected with the blood bank through the FBBA – have greater access to the resources accumulated (primarily by replacement donors) than the wider public. A similar concern was echoed by stakeholders in the transfusion system regarding the flow of blood from the public blood banks to the private hospitals, associated with a perception of lack of transparency to this practice.

Any unwillingness to donate except as a replacement donor is perceived by those who do donate voluntarily as a lack in "altruistic" and "humanitarian" motives. A general tendency was to brand the populace as having a "lack of volunteerism" and as being "selfish," implicitly the opposite of altruistic. The concept that voluntary donation was giving for the common good was directly or indirectly referenced as well. Commonly expressed understandings included:

> People here not educated about the blood donation, they too ignorant and selfish and wouldn't give [blood] just so.

> The whole of the Caribbean, we are a laid back people ... and selfish. You have to come to us and tell us you want something. For you to go to the blood bank that is a big, big thing.

> There are very humanitarian people, who for the good and benefit of humanity, if you are strong and good [healthy], you go to the blood bank and you give people the amount of blood. Nobody have to tell you, so when somebody is in need of it with the blood type, it is there.

Of the voluntary donors interviewed, three described their motivation as altruistic in that it gave them a feeling of "giving something back to society" and thus a sense of well-being.

A crisis of collection

On June 13, 2010, the Ministry of Health of the Government of Trinidad and Tobago held a walkathon to commemorate World Blood Donor Day, which was hosted annually by the NBTS and FBBA. Also present on this occasion were the President of Trinidad and Tobago, Cabinet Ministers and Members of Parliament, the PAHO and WHO Country Representative, as well as various other officers of the Regional Health Authorities. The President, His Excellency Professor George

Maxwell Richards, expressed his support for the advocacy work of the FBBA and encouraged an increase in public awareness of voluntary donation. In her speech after the walkathon, the Minister of Health Therese Baptiste-Cornelis acknowledged the very low rate of blood donation in Trinidad. She made an appeal for increased blood donation by "all persons eligible to donate blood" and pledged that "every citizen that requires a blood transfusion [would have] free access to it – regardless of whether you would have donated in the past." She also announced that the Ministry planned to institute a "100 percent voluntary blood donation system" (Minister's Speech, World Blood Donor Day 2010).

According to stakeholders in the transfusion services, the decision to transition to solely voluntary, non-remunerated blood donation was not mandated by any external international organization, local governmental memorandum, legislation, or decision. As delineated above, long-standing tensions existed among the hospital blood banks, NBTS, FBBS, and the Ministry of Health over the implementation of replacement donation, the circulation of national blood resources, and the continuation of the replacement donation system. Most biomedical personnel considered a transition necessary to meet international standards of care, but some doubted whether this could be achieved in Trinidad given the entrenchment of the replacement donation system and perceptions of general "unwillingness to donate" on the part of all segments of the population. In addition, there were widely divergent opinions about a realistic timeline for the transition. Persons interviewed from within the FBBA considered that a heavily funded, Ministry-backed, blanket public education campaign of three to five years' duration would be necessary before any attempt was made to transition, while some in the NBTS considered that legislative action alone would achieve the goal. The Ministry of Health's decision appeared to be primarily influenced by the perspective that a top-down change in policy to the medical good of the country as a whole would achieve this transition. One of the main advisors to the then Minister of Health described his perspective as "having faith that the people of Trinidad and Tobago would do what is right, when it came down to it." Over the latter half of 2010, notices of the upcoming change in blood bank policy were sent from the Ministry of Health to the Chief Medical Officers and heads of staff of all public hospitals. Then, on December 31, 2010, the chit-based, replacement donation system was formally abandoned.

Despite notices having been sent out, in January 2011, there was what blood bank workers and clinicians described as "a state of utter confusion." Doctors were informed that they no longer needed to advise patients to obtain replacement donors since blood would automatically be available on an as-needed basis. At all of the national blood collection centres there was a sudden decrease in donations over the months of January to March. Replacement donations fell off without any increase in voluntary donations, and blood bank staff described their increasing worry. "We were not sure what to do when we realized that instead of lines of people waiting on a morning there were only a handful, and then only one or two. We have some blood and blood product stocks, but [packed red blood cells] only last for 30 days and we felt there was going to be a crash if something drastic didn't happen," said a technician. The donations at two of the centrally located, historically busy blood donation centres decreased, from 30 to 50 donations a day to single digits, and the donation centre at the headquarters of the National Blood Transfusion Service lost up to 500 units of blood per month (Trinidad and Tobago [TT] Newsday Newspaper, March 27, 2011).

Some people were still sent to the blood banks as replacement donors during this period, recommended by uninformed doctors or by those who wanted to ensure that their patients received blood for crucial surgical interventions. Yet individuals who donated blood as replacement donors sometimes received no blood chits in return. One was told at the blood bank that if she donated without receiving a blood chit, it was likely that her blood would go to a patient in the emergency department rather than to her relative, who needed non-emergency surgery. It is worth noting that over the entire period between December 2010 and March 2011, no mention was made in the print media either of the transition from replacement to voluntary donation or of any blood collection drives. It is not clear whether any efforts were being made at a public education campaign at this time, despite rapidly depleting blood stocks.

On March 10, 2011, Chief Medical Officer of Health (CMOH) Dr. Anton Cumberbatch issued a press release urging people to "continue to give blood freely." This request, however, was accompanied by an ambiguous statement, phrased in terms more consistent with replacement donation: "We would like, if your family is going to do an operation, you would see it as your civic duty to give blood" (Trinidad and Tobago [TT] Express Newspaper, March 10, 2011). On Friday, March 11, 2011, all surgeries were cancelled in the obstetrics and gynecological departments of SFGH due to the heightened risk of performing surgeries without blood available for intra- or post-operative transfusion. When questioned about this, the Minister of Health denied that there was a blood shortage, stating, "There is no blood shortage at the public health institutions," but added that "There is just not as much blood as people would like" (Trinidad and Tobago [TT] Guardian Newspaper, March 12, 2011). A contradictory statement was, however, issued on the same day by the Acting Medical Director of the SFGH, who noted that problems with blood availability were making it necessary to postpone surgeries. He also stated that the CMOH was aware of the problem and had recommended that SFGH initiate a blood transfusion committee for mounting a voluntary blood drive in the region served by that hospital (TT Guardian Newspaper, March 12, 2011).

In the media, Minister Baptiste-Cornelis defended the transition to solely voluntary donation by stating that the chit system "facilitated some corruption" and was being "abused" (TT Express Newspaper, April 7, 2011). She cited instances of counterfeit chits, patients not getting the blood which had been donated in their name, and demands for remuneration at prices of up to TT$1,100.00 per pint (US$170). She also described the chit system as "not in keeping with the WHO standards" (TT Guardian Newspaper, April 29, 2011). In the face of the worsening shortage, blood became even more "expensive" and the Minister reported demands for TT$2,000.00 (US$308) per pint (TT Newsday Newspaper,

April 9, 2011). Despite the increasing demand for blood, its consequent commodification, and the publicizing of the high prices being elicited by donors, the donations at the blood banks continued to fall precipitously. An emergency national blood collection drive spearheaded by the Ministry of Health was launched in March 2011 in an attempt to raise the profile of voluntary blood donation by involving local entertainment personalities. The opening hours of the blood collection centres were also extended from 7 a.m. to 5 p.m., and they began to open on Saturdays as well.

Despite these efforts, however, by mid-April 2011 it was clear that all the public health institutions in the country were operating under a severe blood shortage. This was a terrifying situation, and multiple healthcare personnel have since advanced the opinion that, either directly or indirectly, people died as a consequence of the shortage. The Minister of Health then stated that there was no limit placed on blood being donated for specific persons in need, such as relatives undergoing surgery, but was unable to articulate how there could be certainty that the patient in question would in fact receive blood in the absence of a chit system, given that there was an existing shortage (TT Newsday Newspaper, April 9, 2011). On April 17, an appeal to the public to increase donations was made by the South West Regional Health Authority (SWRHA) and the other health facilities in the southern half of Trinidad. From an estimated daily low of 30, donations had dropped to a maximum of 15 units per day. Blood was now in extremely high demand, yet there was no sudden upsurge in donations concomitant with its commodification.

By April 29, the Cabinet decided to reinstate the chit system for an unquantified but purportedly "limited time." The Cabinet also authorized the purchase of six new four-bed mobile units for blood collection to allow for a much wider range of collection than had previously been possible (TT Guardian Newspaper, April 20, 2011). The Minister also stated that unspecified measures would be taken to deal with the "illegal sale of blood chits ... [and] the proper detection of the bogus chits" consistent with the Human Tissue Transplant Act of 2001. Enforcing this, however, was highly impractical in the absence of any mechanisms in place to detect such transactions.

The reinstatement of the chit donation system prompted an outpouring of media reports and opinions expressing overall relief at having returned to a system that had been "tried and tested" and proved proficient. Yet many of these layperson reports echoed common misconceptions regarding the mechanics of blood donation uncovered during my own research in 2009. What was highlighted in particular was a general lack of awareness of the chronic blood shortage within Trinidad and Tobago, the reasons for the existence of the replacement donation system in the first place, and any analysis of the exchange relations underwriting blood donation, whether of the voluntary replacement or remunerative replacement type. Individuals in the transfusion services expressed relief but were also highly critical of the lack of public education campaigns prior to the cessation of replacement donation. Still other stakeholders expressed dismay at what they perceived as a moral failure of the populace to "step up to the plate and make a difference when it counted."

Conclusion

This overview of the blood donation system in Trinidad and the national failure to transition to non-remunerated voluntary donation in 2011 reveals that top-down regulatory and policy changes alone are insufficient to transform the donation practices of a country. Transfusion medicine in Trinidad and Tobago continues to grapple with low rates of donation and a system of procurement considered unsafe and outmoded by the international arbiters of transfusion. The perspectives advanced by biomedical personnel and stakeholders in this research, however, revealed a lack of interrogation of the principles underlying the current system of blood procurement in Trinidad and its historical antecedents.

It is clear that this attempted transition failed, and that this failure is blamed by some in the transfusion services on the absence of a large public education campaign. However, in a context where replacement donation has been the main mode of blood procurement since the inception of transfusion, and where it is discursively entangled with the prevailing notions of reciprocity and kinship that facilitate social cohesion, I question what type of public education campaign would have been successful. Would a public education campaign that draws upon the international discourse of "altruism" and "voluntarism" be effective in this setting? Drawing upon these research findings, I suggest a campaign that contextualizes blood in terms of local social meanings, as an inalienable substance that is not anonymous but promotes community cohesion through the act of giving.

The failure of transition also threw into stark relief structural inadequacies in the health sector. Successive governments have failed over decades to formulate and pass legislation that would allow for a fully integrated national blood transfusion system and for blood to be managed as a national resource. This lack of political will, as was also noted in other Latin American countries by Martinez and Sanchez,[7] suggests both a deep-seated institutional inertia within the public health sector against "rocking the boat" as well as a lack of long-term vision and planning for the sustainable well-being of the nation. The paucity of documentation and information available about assessments of the blood donation system at the Ministry of Health also suggests a lack of institutional memory consistent with short-term planning. Is this attributable to a highly bureaucratic civil service? To an ignorance of the fundamental necessity of blood to a modern health sector? Or to a generally *laissez-faire* attitude common to post-colonial contexts within both the public and private health sectors? This context should be considered not as a discrete local "cultural system" but, rather, as Eric Wolf (2010, 17) has explicated, subject to "*processes* [like colonialism] that transcend separable cases, moving through and beyond them and transforming them as they proceed."

As of 2015, the FBBA and NBTS continue to share both the premises and the responsibility for the management of the local transfusion service, while the Ministry of Health maintains oversight over their function. The question of the percentage of replacement donation that is actually remunerated arose over the course of this research, but lay outside its scope. This remains a fruitful avenue for future exploration. The perceived failure of "voluntary blood donation" in 2011 has caused deep-seated public and institutional distrust of this system, despite recognition that it was poorly implemented. Chit-based replacement donation continues to be the primary procurement practice within Trinidad and Tobago.

Notes

1 A previous version of this chapter has been published in Johanne Charbonneau and Nathalie Tran (eds). 2012. *Les Enjeux du Don de Sang dans le Monde*. Rennes: Presses de l'EHESP. However, this chapter, originally published in French, has been updated, and additional ideas have been included in the analyses and conclusions.
2 All names have been anonymized to maintain the confidentiality of study participants.
3 The population consists of approximately 40 percent citizens of Indian and African ancestry, with smaller percentages of European, Chinese, Syrian, and Lebanese descent. Christianity is the predominant religion, with Roman Catholics constituting the largest single denomination. The second largest religious denomination is Hindu, while Islam is also a significant block.
4 See Chapter 10.
5 For example, the Water and Sewage Authority of Trinidad and Tobago (WASA), secondary schools, the University of the West Indies, or churches and the Hindu Student Council of Trinidad and Tobago.
6 See also Chapters 2 and 10.
7 See Chapter 10.

References

Bourdieu, P. 1977. *Outline of a Theory of Practice.* Translated by R. Nice. Cambridge: Cambridge University Press.

Charles, K.S., Hughes, P., Gadd, R., Bodkyn, C.J., and Rodriguez, M. 2010. "Evaluation of Blood Donor Deferral Causes in the Trinidad and Tobago National Blood Transfusion Service." *Transfusion Medicine* 20(1): 11–14.

Cohen, L. 1999. "Where It Hurts: Indian Material for an Ethics of Organ Transplantation." *Daedalus* 128(4): 135–165.

Cohen, L. 2001. "The Other Kidney: Biopolitics Beyond Recognition." *Body and Society* 7(2–3): 9–29.

Copeman, J. 2009. *Veins of Devotion: Blood Donation and Religious Experience in North India.* New Brunswick, NJ: Rutgers University Press.

Cruz, J.R. and Perez-Rosales. M.D. 2003. "Availability, Safety and Quality of Blood for Transfusion in the Americas." *Pan American Journal of Public Health* 13: 103–110.

Lévi-Strauss, C. 1966. *The Savage Mind.* Chicago, IL: University of Chicago Press.

Lock, M. 2002. *Twice Dead: Organ Transplants and the Reinvention of Death.* Berkeley: University of California Press.

McCollin, D. 2009. "The History of Health and Healthcare in Trinidad and Tobago 1938–1962." Ph.D. dissertation, University of the West Indies, St. Augustine.

Mauss, M. [1923] 1990. *The Gift: The Form and Reason for Exchange in Archaic Societies.* Translated by W. Halls. London: Routledge.

Pan American Health Organization (PAHO). 1997. "Blood Bank Situation in the Region of the Americas, 1996." *Epidemiological Bulletin* 18: 11–12.

Pan American Health Organization (PAHO). 2008. "Health Systems Profile: Trinidad and Tobago." Washington, DC: PAHO.

Rabinow, P. 1999. *French DNA: Trouble in Purgatory*. Chicago, IL: University of Chicago Press.

Rudmann, S. 2005. *Textbook of Blood Banking and Transfusion Medicine*. London: Elsevier Health Sciences.

Sampath, S., Ramsaran, V., Parasram, S., Mohammed, S., Latchman, S., Khunja, R., Budhoo, D., King, P., and Charles, K. 2007. "Attitudes towards Blood Donation in Trinidad and Tobago." *Transfusion Medicine* 17(2): 83–87.

Scheper-Hughes, N. 2000. "The Global Traffic in Human Organs." *Current Anthropology* 41(1): 191–224.

Scheper-Hughes, N. 2001. "Bodies for Sale – Whole or in Parts." *Body and Society* 7(2–3): 1–8.

Scheper-Hughes, N. and Lock, M. 1987. "The Mindful Body: A Prolegomenon to Future Work in Medical Anthropology." *Medical Anthropology Quarterly* 1(1): 6–41.

Strathern, M. 1992. *After Nature: English Kinship in the Late Twentieth Century*. Cambridge: Cambridge University Press.

Street, A. 2009. "Failed Recipients: Extracting Blood in a Papua New Guinean Hospital." *Body and Society* 15: 193–215.

Titmuss, R. [1971] 1997. *The Gift Relationship: From Human Blood to Social Policy*. London: London School of Economics and Political Science.

Wolf, E. 2010. *Europe and the People Without History*. Berkeley: University of California Press.

Conclusion

Blood donation in the social world: toward a critical, contextualized paradigm of understanding

André Smith and Johanne Charbonneau

As we indicated in the Introduction to this volume, much of the social science literature on blood donation has focused primarily on identifying individual-level factors that may explain why some individuals readily donate blood while others are reluctant or unwilling to do so. Numerous studies have sought to understand the psychological triggers of blood donation, and this research is a staple in the marketing departments of many blood agencies (Grant 2010; Masser *et al.* 2008; Starr 2000). Studies of the technical issues of risk, safety, and efficiency of blood systems, as well as mostly descriptive analyses of blood system policies, are also quite prevalent in the literature. The combined predominance of this type of research has seemingly resulted in a diminished appreciation of the impact of social context on blood donation and of the influence of varied cultural norms on donor behaviour. It has also decontextualized blood donation from the historical and political dynamics that have shaped its emergence as an important aspect of healthcare.

One notable exception is Kieran Healy's (2000) comparative analysis of both the donor recruitment practices of various blood collection regimes in the European Union and the manner in which they impart different social meanings to blood donation. This research demonstrates the value in considering the combined influences of organizational factors, culture, and socio-economic structures on both donor rates and the nature of donor bases. In Healy's view, donor altruism is less intrinsic than it is the consequence of blood collection agencies' emphasizing the value of this trait in their efforts to recruit donors. This argument is captured in the author's oft-quoted statement, "blood can be seen not as something that individuals donate but as something that organizations collect" (Healy 2000: 71). Unfortunately, this type of research remains under-represented in this field of research, where a noticeable dearth of attention is paid to the institutional aspects of blood donation, and critical analyses of blood donation remain few and far between, and their currency outside of the social sciences is quite limited.

This book represents a new agenda for blood donation research – one that is concerned with the diverse historical and contemporary undercurrents that shape how blood donation takes place and the social meanings people attribute to the act of giving blood. The book's chapters turn our attention to key political factors that have shaped blood collection and transfusion practices worldwide. These remarkable analyses trace the evolution of blood donation, presenting it as both the result of technological advances and the consequence of important policy decisions which made it possible for blood to be both anonymously banked and readily transformed into pharmaceutical products. Yet, as several authors remind us, although the practice of anonymous donation is widespread, it is not universal. They point out that direct, family-based blood donation remains entrenched in some parts of the world due to local cultural traditions. The authors also bring their own unique insights, theoretical or otherwise, to bear upon the social-institutional aspects of blood donation.

We begin this conclusion by examining the relevance of the institutionalist analytical framework in relation to the insights and varied findings that are presented in this book. In our Introduction, we maintained that field efficiency is tied to the set of decisions and viewpoints that those dominating this field are able to impose in connection with a number of issues and concerns: risk control, relationships of trust/mistrust between the health and political systems and the population, the defining of social solidarity and of the donation dynamic, and body commodification. In the second part of this conclusion, we use the findings of the previous chapters to better understand this dynamic and to open the discussion toward new issues in blood donation. We conclude by advocating for greater emphasis to be placed on understanding the complex social dynamics that influence and transform the institutional organization of blood donation.

Intersecting organizational fields

Interrelated organizational fields constitute the fundamental building blocks of society (Powell 2007), which is itself structured in terms of the economy, civil society, and the state. All collective actors who constitute a given field, such as a government or a social movement, are themselves part of other fields, such as government ministries or factions in a social movement. Organizational fields can be structured hierarchically, when power in the field is distributed unequally, or horizontally, when power is distributed relatively equally and actors interact as equals and vie for democratic consensus (Emirbayer and Johnson 2008; Martin 2003). Organizational fields operate according to actors' shared understandings of the purpose of the field to which they belong (Scott 2001). However, these actors can also oppose one another in their attempts to gain privileges (Mahoney and Thelen 2009). Organizational fields can transform radically or simply cease to exist if they are destabilized by external shock or by the action of institutional entrepreneurs (DiMaggio 1988; Powell 2007).

While most chapters in this book illustrate the intersectionality of organizational fields, the chapters in Part I do so more prominently than the others, because they focus on the institutional history of blood donation. These chapters show how blood donation and transfusion fields are affected both by the ties they maintain or develop to other fields and by the macrostructures they intersect.

In Chapter 1, Jean-Paul Lallemand-Stempak highlights the Russian-doll quality of the various fields that have shaped both the history of blood donation in the USA and its gradual evolution into a system of voluntary, anonymous, non-remunerated donation. He underlines the gradual and reluctant involvement of the state in regulating blood donation, and traces this involvement to several crises, beginning with World War II, during which the federal government promoted blood collection programs in support of the war effort, imbuing blood donation with patriotic meaning. After World War II, the American blood system involved a patchwork of blood donations, including non-remunerated donation to the American Red Cross, semi-commercial donation to blood banks regulated by the American Association of Blood Banks, and remunerated donation to commercial blood banks. This system remained in place until the early 1970s, when the Nixon administration declared blood to be a national resource that should be managed by the Food and Drug Administration. The author explains how this action emerged from strategic activity in other fields, including the media's reporting on how some commercial blood banks collected blood from at-risk populations, such as drug addicts and prison inmates; the scientific community's favouring of a system of voluntary, non-remunerated donation; and health practitioners' growing concerns about the possibility of lawsuits brought by blood recipients infected by hepatitis-contaminated blood. US racial politics also permeated the field of blood donation, as evidenced by efforts to segregate the blood collected from black donors. In the end, a combination of civil rights legislation and federal-level intervention unified these conflicting fields and facilitated the adoption of a voluntary, non-remunerated, anonymous blood donation system in the USA.

In Chapter 2, William Schneider argues that blood donation systems in Africa evolved in markedly different ways from their counterparts in colonial Europe. Reasons include economic upheavals, political instability, a lack of medical supplies, the unavailability of safe places to store blood, and the HIV/AIDS epidemic starting in the 1980s. The French colonial administration compensated donors with meals, refreshments, and payments (Allain 2010). Blood donation was therefore a source of cash, which was not otherwise readily available to Africans, who responded very well when such payments were offered. In contrast, blood collection in the British African colonies relied on the practice of unpaid, voluntary donation (Titmuss 1971) that had become the hallmark of the worldwide Red Cross blood movement. Following Independence, central coordination became increasingly difficult, and by the mid-1970s, there was a levelling off or, in some places, a decline in the use of transfusions. The author argues that nations across Africa needed to demonstrate both flexibility and strategic thinking to succeed in meeting the blood needs of their populations. The author laments that several African nations continue to lack modern, centralized blood systems and must thus rely on international assistance in managing their blood needs.

In Chapter 3, Vincanne Adams *et al.* explore China's donation system following the public health crisis related to HIV transmission from contaminated blood in the early 1990s. These authors explain why the Public Health Bureau campaign to publicize the marketing of voluntary blood donation was so successful. Relying on the existing social structures of the universities and work units to which the large majority of healthy adult Chinese are affiliated, the Ministry implemented a "planned" (jihua) donation system, in which a quota was established for the work unit. The idea that donors would voluntary sacrifice their blood, and potentially their health, for the work unit, for the larger society, or for the nation, was also met with an expectation that such sacrifice would be compensated. Compensation to the donor was not seen as the same as blood selling for two reasons: (1) workers were asked to voluntarily participate to meet the quota, and compensation was offered as an expression of caring and appreciation for the willing donation of one's valuable essence; and (2) the "profit" motive associated with selling blood to the urban public hospitals was removed. According to the authors, one of the important lessons from China's experiences with blood donation is that it suggests the need for flexibility in defining international standards and strategies for public health when it comes to the safety of blood.

In the fourth and final chapter in this section, Sophie Chauveau analyzes the intersection of commerce and medicine as she examines why France sustained one of the highest rates of HIV- and hepatitis C-contaminated transfusion recipients in Europe. In explaining France's appallingly high infection figures, she singles out the mass production and commercialization of blood products by the pharmaceutical industry and the country's inadequate oversight of this industry. This case study, and the previous one on China, illustrates how an organizational field can be radically transformed in the wake of external crises, particularly when such crises challenge the legitimacy of dominant actors. The tainted blood scandal in France sparked major changes in the economy of blood donation and transfusion, with blood centres becoming bureaucratized and blood products increasingly subjected to a wide range of health, industry, and commercial rules. According to Chauveau, this institutional response to the tainted blood scandal produced an awkward nesting of two fields: on the one hand, a moral economy of the gift (Godbout and Caillé 1992), in which blood donors give blood voluntarily and without being remunerated, and on the other hand, a market economy, which fulfills the growing demand for commercial blood products.

Institutional entrepreneurs, skilled actors, and organizational myth

Organizational fields evolve through the activities of social actors, who come to occupy hierarchical positions within a given field. Dominant actors exercise their influence by setting the rules that make a field work to their advantage, whereas those with fewer privileges and less influence can become institutional entrepreneurs (DiMaggio 1988) who work toward changing field arrangements. As Hoffmann (1999) points out, fields are contested centres of debate. Jockeying for power involves a microfoundation of shared meanings, identities, and values that motivate and facilitate action within the field. This foundation derives from the cognitive ability of social actors to take on the roles of others, to understand these roles in an intersubjective manner, and to mobilize others within chosen frames of actions (Fligstein and McAdam 2011). Divergence of normative orientations between social actors or social groups within the field can result in conflict, which may destabilize the field.

According to Meyer and Rowan (1977), organizational culture did not necessarily correspond with the core everyday activities within an organization. The authors suggested that these structures and rules amount to "myth and ceremony" which give an organization public legitimacy and serve to hide gaps between formal structures and everyday work activity. In this manner, myths and ceremonies help actors maintain a collective sense that their organization functions according to its blueprints, even though they themselves may be operating in a far more improvisational or reactive manner (Elsbach and Sutton, 1992).

The chapters in Part II of this book illustrate that dominant actors in blood systems around the world capitalize on the social networks and belief systems of blood donors to meet an ever-growing demand for blood. They also highlight the value of meeting this objective of adapting donor recruitment practices to the unique local cultures and politics of donor groups.

In Chapter 5, André Smith links the success of one Canadian Blood Services clinic in generating much higher donor rates than comparable clinics with its willingness to tap into a strong local culture of social reciprocity. While effective, some of the clinic's practices contravened formal Canadian Blood Services policies regulating voluntary blood donation, thus challenging the organization's "myths" about donor recruitment and retention. When challenged by Canadian Blood Services dominant actors, employees of the clinic altered some but not all of their practices and publicly reaffirmed their belief that altruism is the key motivation for blood donation.

In Chapter 6, Johanne Charbonneau and Anne Quéniart focus on the factors that have motivated current and former donors in Québec. They suggest that factors such as trust in and familiarity with the blood system, as well as an understanding of the need for blood, reflect the skilled activities of donor recruitment personnel, who have learned to influence donor behaviour with appeals that reinforce the positive aspects of blood donation and the altruistic identity of donors. The authors further argue that institutional conditions favourable to the practice of donation, including conditions that enhance the donation experience, facilitate the adoption of these values among donors. While enormous resources have been invested in industrialized countries toward maintaining safe blood supplies, this chapter highlights that the sufficiency of these supplies remains dependent on social interactions that reinforce the value of blood donation.

In Chapter 7, Jacob Copeman retraces the evolution of blood donation in India since the abolition of paid donation and the phasing out of family-based replacement donation. Devotees of religious orders in the north of India have become nationally recognized as fervent voluntary donors in the past 15 to 20 years. The author highlights the role played by institutional, albeit opportunist, actors in blood donation when he speaks of "the ingenuity of blood bank doctors

... in recognizing the power and intensity of the relationship that exists between gurus and their devotees and enlisting it for their own collection ends" (134). These actors have learned to exploit devotees' belief that blood donation allows the energy of the guru to simultaneously exit and enter the body, thus permitting a deeper connection with the master. However, in discussing this phenomenon, Copeman also points out that the religious movement benefits from this practice, as blood donation enriches the experiential basis of the devotees' religious life in addition to helping blood banks and the community at large. But he also notes the potential risks associated with this practice, including too-frequent donation and the potential for coercion. This chapter demonstrates how blood donation has developed into a site of both striking religious creativity, on the one hand, and controversy and potential risk, on the other.

Power and policy diffusion

The contributions in Part III of the book critically reflect on the actions of government, non-government, and quasi-government agencies and critically engage the norms, beliefs, and technologies associated with donor selection and deferral since the contamination of the blood supply. The authors draw attention to the ways in which blood donation has been intricately intertwined with growing oversight of blood collection practices by the state following the tainted blood scandal of the 1980s. Chapters 8 and 9 articulate the role of regulatory agencies in crafting and enforcing rules that limit how blood is collected and who can donate it. These contributors show that these safety measures aren't the result of a simple logic of precaution but also involve controversial politics of enactment that exclude certain populations from donating on the basis of socially constructed risk profiles. These chapters stress the importance of understanding these policies of exclusion as negotiated responses to the construction of risks rather than as rational procedures devoid of moral or political implications. The two final chapters of the book (Chapters 10 and 11) illustrate situations of permanent instability, when no skilled social actor is capable of dominating the field and imposing ground rules in addition to an institutional logic that could be recognized by all the other actors in the strategic action field.

One important link between the chapters in Part III is the politics of diffusion (Rogers 2003), a process by which "innovation is communicated through certain channels over time among members of a social system" (14). Policy diffusion in government typically involves a protracted learning process characterized by cautious evaluation of the benefits and limitations associated with the policy that is being considered for adoption. As a result, policy diffusion either across governments or within agencies tends to be slow and incremental. However, as Nicholson-Crotty (2009) explains, governments can engage in rapid policy adoption if salient issues threaten the legitimacy of elected officials and undermine public confidence in their ability to manage the affairs of their jurisdiction, which in turn threatens their chance of re-election.

Rapid policy adoption occurred in governments across the world in the wake of the tainted blood scandal, which resulted in dramatic changes to their blood systems. Renaud Crespin and Bruno Danic's detailed account of policy innovations introduced to monitor threats to the French blood supply clearly illustrates this aspect of policy diffusion. While successive governing regimes had already introduced strict standards for the selection of donation candidates, the authors demonstrate that policies implemented after the tainted blood scandal were rooted in a logic of optimal safety and a climate of suspicion that saw the exclusion of an ever-increasing number of "at-risk" populations. The authors also show that the tainted blood scandal involved networks of actors, within and beyond the French blood system, who worked together to formulate and enforce these policies of exclusion. As Rhodes (1996) has previously noted, the adoption of policy in times of crisis can often be reactive and co-optive rather than informed by a cautious assessment and decisions. Indeed, according to the authors, transfusion professionals in France were persuaded into defending these exclusionary policies through an institutional logic of precaution and safety. The authors conclude their chapter with an analysis of the policy of lifetime deferral of men who have sex with men (MSM) from donating blood, one of the most controversial risk management strategies introduced to safeguard the blood supply. They outline the competing interests of challengers and incumbents of the policy in the context of consumer pressure, destabilized knowledge of blood risk, and institutional concerns about public trust in the blood system.

In Chapter 9, Kylie Valentine reminds us of the consequences of rapid policy adoption through an examination of the Australian blood system. As did most developed nations, Australia developed a series of criteria to exclude certain groups of individuals from donating blood in its efforts to protect the blood supply. The author argues that the screening and testing technologies which ensure blood safety introduce social meanings and dimensions of citizenship that extend beyond the donating space. These policies were enforced nationwide and ostracized several populations who had adopted blood donation as a means of expressing social solidarity, civil activity, and altruism. Because race, sexuality, health, and other perennial markers of social status are never eliminated from donation, the act of donation is necessarily about real-life encounters between individuals rather than simply the impersonal implementation of policy. The clinical rationales used to defend deferral policies thus exemplify the ineluctably social and political dimensions of donation.

In contrast, in Chapter 10, Maria Cristina Martínez and Carlo Alberto Sanchez elucidate consequences of a lack of state commitment toward a centralized system of voluntary blood donation in several Latin American countries. The prevalent model of blood donation in Latin America remains one based on independent, hospital-based blood banks where blood donations are obtained primarily from replacement donors rather than through voluntary ones. They attribute this lack of a centralized donation system in many countries to the absence of political will and a deep-seated inertia on the part of health regulatory agencies to assume a dominant role in developing and/or implementing national-level blood transfusion policies and strategies. Their account underlines how the development of a successful voluntary, non-remunerated blood donation system requires effective policy diffusion, good communication, and a culture of innovation.

In Chapter 11, Vishala Parmasad describes what occurred when the Government of Trinidad and Tobago attempted to legislate a ban on family-based replacement donation: hospital blood reserves decreased to critical levels, and government officials became concerned about the emergence of a black market for remunerated blood donation. In the end, government officials reversed their decision and allowed family-based replacement blood donations to coexist with voluntary, non-remunerated donations. Trinidad's failure to transition to a non-remunerated, voluntary blood system shows how top-down regulatory directives are, by themselves, insufficient to transform a country's donation practices. Biomedical personnel and stakeholders interviewed in this study point to a lack of interrogation of the principles underlying the current system of blood procurement and its historical antecedents, in addition to structural inadequacies in the health sector, as being the prime reasons for this failure. This case study illustrates the consequences of inept policy evaluation, and more specifically, according to the author, it illustrates a lack of appreciation of the strong relationship between blood donation and the norm of social reciprocity in Trinidadian-Tobagonian society. Arguably, the lack of "skilled strategic actors" (Fligstein and McAdam 2012) or "institutional entrepreneurs" (DiMaggio 1988) in securing the cooperation of the population was another factor that contributed to the failure to implement an exclusively voluntary, non-remunerated blood donation system in the country.

Issues in the supply of blood products and the circulation of body parts

Meeting the growing demand

In the Introduction, following Meyer and Rowan (1977), we argued the importance for the dominant actors in an organizational field to demonstrate that the system they have put in place is functional and achieves established goals. The foremost issue in this field is the ability to supply safe blood products that meet the growing needs of hospitals. As the previous texts have shown, this goal is certainly easier to achieve in developed countries than in many other parts of the world where equipment is inadequate, resources are insufficient, political systems are unstable, and legislation – when it exists – is seldom applied. But even where organizations are most technologically and legislatively advanced, the system for supplying blood products is not always able to meet the demand, for example, for plasma derivatives. Many Western countries still need to import from abroad (from the United States or Germany, for instance); that is, from countries where plasma is still largely supplied by donors who are "compensated" (remunerated) for their effort (Costa-Font *et al.* 2012; Farrugia *et al.* 2010; Goette *et al.* 2012). Although what is promoted in these importing countries is altruistic and voluntary donation, their populations are generally not informed of the fact that blood product needs are largely being met thanks to these "remunerated" donations. Hospitals in these countries have, for that matter, set up programs to control the use of blood products in an effort to reduce waste and thereby ease pressure on the demand (Carson *et al.* 2011; Tinmouth *et al.* 2008). But in spite of these initiatives, as well as the development of new surgical techniques (bloodless surgery) and the search for blood product substitutes (Hemopure, Biopure, etc.), scientific advances suggest that the demand will only grow in the future. Indeed, trial tests currently underway (Thomson 2014) to determine the effectiveness of transfusing blood from young people in order to reduce the damage caused by Alzheimer's disease and improve the state of patients suffering from this illness suggest that the coming years will see a major rise in the demand for blood products.

In our Introduction, we maintained that the proof of the reference model's efficiency is in fact tied to the set of decisions and viewpoints that those dominating the field are able to impose in connection with a number of issues and concerns: risk control, relationships of trust/mistrust between the health and political systems and the population, the defining of social solidarity and of the donation dynamic, and body commodification.

Controlling health risks

The issue of risk control was primarily documented in the text by Crespin and Danic, as well as that of Valentine, but in fact it has been mentioned by all the contributors to this volume. The historical texts in the first part of the book clearly show that blood transfusion history is a history of risk control. The first transfusions were performed under very hazardous conditions, but they were nevertheless better than no transfusions at all. Scientific and technological advances have contributed to developing better conditions for transfusions and have helped to supply tools by which to better understand the risks involved in this regard one might cite the example of screening tests for infectious diseases. Immediately following World War II, as various forms of legislation and regulation attest, authorities began to consider donors themselves as the greatest potential source of risk. As Crespin and Danic remind us, the bond of trust between institutions and donors was forever broken, ushering in a persistent climate of mistrust. Recruitment from the army and prisons, which had been valuable sources of donors, came to an end as a result of high risk levels. Furthermore, Titmuss' arguments ultimately convinced a number of states – and the major international organizations – that poor populations, attracted by the "financial gain" of paid donation, jeopardized the supply of blood products.

The contaminated blood affair marked a turning point in the history of risk control associated with blood donation. As Chauveau has noted, the affair led to a complete overhaul in the supply of blood products. According to Smith, following this event, the new regulatory arrangements of blood systems transformed the "gift of life" into a scarce commodity that constantly raises concerns over safety and supply. The authorities in charge resolved to prevent even "theoretical" risks. This new orientation was made very clear in the recommendations of the Krever Commission, which was tasked with unravelling the contaminated blood affair in Canada. Krever recommended that the Canadian blood system adopt a precautionary approach to risk-related decision-making. This recommendation stipulated that consideration be given to actual as well as theoretical risks in the event that "a potential disease-causing agent is or may be blood borne, even when there is no evidence that recipients have been affected."

As Crespin and Danic have shown, under the precautionary principle, the blood supply system came to be "healthicized" through the definition of increasingly restrictive selection and exclusion criteria, as well as the introduction of increasingly intrusive questions. Giving blood thus became less of a risk for a donor who was now at risk than for a recipient whose health and safety were the new priority of a transfusion system that needed to ensure its own sustainability. The new "hierarchy of knowledge" (Crespin and Danic), dominated by epidemiology and biology, established a process of harmonizing practices and of disseminating standardized and objective rules and best practice guides that were defined essentially in Western countries and circulated through various international authorities, such as professional and academic associations.

As shown by Crespin and Danic, as well as by Valentine, public debates on exclusion criteria do take place – often at the initiative of homosexual rights associations – in which various groups are invited to express their views on the rules imposed by institutions. But at the end of the day, scientific expertise continues to predominate. According to Crespin and Danic, the democratization of health-related decisions results directly from the effects of the publicity now accorded to debates between experts. Various political actors stand to obtain undeniable political gain by this public "staging" of debates which offers a way of ensuring acceptance of a decision. It allows these actors to appear responsive to the demands made by associations while presenting themselves as being at the forefront of a struggle against discrimination. But, by basing themselves on epidemiological expertise, it also authorizes them to show themselves to be guarantors and protectors of health – which constitutes a powerful legitimizing tool in political action. As Charbonneau and Quéniart show, blood donors, for their part, remain ambivalent: they are aware of the severity of selection criteria which is intended to guarantee blood products' safety, but they also question these rules when they themselves, or those close to them, are targeted.

In many parts of the world, safe blood products are far from sufficient to meet the needs of local populations. Martinez and Sanchez have identified many factors behind this problem, including a lack of resources and political will, but also the fact that certain countries are more strongly affected by the presence of infectious diseases than others. As Smith reminds us, with the increase in restrictions, the pressure to recruit donors is constantly on the rise. Copeman nevertheless shows the limitations of trying to recruit donors at all costs: in India, the alliance with religious gurus has attracted numerous donors who consider that the risk to which they expose themselves when giving blood (without respecting established criteria) makes their sacrifice more valuable.

It is highly likely that the influence of the precautionary principle will continue to grow in the coming years. Within this context, all emerging threats are today translated into transfusion risks, as is the case of prion, the West Nile virus, Severe Acute Respiratory Syndrome (SARS), dengue fever, chikingunya fever, H1N1 flu, etc. Will these growing restrictions, in a context of rising demand, lead the authorities in charge to show greater openness to groups who, for their part, demand the right to donate blood? It is important to bear in mind that such associations increasingly base themselves on scientific expertise. A "sense of biological citizenship," as Rose and Novas (2006) put it, has developed in recent years in step with the idea that it is important for populations to be educated about science and technology. Thanks to the Internet, everyone today not only has access to a vast storehouse of scientific information but also has the ability to create active communities of citizens. Alliances between these communities and scientists are becoming more and more common. It is not surprising that discussions regarding selection criteria for blood donations are turning into expert debates. Over the past years, a few countries, such as the United Kingdom (SaBTO 2011; Waygood 2011), Canada (Andreatta 2013), and New Zealand (Flanagan 2014), have revised their legislation to allow homosexuals to donate blood. In reality, however, the restrictions in this regard still remain very stringent.

Building public trust

All of these debates about controlling health risks are directly connected to the responsible institutions' ability to build a population's trust in order to lead citizens to voluntarily come out and donate blood. The voluntary and altruistic donation system is very much dependent on this issue of trust. In the early history of blood transfusion, much time was needed to convince individuals that transferring a stranger's blood into one's own body could improve health (Danic and Lefrère 2010; Murray 1991; Rousseau 2005). The racial barrier subsequently proved to be another difficult obstacle to overcome, given that, as Lallemand-Stempak shows, the media itself fuelled public fears regarding the mixing of blood. Some cultures still continue to resist the practice of blood donation, and scientific arguments are not always able to convince them that no permanent bodily losses will ensue as a result (Zaller *et al.* 2005; Maher and Ho 2009). Copeman notes that if certain Indians, whose practices he has studied, willingly accept to donate blood, it is not that these devotees differ from the majority of Indians in viewing blood donation as a safe activity but rather that they see themselves as being exempt from the ill effects that would ordinarily ensue. This author has taken up Cohen's (2004) idea of "as-if modernity." In donating their blood, devotees appear to evince confidence in the claims of medical science about the harmlessness of blood donation to the donor. Adams *et al.* demonstrate how the Public Health Bureau in China took advantage of the media, the established relationships that people had with their work unit, and the knowledge that in order for citizens to trust in the state's demands for blood donation, they would have to be convinced of not only its safety but its worthiness, as a contribution to the national good.

The contaminated blood affair profoundly undermined public trust in the institutions responsible for supplying blood products. This crisis of confidence prompted a decline in blood donations, and in its wake, institutions worked very hard to mend their reputations. Valentine as well as Charbonneau and Quéniart have noted that although this trust has been restored in many countries, it is sometimes shaken when institutions are considered to go too far by imposing criteria perceived as sources of discrimination and social exclusion. As mentioned earlier, it is now institutions that have lost their trust in donors. However, in many countries, the crisis of confidence in institutions has never been resolved. Parmasad has pointed out that in Trinidad, the population even has the sense that the voluntary system which some are trying to impose is being developed solely for the country's elite, who would be its only beneficiaries. In short, in countries where no actor has truly succeeded in dominating the field of blood donation and transfusion, it is not surprising to observe a lack of trust in the system.

Today, thanks to technological advances, many other parts of the body (oocytes, sperm, bone marrow, breast milk, etc.) can be exchanged and donated within society. In some cases, the parties involved in these exchanges prefer to trust only each other (Swanson 2014). An example may be seen in breast milk networks that have been created and are taking advantage of Internet resources to make themselves known. Informal agreements, too, have emerged, for example, to allow gay or lesbian couples to have children. Unlike blood, certain bodily fluids can circulate without the intervention of an intermediary. Citing arguments of risk control, the public authorities in charge generally attempt to retake control of the "circulation" of such fluids.

Disseminating the model of altruistic, voluntary, and anonymous donation

The authorities in charge consider that establishing public confidence depends on their ability to impose the rules that ensure blood products' safety. The model that is judged to be the safest by experts, and that is promoted by scientific authorities, is the one based on altruistic, voluntary, and anonymous donation. Paradoxically, even though the contaminated blood affair revealed that voluntary donation itself could be a vehicle for contamination, the principle of voluntary, anonymous, and non-remunerated donation emerged strengthened from the crisis.

As several authors have observed in this book, recruiting donors consistent with these principles does not sit well with some of the dominant cultural models prevailing in many parts of the world. In countries fraught with political instability and often limited social protection from the state, mutual aid among family, friends, and within local communities is the only type of solidarity that has been able to support populations over the decades. As Parmasad relates, people may be justified in wondering, "If I volunteer to give blood and my child needs some tomorrow, what will he do if I am unable to give him blood?" The social values of family obligation, religious duty, and patriotic sentiment have not disappeared from our societies to the exclusive benefit of altruism toward the strangers along-side whom we live (Charbonneau and Tran 2012), even if this is what Titmuss believed. With increasing international migration, the cultures of donation and social solidarity are becoming intermingled. Researchers have observed that populations of immigrant origin and ethnic minorities in Western countries (Charbonneau and Tran 2012; Glynn *et al.* 2006; Murphy *et al.* 2009) are often less active as blood donors. In some cases, they have kept the memory of the blood supply systems of their countries of origin, or perhaps of certain cultural restrictions associated with the symbolism of blood and blood donation.

Furthermore, as shown by the analyses of Smith as well as Charbonneau and Quéniart, even in a country as developed as Canada, those responsible for coming up with strategies to boost recruitment in order to meet growing needs are adept at using many arguments other than altruism to convince people to donate blood. They do not hesitate to recruit from businesses, schools, or public organizations; to join forces with local associations in order to take advantage of peer pressure; or to heighten donors' sense of obligation by constantly remind-ing them that it is time to come back to make another donation.

The model of altruistic, voluntary, and anonymous donation also implies that citizens give blood irrespective of their social, ethnic, or religious backgrounds. As Lallemand-Stempak shows, debates about the circulation of blood between people of different races have been arduous, yet the universal vision has ulti-mately prevailed. The development of "personalized medicine" (Hood *et al.* 2012; PCAST 2008) nevertheless brings into question some of the achievements in this regard.

For a number of years, those services in charge of donor recruitment have been drawing up plans that directly target certain ethnic minorities. For medical reasons, certain specific ethnic groups may have needs that can be met only by blood donations from other community members; for example, in the context of treating certain diseases prevalent in specific communities (Duboz *et al.* 2012; Grossman *et al.* 2005; Price *et al.* 2009). This is the case with sickle-cell anemia, a genetic disease that is inherited from two parents carrying a mutant gene and that results in a malformation of red blood cells and multiple related complica-tions. Some patients, including severely affected children, will require blood transfusions every eight weeks, and sometimes as often as every two weeks. This disease is found in Africa, North America, and the Caribbean, but also in the Middle East, West Asia, or Mediterranean countries such as Turkey, Greece, and Italy, in addition to South America. The fact remains that the black population is the one most affected by this disease. A number of researchers, including Price *et al.* (2009), note the greater likelihood of finding similar phenotypes within the same population based on geographical ancestry, which can lower alloimmuni-zation risks. In several Western countries, institutions have stepped up efforts to recruit more donors from black communities. Scientists in the biomedical field have therefore brought back the issue of the importance of race, though associating it with a positive connotation.

This is precisely the direction being taken by personalized medicine, which is based on the observation of individuals' biological differentiation. Personalized medicine is presented as an approach aimed at choosing the medical treatment best adapted to patients' biological profiles and the molecular characteristics of their diseases (Hood *et al.* 2012; PCASC 2008). This medical approach was developed in connection with the Human Genome Project (Andrews and Nelkin 2001), which, among other things, sought to collect blood from populations considered to be isolated and genetically distinct from others. The underlying idea was that some groups might have pure types of genes; the approach was therefore to classify populations into biological groups. The project stirred up considerable controversy, since it revived the idea of human races. Indeed, it was not long before race, in genetic research, came to be viewed as worthy of investigation. Even so, the results of research performed as part of the Human Genome project show that 99.9 percent of human beings' genetic sequences are identical and that, of the remaining 0.1 percent, only 3 to 10 percent are associated with a geographical ancestry (Koenig *et al.* 2008). A meta-analysis of 335 articles published in the field of population genetics has confirmed that pure races do not exist, that most genetic variations observed to date involve intragroup variations, that these variations are not necessarily based on continental ancestry, that the categories used by researchers (e.g., blacks) are defined differently from one study to another, and that the most frequently used variable (skin color) is not a good criterion for defining specific groups when it comes to phenotypic traits (Outram and Ellison 2010). In spite of these results, medication specifically targeting the black population has emerged in the past decade (March 2000; Koenig *et al.* 2008).

In such a context, it is not surprising that blood organizations do not hesitate to develop targeted strategies for ethnic communities, and especially black communities (Charbonneau and Tran 2015). More recently, we have also witnessed pleas addressed to a specific ethnic community, namely the Vietnamese community, in order to find a stem cell donor compatible with a Vietnamese woman suffering from leukemia (Lacoursière 2014). Social media were widely used to broadcast the pleas, thus serving as a reminder that members of ethnic minorities are less likely to join stem cell donor registries.

Protection against the commercial exploitation of body parts

Although organizational strategies and donor motivations are more diversified than the altruistic and voluntary donation model would suggest, few today agree with the remuneration of donors. Still, as Schneider and Adams *et al.* point out, in poor countries, supplying food has a different meaning than providing compensation for the inconvenience and travel required of donors in order to attend blood clinics, as is customary in Germany or in the United States. Even in developed countries, however, the debate between donation and commerce is far from settled. Several countries' dependence on the importation of plasma deriv-atives obtained from paid donors constantly stokes this debate (Costa-Font *et al.* 2012; Farrugia *et al.* 2010; Goette *et al.* 2012). As Chauveau observes, the cost-free nature of blood products is in fact somewhat fictitious, considering the real costs involved in preparing these products. It is state control over the fees paid to the plasma industry, or the fact that the state itself handles the processing, that offers protection against the genuine commercial exploitation of blood. Donors are motivated by the fact that their blood donations meet concrete needs. Although they themselves have a rather disenchanted vision (Attali 2004) of this "bodily product" that is used to save lives, Parmasad points out that blood appears to be less implicated in the commodification process than other body parts that are bought and sold on the black market across the world (Andrews and Nelkin 2001; Lock and Nguyen 2010; Scheper-Hugues 2001; Waldby and Mitchell 2006). This commodification process brings to light a general flow of products from the poor to the rich, from the countries of the Global South to the Global North, and from women to men (Cohen 1999; Scheper-Hugues 2000), thus pointing to the presence of significant inequalities in access to care and to medical products.

In rich countries, the commerce of parts of the body has also found its way into the system through the development of private sperm, oocyte, or even stem cell banks. Umbilical cord blood has become established as an increasingly viable clinical alternative to bone marrow in the treatment of leukaemia. Some banks offer the opportunity to retain stem cells privately. In fact, international private umbilical cord blood banking has expanded rapidly in recent years. Private companies offer parents the opportunity to store umbilical cord blood for the possible future use by their child or other family members. The private cord blood industry has been criticized (Brown 2013; De Lora 2009; Hollands and McCauley 2009), and a network of public banks also exists based on the prin-ciple of anonymous donation to strangers. These new domains in which body parts circulate exhibit the same power plays as those observed in the first decades of blood supply systems. The field of bodily products' circulation appears, in fact, to be far from stabilized.

Charting a research agenda

We believe that this book represents a clarification and reconsideration of the meaning of blood donation in diverse and complex social environments. An inter-pretation of these contributions through the lens of the theory of fields further high-lights the embeddedness of blood donation in history, culture, politics, conflict, law and ethics, and organizational dynamics, as well as in the interactions and meaning-making of everyday life. This is important because, as several authors remind us, blood has been socially decontextualized both through technology and by research centred on the value of blood as a health commodity.

We also need to consider a research agenda that disentangles blood from tech-nology and technical discourse, and reinserts it into the lived experience of donors and non-donors, into the complex organizational and regulatory dynamics of blood systems, and ultimately, into the social structure itself. Titmuss' ground-breaking analysis of blood donation systems in England and the United States in the early 1970s was the first to underline the value of the social sciences in understanding the socio-organizational aspects of blood donation. The theoretical insights of the prominent social scientists cited in this book, such as Pierre Bourdieu and Michel Foucault, allow us to understand blood at the nexus of interactional, institutional, and structural social forces.

Why does such an approach matter? It matters first because it opens the door to situating blood donation within broader political and social undercurrents that have been largely obscured by scientific and behavioural analyses of the practice. The works of Lallemand-Stempak, who ties blood donation and transfusion to US racial politics, and Schneider, who situates the emergence of African blood systems within a colonial political context, illustrate the value of such critical analyses. Next, critical appraisals of the role of the state in governing blood and regulating its donation, like those of Valentine, Crespin and Danic, and Chauveau, inspire us to strive to consider the social justice implications of having groups of individuals excluded from participating in this socially valued activity. Parmasad's, and Martinez and Sanchez's analyses also provide welcome nuance to these appraisals by emphasizing that the absence of adequate governance impacts upon the availability and quality of blood. Thus, blood systems cannot be seen simply as technical organizations; they are subject to the external pressures of stakeholders and to the dynamics of state–society relations.

Blood, culture, and society are intricately intertwined throughout this book. As the contributed chapters suggest, we ought to turn our critical attention beyond behavioural accounts of blood donation as the predominant paradigm in this field of research. They form part of an emerging critical field that conceptualizes blood donation in terms of its structural embeddedness. While blood resides in the individual, donating it to others is a fundamentally intersubjective and social act that is linked to diverse personal, political, and cultural meanings, which are themselves intersected by structural constraints that influence the willingness of some to donate and limit the legitimacy and ability of others to do so. Further research in the field would improve our understanding of the socio-political context of blood donation and the ramifications of sociological dynamics on the gift of life.

References

Advisory Committee on the Safety of Blood, Tissues and Organs (SaBTO). 2011. *Donor Selection Criteria Review.* Department of Health, and SaBTO, Blood Donor Selection Steering Group.

Andreatta, D. 2013. "Ban Lifted on Gay Men Giving Blood, but Tough Restrictions Remain." *The Globe and Mail.*

Andrews, L. and Nelkin, D. 2001. *Body Bazaar. The Market for Human Tissue in the Biotechnology Age.* New York: Crown Publishing.

Attali, J. 2004. "La symbolique du sang dans la société." *Transfusion Clinique et Biologique* 11(5–6): 271–273.

Brown, N. 2013. "Contradictions of Values Between Use and Exchange in Cord Blood Bioeconomy."*Sociology of Health and Illness* 35(1): 97–112.

Carson, J.L., Terrin, M.L., and Noveck, H. 2011. "Liberal or Restrictive Transfusion in High-risk Patients after Hip Surgery." *The New England Journal of Medicine* 365(26): 2453–2462.

Charbonneau, J. and Tran, N. 2015. "The Paradoxical Situation of Blood Donation in the Haitian-Quebec Community." *Canadian Ethnic Studies* 47(2): 71–96.

Cohen, L. 1999. "Where It Hurts: Indian Material for an Ethics of Organ Transplantation." *Daedalus* 128(4): 135–165.

Cohen, L. 2004. "Operability: Surgery at the Margin of the State." In *Anthropology in the Margins of the State*, edited by V. Das and D. Poole, 165–190. Santa Fe: School of American Research Press.

Costa-Font, J., Jofre-Bonet, M., and Yan, S.T. 2012. *Not All Incentives Wash Out the Warm Glow: The Case of Blood Donation Revisited*. London: Centre for Economic Performance, London School of Economics and Political Science, no. 1157.

Danic, B. and Lefrère, J.J. 2010. "Le sang dans l'art, l'art dans le sang." *Transfusion Clinique et Biologique* 17(5–6): 382–385.

De Lora, P. 2009. *In Cord Blood. Are the Stem Cells from the Umbilical Cord Private Property?* Report. Universidad Autonoma de Madrid/Harvard University.

DiMaggio, P.J. 1988. "Interest and Agency in Institutional Theory." In *Institutional Patterns and Culture*, edited by L. Zucker, 3–22. Cambridge, MA: Ballinger Publishing.

Duboz, P., Lazaygues, C., and Boëtsch, G. 2012. "Donneurs de sang réguliers ou donneurs occasionnels: différences sociodémographiques et motivationnelles." *Transfusion Clinique et Biologique* 19(1): 17–24.

Elsbach, K.D. and Sutton, R.I. 1992. "Acquiring Organizational Legitimacy through Illegitimate Actions: A Marriage of Institutional and Impression Management Theories." *Academy of Management Journal* 35: 699–738.

Emirbayer, M. and Johnson, V. 2008. "Bourdieu and Organizational Analysis." *Theory and Society* 37: 1–44.

Farrugia, A., Penrod, J., and Bult, J.D. 2010. "Payment, Compensation and Replacement – The Ethics and Motivation of Blood and Plasma Donation." *Vox Sanguinis* 99(3): 202–211.

Flanagan, P. 2014. *Behavioural Donor Deferral Criteria Review*. Report to the NZ Blood Service.

Fligstein, N. 2001. "Social Skill and the Theory of Fields." *Sociological Theory* 40: 397–405.

Fligstein, N. and McAdam, D. 2011. "Toward a General Theory of Strategic Action Fields." *Sociological Theory* 29: 1–26.

Fligstein, N. and McAdam, D. 2012. *A Theory of Fields*. New York: Oxford University Press.

Glynn, S.A., Schreiber, G.B., and Murphy, E.L. 2006. "Factors Influencing the Decision to Donate: Racial and Ethnic Comparisons." *Transfusion* 46(6): 980–990.

Godbout, J.T. and Caillé, A. 1992. *L'esprit du don*. Paris: La Découverte.

Goette, L., Stutzer, A., and Frey, M. 2010. "Prosocial Motivation and Blood Donations: A Survey of the Empirical Literature." *Transfusion Medicine and Hemotherapy* 37(3): 149–154.

Grant, D.B. 2010. "Integration of Supply and Marketing for a Blood Service." *Management Research Review* 33: 123–133.

Grossman, B., Watkins, A.R., and Fleming, F. 2005. "Barriers and Motivators to Blood and Cord Blood Donations in Young African-American Women." *American Journal of Hematology* 78: 198–202.

Healy, K. 2000. "Embedded Altruism: Blood Collection Regimes and the European Union's Donor Population." *American Journal of Sociology* 105: 1633–1657.

Hoffmann, A.J. 1999. "Institutional Evolution and Change: Environmentalism and the US Chemical Industry." *Academy of Management Journal* 42(4): 351–371.

Hollands, P. and McCauley, C. 2009. "Private Cord Blood Banking: Current Use and Clinical Future." *Stem Cell Review* 5(3): 195–203.

Hood, L., Flores, M.A., Brogaard, K.R., and Price, N.D. 2012. "Systems Medicine and the Emergence of Proactive P4 Medicine: Predictive, Preventative, Personalized, and Participatory." *Handbook of Systems Biology – Concepts and Insights.* Section V, ch. 23, 445–467.

Koenig, B., Lee, S. S-J., and Richardson, S.S. 2008. *Revisiting Race in a Genomic Age.* Princeton, NJ: Rutgers University Press.

Lacoursière, A. 2014. Le SOS d'une cancéreuse. *La Presse.ca, 4 July.*

Lock. M. and Nguyen, V.K. 2010. *An Anthropology of Biomedecine.* Chichester: Wiley-Blackwell.

Maher, L. and Ho, H.T. 2009. "Overdose Beliefs and Management Practices among Ethnic Vietnamese Heroin Users in Sydney, Australia." *Harm Reduction Journal* 6(6): 1–10.

Mahoney, J. and Thelen, K. 2009. "A Theory of Gradual Change." In *Explaining Institutional Change: Ambiguity, Agency, and Power*, edited by J. Mahoney and K. Thelen, 1–37. New York: Cambridge University Press.

March, R. 2000. "Pharmacogenomics: The Genomics of Drug Response." *Yeast* 17: 16–21.

Martin, J.L. 2003. "What is Field Theory?" *AJS* 109(1): 1–49.

Masser, B.M., White, K.M., Hyde, M.K., and Terry, D.J. 2008. "The Psychology of Blood Donation: Current Research and Future Directions." *Transfusion Medicine Reviews* 22(3): 215–233.

Meyer, J.W. and Rowan, B. 1977. "Institutionalized Organizations: Formal Structure as Myth and Ceremony." *AJS* 83(2): 340–363.

Murphy, E.L., Shaz, B., and Hillyer, C.D. 2009. "Minority and Foreign-born Representation among US Blood Donors: Demographics and Donation Frequency for 2006." *Transfusion* 49: 2221–2227.

Murray, T.H. 1991. "The Poisoned Gift: Aids and Blood." In *A Disease of Society: Cultural and Institutional Responses to AIDS*, edited by D. Nelkin, D.P. Willis, and S. Parris, 216–240. Cambridge: Cambridge University Press.

Nicholson-Crotty, S. 2009. "The Politics of Diffusion: Public Policy in the American States." *Journal of Politics* 71: 192–205.

Outram, S.M. and Ellison, G.T. 2010. "Arguments Against the Use of Racialized Categories as Genetic Variables in Biomedical Research: What Are They, and Why Are They Being Ignored?" In *What's the Use of Race?*, edited by I. Whitmarsch and D.S. Jones, 91–124. Cambridge MA: MIT Press.

Powell, W.W. 2007. "The New Institutionalism." *The International Encyclopedia of Organization Studies.* Thousand Oaks, CA: Sage (preprintwww.stanford.edu/group/song/papers/NewInstitutionalism.pdf).

President's Council of Advisors on Science and Technology (PCAST). 2008. *Priorities for Personalized Medecine.* Report. Executive Office of the President of the United States of America.

Price, C.L., Johnson, M.T., and Lindsay, T. 2009. "The Sickle Cell Sabbath: A Community Program Increases First-time Blood Donors in the African American Faith Community." *Transfusion* 49: 519–523.

Rhodes, R.A.W. 1996. "The New Governance: Governing without Government." *Political Studies* 44: 652–667.

Rogers, E. 2003. *Diffusion of Innovation*, 5th edn. New York: Free Press.

Rose, N. and Novas, C. 2006. "Biological Citizenship." In *Global Assemblages. Technology, Politics and Ethics as Anthropological Problems*, edited by A. Ong and S.J. Collier, 439–463. Oxford: Blackwell.

Rousseau, V. 2005. *Le goût du sang: croyances et polémiques dans la chrétienneté occidentale*. Paris: Armand Colin.

Scheper-Hughes, N. 2000. "The Global Traffic in Human Organs." *Current Anthropology* 41(1): 191–224.

Scheper-Hughes, N. 2001. "Bodies for Sale – Whole or in Parts." *Body and Society* 7(2–3): 1–8.

Scott, W.R. 2001. *Institutions and Organizations.* Thousand Oaks, CA: Sage.

Starr, D. 2000. *Blood: An Epic History of Medicine and Commerce*. London: Harper Perennial.

Swanson, K.W. 2014. *Banking on the Body*. Cambridge, MA: Harvard University Press.

Thomson, H. 2014. "Young Blood to be Used in Ultimate Rejuvenation Trial." *New Scientist.* www.newscientist.com/article/mg22329831.400-young-blood-to-be-used-in-ultimate-rejuvenation-trial.html#.VT6csWB0y70 (last accessed December 11, 2014).

Tinmouth, A., McIntyre L.A., and Fowler, R.A. 2008. "Blood Conservation Strategies to Reduce the Need for Red Blood Cell Transfusion in Critically Ill Patients." *CMAJ* 178(1): 49–57.

Titmuss, R.M. 1971. *The Gift Relationship: From Human Blood to Social Policy*. New York: Pantheon Books.

Waldby, C. and Mitchell, R. 2006. *Tissue Economies. Blood, Organs, and Cell Lines in Late Capitalism*. Durham, NC: Duke University Press.

Waygood, J. 2011. "UK Government Lifts Lifetime Ban on Gay Blood Donation." *So So Gay.* http://sosogay.co.uk/2011/government-announces-end-of-lifetime-ban-on-gay-blood-donation/ (last accessed December 11, 2014).

Zaller, N., Nelson, K.E., and Ness, P. 2005. "Knowledge, Attitude and Practice Survey Regarding Blood Donation in a Northwestern Chinese City." *Transfusion Medicine* 15(4): 277–286.

Index

Page numbers in *italics* denote tables.